Case Based Oral Mucosal Diseases

Qianming Chen • Xin Zeng
Editors

Case Based Oral Mucosal Diseases

PMPH PEOPLE'S MEDICAL PUBLISHING HOUSE
Springer

Editors
Qianming Chen
West China Hospital of Stomatology
Sichuan University
Chengdu
Sichuan
China

Xin Zeng
West China Hospital of Stomatology
Sichuan University
Chengdu
Sichuan
China

ISBN 978-981-13-0285-5 ISBN 978-981-13-0286-2 (eBook)
https://doi.org/10.1007/978-981-13-0286-2

The print edition is not for sale in China Mainland. Customers from China Mainland please order the print book from: People's Medical Publishing House

Library of Congress Control Number: 2018952230

Printed on acid-free paper

This Springer imprint is published by the registered company Springer Nature Singapore Pte Ltd.
The registered company address is: 152 Beach Road, #21-01/04 Gateway East, Singapore 189721, Singapore

Preface

The catch-all term, oral mucosal diseases, refers to various diseases of the oral mucosa and related soft tissues. Aside from certain individual cases that can be attributed to local factors, a majority of oral mucosal diseases occur due to a combination of both local and systemic factors. In recent years, the model of biological-psychological-social medicine has become especially significant in studying the pathogenicity and management of oral mucosal diseases.

Since an increase has been recorded in the incidence rate and the number of complicated cases of oral mucosal diseases, the Department of Oral Mucosal Diseases has been tasked with the regular development of novel diagnostic and treatment methods. As a result, we have left no exceptions in exploring clinical cases. In addition to a large number of common cases, an increasing number of rare, anomalous cases of oral mucosal diseases have been recorded. Often, it is difficult to provide immediate and definitive diagnoses for the latter type of cases. In order to provide definitive diagnoses, as well as out of curiosity, we took the initiative to review pictures, books, and other literature, as well as communicate with experts in relevant disciplines. Based on the information from such data and communications, we further examined patients to provide an accurate diagnosis and treatment. We feel gratified and accomplished because our expertise has allowed us to help patients who seek medical attention from us. Such experiences have left us even more intrigued by the complexity of oral mucosal diseases, further igniting our strong interest in this discipline.

"A picture is worth a thousand words." This is an inspirational quote that comes to our mind every time we review the collected images of clinical cases. Looking back at medical records and recalling the situation of each patient, the educational process of diagnosis and treatment, as well as our experiences after reaching a definitive diagnosis on the disease, we realize that each picture has a story. Therefore, we have also gained a deeper insight into two criteria that need to be fulfilled to be a good physician: (1) medical skills and (2) empathy toward patients. This brings to memory the epitaph of an American physician, Dr. Edward Livingston Trudeau: "To Cure Sometimes, To Relieve Often, To Comfort Always." Truly, this is particularly the case with medical practitioners working on rarely studied oral mucosal diseases.

We are passionate about this profession. We enjoy the ideas and discoveries in the diagnosis and treatment of each patient. Besides, we also enjoy the recognition of our careers, as well as the sentiment behind the story of each patient.

Due to the abovementioned reasons, we desired to write a reference book on the clinically common and rare cases of oral mucosal diseases. One of our students, Jin Xin, also repeatedly suggested, while arranging the image resources of clinical cases, that we should not leave them as they are. After careful consideration, we began to write a book about oral mucosal diseases based on those pictures of clinical cases with the involvement and support of Dr. Jin Xin, Assoc. Prof. Jiang Lu, Assoc. Prof. Zhou Yu, and Assoc. Prof. Dan Hong-Xia from the Department of Oral Mucosal Diseases; Professor Wu Lan-Yan and Assoc. Prof. Geng Ning from the Department of Oral Pathology; as well as Assoc. Prof. Li Wei from the Department of Dermatology, West China College of Stomatology, Sichuan University. We look forward to seek an appropriate way to reveal, share, and discuss with our colleagues and students the clinical manifestations of oral mucosal diseases and the process of diagnosis and treatment for such cases. Besides, we also aim to provide a desk reference book for freshmen in this discipline.

On the occasion of completing this book, we would like to thank our mentor, Prof. Li Bing-Qi, for his care, support, and enlightenment. We would also like to express our gratitude to Dr. Jin Xin for his participation and great effort throughout the entire writing process, as well as Li Xiao-Ying (Deputy Chief Nurse) and Wu Yuan (Nurse) from the Department of Oral Mucosal Diseases, West China College of Stomatology, Sichuan University, for the photography of all the clinical pictures used in the book. Last but not least, we would also like to express our appreciation to all colleagues at the Department of Oral Mucosal Diseases, West China College of Stomatology, Sichuan University.

Chengdu, China

Qianming Chen
Xin Zeng

Contents

Oral Infectious Diseases

1

Xin Jin, Xin Zeng, and Qianming Chen

Keywords
Herpes Simplex · Acute Herpetic Gingivostomatitis · Herpes Labialis · Herpes Zoster · Varicella · Hand-Foot-Mouth Disease · Herpangina · Oral Candidosis · Pseudomembranous Candidosis · Acute Erythematous Candidosis · Chronic Erythematous Candidosis · Chronic Hyperplastic Candidosis · Coccigenic Stomatitis · Oral Tuberculosis

X. Jin
College of Stomatology, Chongqing Medical University, Chongqing Key Laboratory of Oral Diseases and Biomedical Sciences, Chongqing, China

X. Zeng
State Key Laboratory of Oral Diseases, National Clinical Research Center for Oral Diseases, Department of Oral Medicine, West China Hospital of Stomatology, Sichuan University, Chengdu, Sichuan, China

Q. Chen (✉)
Changjiang Scholars Program, Ministry of Education, Beijing, China

State Key Laboratory of Oral Diseases, National Clinical Research Center for Oral Diseases, Department of Oral Medicine, West China Hospital of Stomatology, Sichuan University, Chengdu, Sichuan, China
e-mail: qmchen@scu.edu.cn

1.1 Herpes Simplex

Case 1 Acute Herpetic Gingivostomatitis (Children)

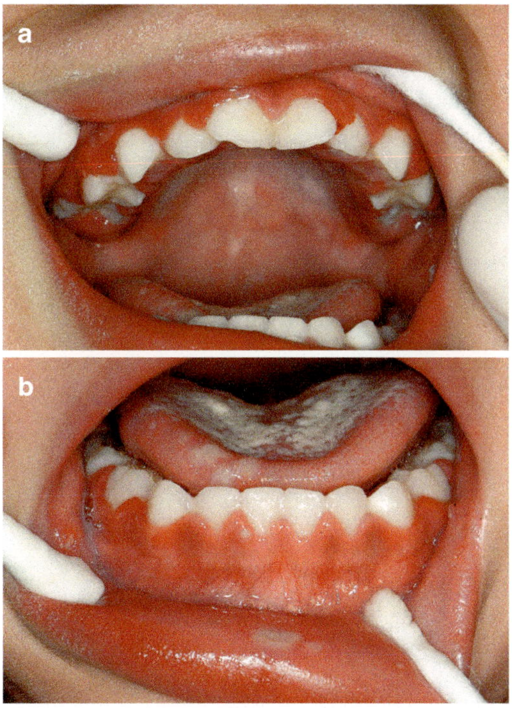

Fig. 1.1 (**a**) Red and swollen gums with erosions in clusters on the gingiva. (**b**) Red and swollen gums with erosions in clusters on the gingiva and tongue

Q. Chen, X. Zeng (eds.), *Case Based Oral Mucosal Diseases*,
https://doi.org/10.1007/978-981-13-0286-2_1

Age: 23 months
Sex: male
Chief Complaints:
23-month-old boy with a fever for 7 days, with ulcers in the mouth for 3 days
History of Present Illness:
A 23-month-old boy had a fever 7 days ago, and his maximum body temperature is 40 °C. The body temperature decreased after intravenous infusion (detailed drugs were unknown). He was taken in local hospital, but still running a low-grade fever. Vesicles and ulcers were observed in his mouth, with swollen gums 3 days ago. He had a difficulty of eating due to oral pain.
Past Medical History: None.
Allergy: None.
Physical Examination:
Red and swollen gums were detected, and erosions in clusters could be seen on the gingiva, labial mucosa, and front dorsum of the tongue (Fig. 1.1).
Laboratories and Imaging Studies: None.
Diagnosis:
Acute Herpetic Gingivostomatitis
Diagnosis Basis:

1. Fever history.
2. Oral lesions were characterized by red and swollen gingiva and erosions distributed in clusters.

Management:

1. Medication
   Rp.: Kouyanning granules 3 g × 10
   Sig.: 1.5 g p.o.t.i.d.
   Vitamin C 0.1 g × 100
   Sig.: 0.05 g p.o.t.i.d.
   Compound chlorhexidine solution 300 ml × 1
   Sig.: 1:1 diluted and topical use t.i.d.
   Recombinant human epidermal growth factor hydrogel 20 g × 1
   Sig.: topical use t.i.d.
2. Drink extra fluids and take more breaks

Case 2 Acute Herpetic Gingivostomatitis (Adult)

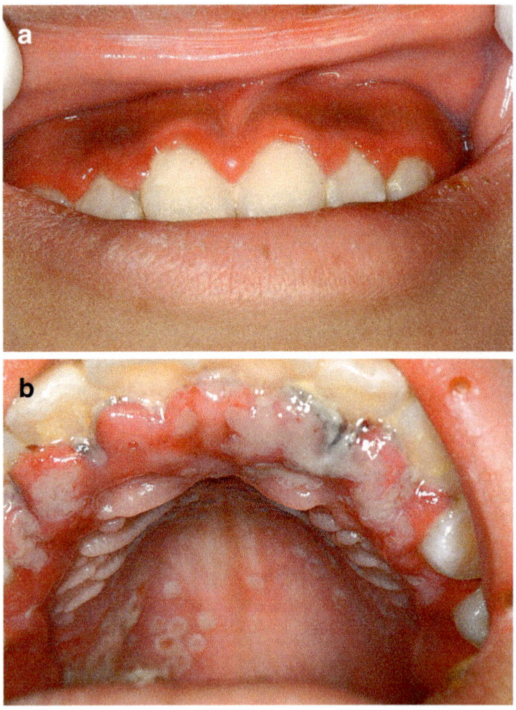

Fig. 1.2 (**a**) Widespread red and swollen gums. (**b**) Widespread red and swollen palatal gingiva, vesicles and ulcers distributed in clusters on the palate and palatal gingival mucosa

Age: 22 years
Sex: male
Chief Complaints:
Oral pain for 4 days
History of Present Illness:
A 22-year-old man presented to our clinic with inflamed, erosive, and painful gingiva for 4 days. He had a cold and cephalosporins were taken before the onset of oral lesions.
Past Medical History: None.
Allergy: None.
Physical Examination:
Generalized inflamed and swollen gingiva was detected, with vesicles and ulcers distributed in clusters on the palate and palatal gingival mucosa (Fig. 1.2).

Laboratories and Imaging Studies: None
Diagnosis:
Acute Herpetic Gingivostomatitis
Diagnosis Basis:

1. History of cold.
2. Oral lesions were characterized by red and swollen gingiva, with vesicles and ulcers distributed in clusters.

Management:

1. Aerosol therapy
   Rp.: Dexamethasone sodium phosphate injection 1 ml × 1
   Gentamycin sulfate injection 2 ml × 1
   Vitamin B12 injection 1 ml × 1
   Vitamin C injection 2.5 ml × 1
   Sig.: aerosol therapy q.d.-b.i.d. for 3 days
2. Medication
   Rp.: Valaciclovir hydrochloride tablets 0.3 g × 12
   Sig.: 0.3 g p.o. b.i.d.
   Kouyanning granules 3 g × 10
   Sig.: 6 g p.o. t.i.d.
   Vitamin C 0.1 g × 100
   Sig.: 0.2 g p.o. t.i.d.
   Compound chlorhexidine solution 300 ml × 1
   Sig.: rinse t.i.d.
   Dexamethasone sodium phosphate injection 1 ml × 5
   Sig.: 1:50 diluted and rinse t.i.d.
   Recombinant human epidermal growth factor hydrogel 20 g × 1
   Sig.: topical use q.d.
3. Drink extra fluids and take more breaks

Case 3 Recurrent Herpes Simplex (Herpes Labialis)

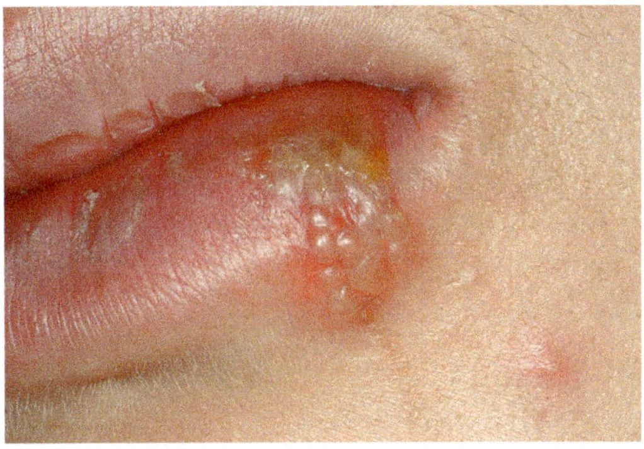

Fig. 1.3 Clusters of vesicles involving the left vermilion border of the lower lip and adjacent skin

Age: 29 years
Sex: female
Chief Complaints:
Vesicles on the lower lip for 1 day
History of Present Illness:
A 29-year-old lady caught a cold 2 days ago, following symptoms such as burning and swelling on the lower lip. Within one day, small vesicles develop in clusters at the same site. She also complained of recurrent vesicles along the vermilion border of the lips once exposure to cold or spicy food, which could heal spontaneously.
Past Medical History: None.
Allergy: None.
Physical Examination:
Small vesicles were observed in clusters involving the left vermilion border of the lower lip and adjacent skin, surrounded by a mild erythematous rim (Fig. 1.3).
Laboratories and Imaging Studies: None.
Diagnosis:
Herpes Labialis
Diagnosis Basis:

1. History of recurrent vesicles along the vermilion border of the lips.
2. Small vesicles distributed in clusters.

Management:

1. Medication
   Rp.: Acyclovir eye drops 8 ml × 1
   Sig.: topical use t.i.d.
   Prednisolone acetate injection 125 mg × 1
   Sig.: topical use (without perioral skin) t.i.d.
2. We advised the patient to keep warm and reduce spicy food

Case 4 Recurrent Herpes Simplex (on the Palate)

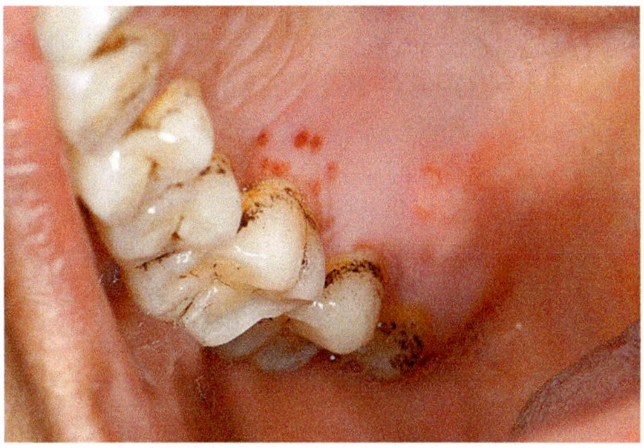

Fig. 1.4 Spotlike erosions in clusters on the right part of palate

Age: 53 years
Sex: female
Chief Complaints:
Repeated vesicles on the lip for 2 years and erosions on the palate for 2 days
History of Present Illness:
A 53-year-old woman presented to our clinic claiming the presence of recurrent vesicles on the lips and vermilion commissures. The clinical course usually lasts for about 1 week. Vesicles quickly rupture, leading to erosions that can heal spontaneously. Two days ago, vesicles appeared and ruptured, resulting in painful erosions.
Past Medical History: None.
Allergy: None.
Physical Examination:
Localized spotlike erosions were distributed in clusters on the right part of palate, with yellow pseudomembrane and hyperemia (Fig. 1.4).
Laboratories and Imaging Studies: None
Diagnosis:
Recurrent Herpes Simplex
Diagnosis Basis:

1. History of recurrent vesicles on the lips and vermilion commissures.
2. Oral lesion was located on the palate.
3. Erosions result from the rupturing vesicles distributed in clusters.

Management:

1. Medication
   Rp.: Compound chlorhexidine solution 300 ml × 1
   Sig.: rinse t.i.d.
   Prednisolone acetate injection 125 mg × 1
   Sig.: topical use t.i.d.

[Review] Herpes Simplex
Herpes simplex is caused by the herpes simplex virus type 1 (HSV-1). Herpes simplex virus (HSV) is a nuclear replicating enveloped DNA virus, with two strains of HSV-1 and HSV-2. Generally, HSV-1 is considered to give rise to infection "above the waist" including oral mucosa, perioral skin, and facial skin and HSV-2 "below the waist," which is associated with genital lesions [1]. In recent years, studies have shown that the predilection site of a specific viral subtype is changing, in part due to varying sexual practices [2–4].

This disease is contagious, especially in a closed community setting such as a daycare center or orphanage nursery. HSV is primarily transmitted by contact with infected oral secretions. Its distribution shows no sex or seasonal differences [5]. Studies reported that the prevalence of HSV-1 antibodies increased steadily with age and reached high levels of about 90% among subjects 40 years of age or older, indicating they had infection history [6]. HSV is thought to spread principally during the prodrome phase of the primary infection and is usually greater in immunocompromised individuals or in those undergoing oral surgery.

In the initial period of infection, HSV-1 infects the oral mucosa and enters the cell. Once inside the cell, virus replication causes plenty of virions produced that ultimately results in cell death, and finally primary infection symptom appears [1]. After primary infection and local replication on the oral mucosa, HSV-1 enters into sensory nerve endings, following transports to the neuronal cell bodies along retrograde axonal. The immune system limits the spread of virus infection at synaptic junctions through the establishment of latency, without neuronal damage. Recurrent infections arise in 30–40% of HSV-1 seropositive patients, which have been associated with exposure to sunlight, stress, fatigue, cold, spicy food, menstruation, and orofacial trauma [2]. When HSV-1 reactivation occurs, newly generated virions spread from the infected neurons to mucocutaneous sites and saliva by anterograde axoplasmic transport, resulting in mild mucocutaneous disorders.

Primary herpetic stomatitis is a primary infection by herpes simplex virus, also known as acute herpetic gingivostomatitis. Onset of it is usually during childhood from 6 months to 3 years old, and the peak incidence appears between 9 months and 28 months of age [7, 8]. The incubation period is about 2–12 days (average 4 days); symptoms such as cold, fever, or cough can arise. One to 3 days later, mucocutaneous vesicle ruptured. It typically affects the lips, tongue, gingiva, buccal mucosa, and palate. The oral lesions manifest as blisters with 1–2 mm in diameter, which rupture rapidly and coalesce to shallow, painful, and usually irregular ulcers. They are often covered by a yellowish-gray pseudomembrane, with surrounding hyperemia. The ulcers gradually heal in 10–14 days, without scarring. The swelling gingiva is one of the gingival features, which may be misdiagnosed as gingivitis caused by dental plaque and calculus. Perioral lesions are found in approximately 2/3 of affected children. Most children have a fever of >38.0 °C for approximately 4 days, with enlarged cervical lymph nodes, increased saliva secretion, dehydration, coated tongue, bad breath, and skin rash. The severity of illness is associated with the host immunoreactions [1]. Virus spread widely or secondary bacteremia is rare [7].

Recurrent herpes simplex typically affects the lips, vermilion commissures, and perioral skin, termed as recurrent herpes labialis (RHL) [9]. RHL is preceded by premonitory symptoms such as burning, tingling, soreness, or swelling at the site where the lesions will occur [2]. In about 6 h, the lesions are usually red macules that rapidly become vesicular, following scabs and ulcers. Healing happens in 10 days from initial symptom onset, without scarring [1, 2]. The intraoral recurrent herpes simplex often occurs on the palate and gingival mucosa, which is characterized by erosions in clusters.

The diagnosis of herpes simplex is based on the clinical history and features [7]. Laboratory tests such as tissue culture techniques and detection of viral DNA are not the conventional diagnostic methods. All the cases of this unit are diagnosed by the typical history and clinical features.

Treatments of acute herpetic gingivostomatitis include systemic therapy and topical treatment. Topical treatment is mainly applied in recurrent herpes simplex.

Oral drugs include antiviral drugs (acyclovir and valaciclovir), Kouyanning granules, and vitamin C. If the course of disease is more than 5 days, antiviral drugs are not recommended. The usage of acyclovir is as follows: for children younger than 2 years old, 100 mg orally, five times per day, for 5 days, is the course of treatment, and for children older than 2 years old, 200 mg orally, five times per day, for 5 days, is the course of treatment [10]. Because it is a self-limiting illness with short disease course, acyclovir is not recommended if the symptom is mild. For adults, 200 mg orally, five times daily, for 5–7 days, is the course of treatment. Adult patients can also take valaciclovir hydrochloride tablets orally, 300 mg, on an empty stomach before meal, twice a day, for 7 days. Kouyanning granules should be taken as follows: 3–6 g, three times a day, for 3–5 days, with a gradual dosage reduction according to weight and age in children.

Topical treatments include gargarism (compound chlorhexidine solution, three times a day, 1:1 diluted for children use), topical-use drug (recombinant human epidermal growth factor hydrogel, once daily, compound ulcer paste or glucocorticoids such as 0.1% triamcinolone acetonide dental paste, 0.1% dexamethasone ointment, prednisolone acetate injection, triamcinolone acetonide injection, 1:5 diluted or dexamethasone paste, three times a day), and spray (stomatitis spray, three times a day). Acyclovir eye drops can be topically used on herpes labialis three times a day. Glucocorticoids should be used with caution for children under 6 years because they can cause growth retardation and bone loss, even the topical application is not suitable for long-term and extensive use. Moreover, glucocorticoids for herpes labialis should not be used on the perioral skin to avoid hyperpigmentation on the orofacial skin.

Aerosol therapy could have additional use for serious cases, including dexamethasone sodium phosphate injection, gentamycin sulfate injection, vitamin C injection, and vitamin B12 injection, once or twice a day. For children younger than 6 years old, gentamycin sulfate injection is not recommended for aerosol therapy.

1.2 Herpes Zoster and Varicella

Case 5 Herpes Zoster (Lip, Buccal Mucosa, Tongue and Skin)

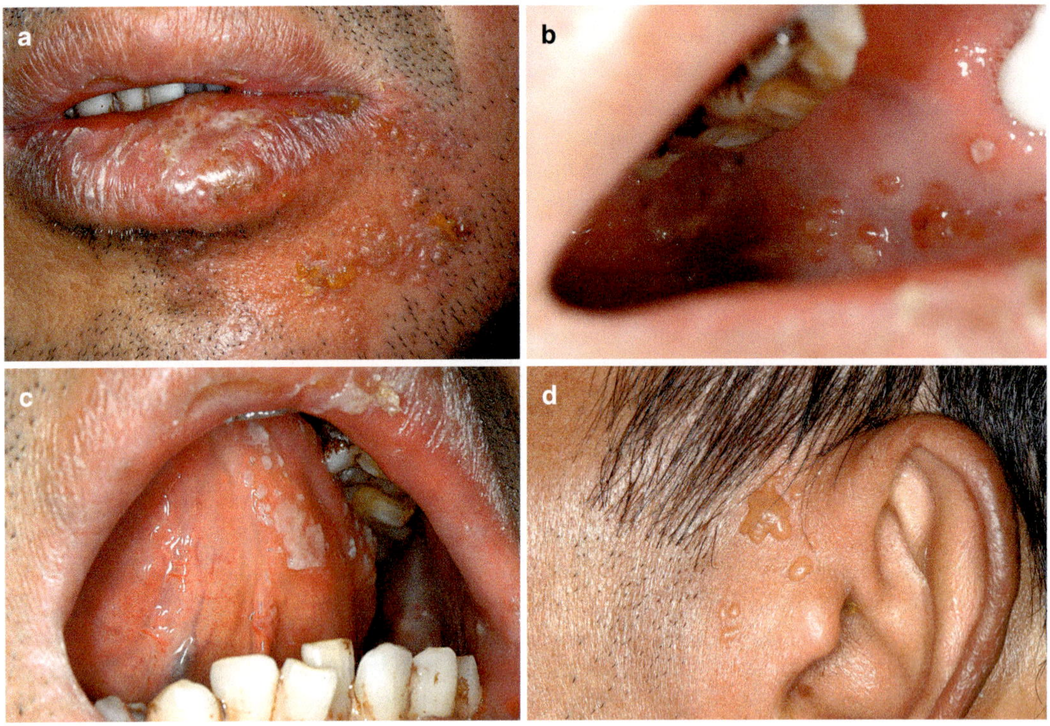

Fig. 1.5 (**a**) Vesicles in clusters involving the left vermilion border of the lower lip and adjacent skin. (**b**) Multiple blisters distributed on the left buccal mucosa. (**c**) Multiple erosions on the left lateral and ventral tongue, covered by a yellowish pseudomembrane, and the rash does not cross the midline. (**d**) Vesicles on the left preauricular region

Age: 46 years
Sex: male
Chief Complaint:
46-year-old man with oral ulcers for 1 week
History of Present Illness:
A 46-year-old man presented to our clinic with painful ulcers on the oral mucosa for 1 week after a cold, and painful blisters on the preauricular region appear 3 days ago.
Past Medical History: None.
Allergy: None.
Physical Examination:
Multiple blisters and erosions were distributed on the left dorsum, lateral and ventral tongue, left buccal mucosa, and the left mandibular lingual gingiva, and part of them coalesced covered by a yellowish pseudomembrane. Many vesicles appeared on the left lower lip and perioral and preauricular region (Fig. 1.5).
Laboratories and Imaging Studies: None.
Diagnosis:
Herpes Zoster
Diagnosis Basis:

1. Oral and cutaneous lesions are unilateral and do not cross the midline.
2. Multiple blisters and erosions are observed.

Management:

1. Aerosol therapy
   Rp.: Dexamethasone sodium phosphate injection 1 ml × 1
   Gentamycin sulfate injection 2 ml × 1
   Vitamin B12 injection 1 ml × 1

Vitamin C injection 2.5 ml × 1
Sig.: aerosol therapy q.d. or b.i.d. for 3 days

2. Medication
   Rp.: Acyclovir 100 mg × 48
   Sig.: 200 mg p.o. 5 times a day
   Pidotimod 0.4 g × 12
   Sig.: 0.4 g p.o. b.i.d.
   Zhongtong'an capsules 0.28 g × 72
   Sig.: 0.56 g p.o. t.i.d.
   Vitamin C 0.1 g × 100
   Sig.: 0.2 g p.o. t.i.d.
   Compound chlorhexidine solution 300 ml × 1
   Sig.: rinse t.i.d.
   Dexamethasone sodium phosphate injection 1 ml × 5
   Sig.: 1:50 diluted and rinse t.i.d
   Prednisolone acetate injection 125 mg × 1
   Sig.: topical use t.i.d.
3. Advising to the dermatological department for local treatment of cutaneous lesions.

Case 6 Herpes Zoster (Lip and Palate)

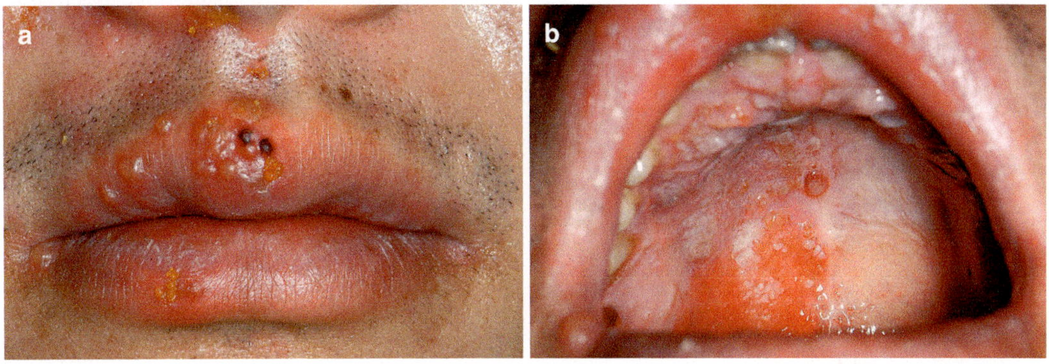

Fig. 1.6 (**a**) Clear vesicles in clustered at the right perioral skin and lips, and do not cross the midline. (**b**) Blisters and erosions on the right palate, and do not cross the midline

Age: 23 years
Sex: male
Chief Complaint:
23-year-old man with oral and facial blisters for 2–3 days
History of Present Illness:
A 23-year-old man presented to our clinic with oral and facial blisters for 2–3 days, with unbearable pain. He caught a cold 1 week ago.
Past Medical History: None.
Allergy: None.
Physical Examination:
The clear vesicles were clustered at the right nose, perioral skin, and lip; bead-like blisters on the right palate can also be noticed. All the vesicular rashes were unilateral and do not cross the midline. There were erosions in clusters on the right buccal mucosa covered by a yellowish-white pseudomembrane (Fig. 1.6).
Laboratories and Imaging Studies: None.
Diagnosis:
Herpes Zoster
Diagnosis Basis:

1. Oral and cutaneous lesions are unilateral and do not cross the midline.
2. Multiple blisters and erosions are observed.

Management:
The same as Case 5

Case 7 Varicella (Adult)

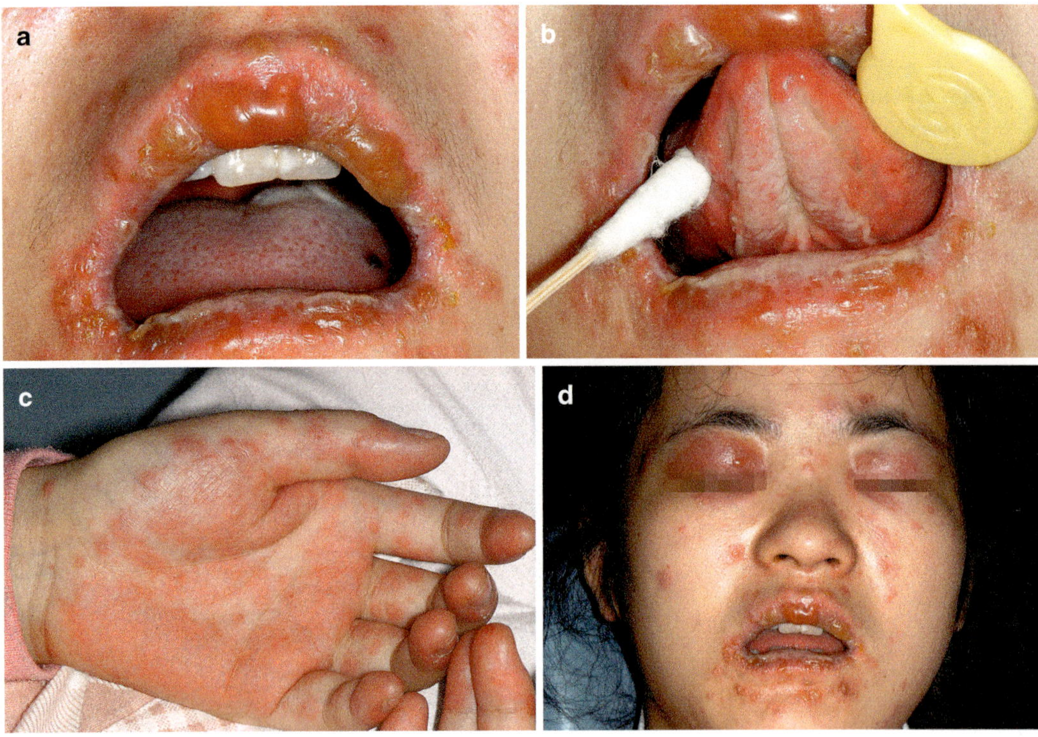

Fig. 1.7 (**a**) Widespread fluid-filled vesicles of different sizes on the lips. (**b**) Multiple erosions coalesced on the ventral tongue, covered by a yellowish pseudomembrane. (**c**) Miliary blisters and erythematous macules spread all over the palms. (**d**) Erythematous macules and vesicles on the face

Age: 20 years
Sex: female
Chief Complaint:
20-year-old woman with widespread oral ulcers for 3 days
History of Present Illness:
A 20-year-old woman presented to our clinic with widespread oral ulcers and unbearable pain for 3 days after a fever. The erythematous lesions and fluid-filled vesicles were observed involving the face, chest and palms. No medicine was taken prior to the illness onset.
Past Medical History: None.
Allergy: None.
Physical Examination:
Widespread small, fluid-filled vesicles with 1–8 mm in diameter involved the face, perioral skin, lips, dorsum and ventral tongue, buccal mucosa, and palate, with some of them ruptured to form irregular ulcers. Miliary blisters and erythematous macules were spread all over the face, neck, and palms (Fig. 1.7).
Laboratories and Imaging Studies: None.
Diagnosis:
Varicella
Diagnosis Basis:

1. The case begins with a prodrome of fever.
2. Erythematous macules and vesicular lesions appeared involving the scalp, face, and trunk 1–2 days after the fever.

Management:

1. Aerosol therapy
   Rp.: Dexamethasone sodium phosphate injection 1 ml × 1
   Gentamycin sulfate injection 2 ml × 1

Vitamin B12 injection 1 ml × 1
Vitamin C injection 2.5 ml × 1
Sig.: aerosol therapy q.d. or b.i.d. for 3 days

2. Medication
   Rp.: Compound chlorhexidine solution 300 ml × 1
   Sig.: rinse t.i.d.
   Dexamethasone sodium phosphate injection 1 ml × 5
   Sig.: 1:50 diluted and rinse t.i.d.
   Prednisolone acetate injection 125 mg × 1
   Sig.: topical use t.i.d.
3. Hospitalization in the dermatological department is recommended due to her severe condition. Exclusion from others in order to avoid infection.

Case 8 Varicella (Children)

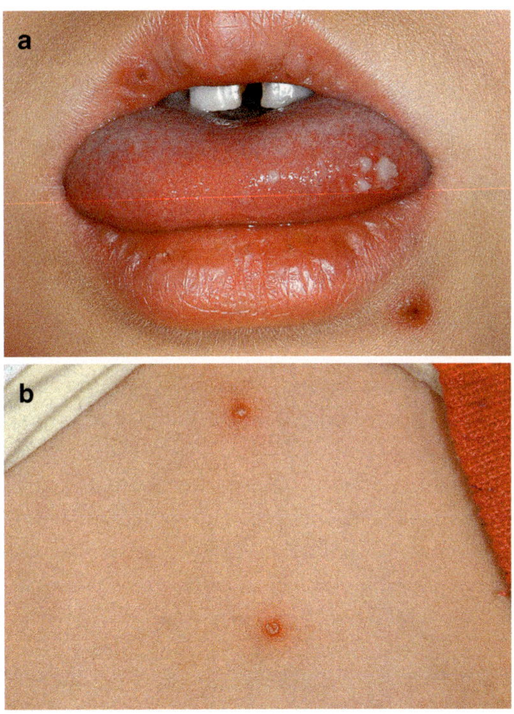

Fig. 1.8 (**a**) Several erosions covered by white pseudomembranes on the tip of the tongue, with crusting on the left perioral skin. (**b**) Erythema and vesicles on the skin of chest and abdomen

Age: 5 years
Sex: female
Chief Complaint:
5-year-old girl with oral ulcers for 3 days
History of Present Illness:
A 5-year-old girl presented to our clinic with multiple painful oral ulcers for 3 days after a fever. The fluid-filled vesicles were observed involving the back and abdominal skin.
Past Medical History: None.
Allergy: None.
Physical Examination:
Several blisters and erosions covered by white pseudomembranes appeared on the right side of retromolar trigone and tip of the tongue, with miliary erosions and crusting on perioral skin. Scattered fluid-filled vesicles with 3 mm in diameter were detected on the skin of back, chest, and abdomen. There were no obvious abnormalities on the hands and feet (Fig. 1.8).
Laboratories and Imaging Studies: None.
Diagnosis:
Varicella
Diagnosis Basis:

1. The case begins with a prodrome of fever.
2. Blisters of skins distributed centripetally.

Management:

1. Medication
   Rp.: Kouyanning granules 3 g × 10
   Sig.: 3 g p.o. t.i.d.
   Vitamin C 0.1 g × 100
   Sig.: 0.1 g p.o. t.i.d.
   Compound chlorhexidine solution 300 ml × 1
   Sig.: rinse t.i.d.
   Recombinant human epidermal growth factor hydrogel 20 g × 1
   Sig.: topical use q.d.
2. Hospitalization in the dermatological department is recommended. Exclusion from childcare in order to avoid infection until the blisters disappeared.

[Review] Herpes Zoster and Varicella

Herpes zoster is the manifestation of herpes varicella-zoster virus (VZV) infections. It occurs when the varicella-zoster virus, which causes both varicella and herpes zoster, is reactivated and spreads through the afferent nerve to the skin, with intense pain [11]. Herpes zoster can develop in anyone who has had varicella, and the frequency increases with increasing age [12]. Some patients, who have not suffered varicella in childhood, may manifest when varicella when infected with VZV as adults.

Primary VZV infection (varicella) causes VZV-specific antibody to be produced and VZV-specific T cell-mediated immune response, which can be detected within 1–2 weeks after appearance of lesions. The response is essential for recovery from varicella, due to both CD4 and CD8 effectors and memory T cells included. The memory T cell response during varicella will protect against infection during reexposure to VZV [13]. Varicella also results in lifelong latency of VZV in neurons of cranial nerve and dorsal root ganglia [14]. VZV-specific T cell-mediated immune response is also essential to maintain VZV latency in sensory ganglia at a subclinical state. When these responses are impaired, as occurs with aging or immunosuppression, the latent VZV will be reactivated. It will cause a ganglionitis with associated dermatomal neuropathic pain and following painful dermatomal vesicular rash, leading to herpes zoster [13].

Incubation period of varicella is generally ranging from 14 to 16 days. The initial cutaneous manifestations often involve the scalp, face, and trunk. They are pruritic erythema, with systemic symptoms of fever, fatigue, and anorexia. Then the maculopapular phase progresses to a vesicular phase, during which small fluid-filled vesicles occur with the range of number from 100 to 300 lesions. Approximately 24–48 h after the appearance of each lesion, crusting phase begins. Hypopigmentation is common and scarring is rare during healing. The cutaneous rash is centripetally distributed, starting with the face, following the trunk and limbs. Ulcerative and painful lesions appear on mucous membranes, such as the oropharynx and conjunctivae [15]. Varicella lesions in adult are more serious than in children; the specialist should be alert to complications such as pneumonia, neurologic disease, and bacterial infection. Hospitalization for further treatment is required if serious complications are noticed.

Herpes zoster is characterized by a band-like rash in the skin that corresponds to the affected nerve. The rash is unilateral and does not cross the midline. Chest herpes zoster is most commonly involved, followed by trigeminal herpes zoster. Localized sensations are ranging from mild itching or tingling to severe pain that precedes the development of the skin lesions by 1–5 days. As the cutaneous disease progresses, vesicles usually coalesce into larger fluid-filled lesions, following postulation and scabbing. Unilateral blisters are common oral lesions, which break down and coalesce to form extensive ulcers covered by a thick pseudomembrane. The lesions usually heal within 2–4 weeks, with complications of fatigue, headache, and photophobia; fever is unusual [11].

The Ramsay Hunt syndrome is a rare disease caused by an infection of the geniculate ganglion by the varicella-zoster virus. The main clinical features of the syndrome are as follows: Bell's palsy, unilateral or bilateral, vesicular eruptions on the ears, and ear pain [16].

The diagnosis of herpes zoster is usually based on the clinical history and features. All the cases of this unit are diagnosed by the typical history and clinical features.

Systemic treatment in the dermatological department is recommended due to band-like rash presenting as the typical cutaneous lesions. The treatment agents include antiviral drugs, immunomodulatory drugs, painkillers, and neurotrophic drugs. Acyclovir (200 mg orally, five times a day, for 5–10 days, or 400 mg orally, three times a day, for 5 days), valaciclovir (300 mg orally, twice a day for 7 days), and famciclovir (250 mg orally, three times a day for 7 days) are all effective antiviral drugs for treating herpes zoster. For patients with renal impairment, dose reduction is required. Immunomodulatory drugs include pidotimod (0.4 g orally, twice a day), transfer factor capsules (6 mg orally, three times a day), and thymopetidum enteric-coated tablets (20 mg orally, one to three times a day). Neurotrophic drugs include vitamin B1 (10 mg orally, three times a day), vitamin B12 injections (0.025–0.2 mg, intramuscular injection, q.o.d.), and mecobalamin (0.5 mg orally, three times a day).

Topical treatment of oral lesions for varicella and herpes zoster includes gargle, coated drugs, and spray. Gargle includes compound chlorhexidine solution, three times a day (1:1 diluted for children). Coated medicine includes recombinant human epidermal growth factor hydrogel or recombinant bovine basic fibroblast growth factor gel, once daily, or compound ulcer paste and glucocorticoids such as prednisolone acetate injection, triamcinolone acetonide injection (1:5 diluted), triamcinolone acetonide dental paste, and 0.1% dexamethasone ointment or dexamethasone paste, topical use three times a day. Spray such as stomatitis spray can be used three times a day. Painkiller such as compound chamomile and lidocaine hydrochloride gel or compound benzocaine gel can be applied as well, topical use three times a day. For children younger than 6 years old, glucocorticoid is not recommended.

Zostavax is a concentrated formulation of Varivax that the US Food and Drug Administration (FDA) has approved to prevent herpes zoster and its complications in immunocompetent adults aged ≥60 years. The vaccine was designed to boost cell-mediated immune responses, which should keep latent varicella-zoster virus from reactivating and thus prevent herpes zoster [17]. A randomized, double-blind, placebo-controlled trial of 38,546 adults 60 years of age or older discovered that the zoster vaccine markedly reduced morbidity from herpes zoster and postherpetic neuralgia among older adults, with a median of 3.12 years of follow-up [18]. Varicella vaccine is an effective means for prevention, and it plays a vital role in controlling the outbreaks for varicella. Therefore, the vaccine is recommended to prevent varicella in all children and adults who are seronegative for antibodies to varicella-zoster virus [11]. The great majority of vaccine recipients were under prolonged protection, which were supervised for 7 years from clinical trial. Some subjects with vaccine injected develop mild infections after exposure to natural virus, but the rashes are fewer with no fever in most cases [19]. However, it is unclear if the vaccine can affect the morbidity and severity of herpes zoster.

1.3 Hand-Foot-Mouth Disease

Case 9 Hand-Foot-Mouth Disease

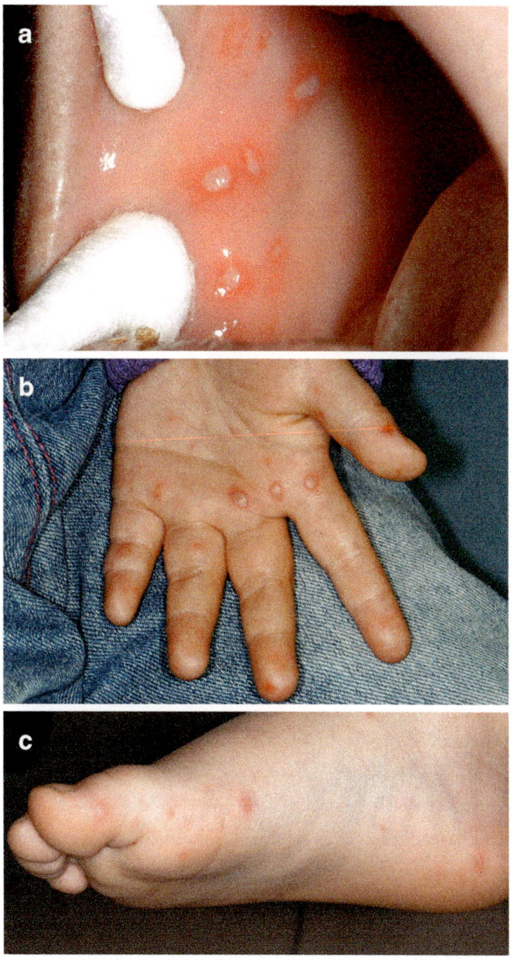

Fig. 1.9 (**a**) Scattered ulcers or erosions on the right buccal mucosa. (**b**) Blisters on the palms and fingers. (**c**) Blisters on the toes and soles

Age: 7 years
Sex: female
Chief Complaints:
Oral ulcers and red spots on the hands for 1 day

History of Present Illness:
The parents found oral ulcers accompanied with slight pain and red spots on her hands for 1 day. She had a history of cold before any symptoms.
Past Medical History: None.
Allergy: None.
Physical Examination:
There were scattered ulcers or erosions on the right buccal mucosa and tip and bilateral ventrum of the tongue, with about 2 mm in diameter. And blisters appeared with 1–3 mm in diameter on the palms, fingers, toes, and soles (Fig. 1.9).
Diagnosis:
Hand-Foot-Mouth Disease
Diagnosis Basis:

1. Little ulcers scattered on the oral mucosa.
2. The ulcers were accompanied with blisters on the hand and foot.

Management:

1. Medication
   Rp.: Kouyanning granules 3 g × 10 packets
   Sig.: 3 g t.i.d. p.o.
   Vitamin C 0.1 g × 100 tablets
   Sig.: 0.1 g t.i.d. p.o.
   Recombinant human epidermal growth factor hydrogel 20 g × 1
   Sig.: topical use, q.d.
2. Exclusion from childcare in order to avoid infection until the blisters disappeared.

[Review] Hand-Foot-Mouth Disease
Hand-foot-mouth disease (HFMD) is a common viral illness of infants and children. It is a syndrome characterized by vesicular stomatitis and cutaneous lesions of the distal extremities, which usually affect children under 10 years of the age. The incidence of HFMD is greatest in summer and early autumn [20]. It is often caused by Coxsackie A virus (A16) but may be caused less commonly by Coxsackie B and enterovirus 71 (EV71). A domestic study showed that the incidence of HFMD was increased year by year. EV71 and Coxsackie virus A16 were both the major etiologic agents of HFMD. The younger ones had higher risk of becoming severe and death cases [21]. Enterovirus 71 is often associated with a worldwide outbreak of HFMD, which can cause severe complications such as meningitis and myocarditis [22–25]. In a study in Thailand, A16 and EV71 strains obtained from outbreaks were characterized. Based on sequence analysis, nucleotide changes were found to cluster in the internal ribosome entry site (IRES) element of the 5′-untranslated region (5-UTR), which indicated the molecular basis of EV71 and CA16 outbreaks [26]. Infection sources of the HFMD are patients or virus carriers. Viruses usually spread through direct contact and droplets. It should be noted that HFMD is not related to foot and mouth disease of animals [27].

The incubation period is 3–6 days, with prodrome of fever, sore throat, and anorexia. One to two days later, red spots and blisters appear on the buccal mucosa, gingiva, and lateral or ventral tongue, which usually easily break into erosions and ulcers. The blisters and skin rash appear in 75% of patients without itchiness, which mainly occurs on the palm, fingers, toes, soles, and buttocks, at the same time or later after the oral lesion. The illness usually lasts 7–10 days. Infection causes immunity to the specific virus, but other enterovirus group could result in a second episode [27]. Most patients are only with oral, hand, and foot lesions; however, if headache, vomiting, cyanosis, abnormal heart rate, or other abnormal symptoms are detected, physicians should be especially alert to the complications such as meningitis or myocarditis.

Adults can also suffer from hand-foot-mouth disease. If the infection occurs late in pregnancy, enterovirus infection can be transmitted to the fetus. Subsequently, the newborn may have meningitis, thrombocytopenia, disseminated intravascular coagulation, myocarditis, or hepatitis, and disease appears to be more severe than if it is postnatally acquired [28].

Diagnosis is usually based on the clinical features alone. Diagnosis of HFMD in Case 9 was based on the typical lesions that occurred on the oral mucosa, hands, and feet.

Different treatments should be applied according to the degree of patients' conditions. Patients with mild symptoms take Kouyanning granules orally, 1.5–3.0 g continuous for 3–5 days, and vitamin C tablets, 0.05–0.1 g orally three times a day; vitamin B tablets can also be taken orally, 0.5–1 tablet a day. Topical medications include rinse (cleansing) solutions, spreads, and sprays. Compound chlorhexidine solution (1: 1 diluted for children) can be used as rinse solution, three times a day. Liniment such as recombinant human epidermal growth factor hydrogel, once a day, or compound ulcer paste can be applied. Stomatitis spray can be selected as the spray, three times a day. At the same time, parents should be especially alert to the general conditions of children; hospitalization for further treatment is required if severe clinical status or serious complications are noticed.

Exclusion from school or childcare is suggested to avoid infecting others.

1.4 Herpangina

Case 10 Herpangina

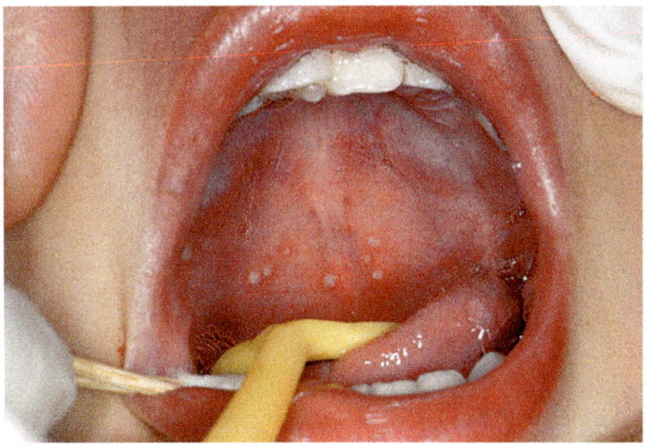

Fig. 1.10 Ulcers and erosions on posterior soft palate

Age: 2 years 8 months
Sex: male
Chief Complaints:
Oral pain for 1 day
History of Present Illness:
The teacher noticed that oral ulcers were located on their child's throat, with pain for 1 day. He had a history of cold 5 days ago.
Past Medical History: None.
Allergy: None.

Physical Examination:
There were several ulcers and erosions with 1–2 mm in diameter on posterior soft palate with mild hyperemia. Gingival redness and swelling were not detected, and there were no obvious abnormalities on the hands and feet (Fig. 1.10).
Diagnosis:
Herpangina
Diagnosis Basis:

1. The history of catching cold.
2. Several superficial round small ulcers were all in the posterior oral cavity.

Management:

1. Aerosol therapy
   Rp.: Dexamethasone sodium phosphate injection 1 ml × 1
   Gentamycin sulfate injection 2 ml × 1
   Vitamin B12 injection 1 ml × 1
   Vitamin C injection 2.5 ml × 1
   Sig.: aerosol therapy q.d. or b.i.d. for 3 days
2. Medication
   Rp.: Kouyanning granules 3 g × 10 packets
   Sig.: 3 g t.i.d. p.o.
   Vitamin C 0.1 g × 100 tablets
   Sig.: 0.1 g t.i.d. p.o.
   Compound chlorhexidine solution 300 ml × 1
   Sig.: rinse t.i.d.
   Recombinant human epidermal growth factor hydrogel 20 g × 1
   Sig.: topical use q.d.

[Review] Herpangina
Herpangina is an oral lesion mainly caused by the infection of Coxsackie virus A (CV-A). The virus types vary with the outbreak year and the area, and the main types are CV-A2, CV-A4, CV-A5, CV-A6, CV-A8, CV-A9, CV-A10, CV-A16, CV-A22, etc. [29–31]. The illness is highly infectious and spreads fast, which usually affects children. The incidence of herpangina is greatest in summer and autumn. It is characterized by an acute onset of fever and sore throat with mild precursory and general symptoms [32]. The clinical features are blisters with 1–2 mm in diameter on

the posterior oral mucosa, which often become erosions or ulcers. The site of lesions is limited to the posterior oral cavity, such as the soft palate, uvula, and tonsil. The disease usually lasts about 7 days. Diagnosis is mainly based on the history of the disease and the typical lesions on the posterior oral cavity.

Systemic treatment of the disease can use Kouyanning granules orally, 1.5–3.0 g continuous for 3–5 days, and vitamin C tablets, 0.05–0.1 g orally three times a day; vitamin B tablets can also be taken orally, 0.5–1 tablet a day. Topical medications include rinse (cleansing) solutions, spreads, and sprays. Compound chlorhexidine solution (1:1 diluted for children) can be used as rinse solution, three times a day. Liniment such as recombinant human epidermal growth factor hydrogel, once a day; or compound ulcer paste, 0.1% triamcinolone acetonide dental paste, and 0.01% dexamethasone compound three times a day; or prednisolone acetate injection and triamcinolone acetonide injection (1:5 diluted), three times a day, can be applied. Stomatitis spray can be selected as the spray, three times a day. Glucocorticoids should be used with caution for children under 6 years because they can cause growth retardation and bone loss, even the topical application is not suitable for long-term and extensive use.

1.5 Oral Candidosis

Case 11 Pseudomembranous Candidosis

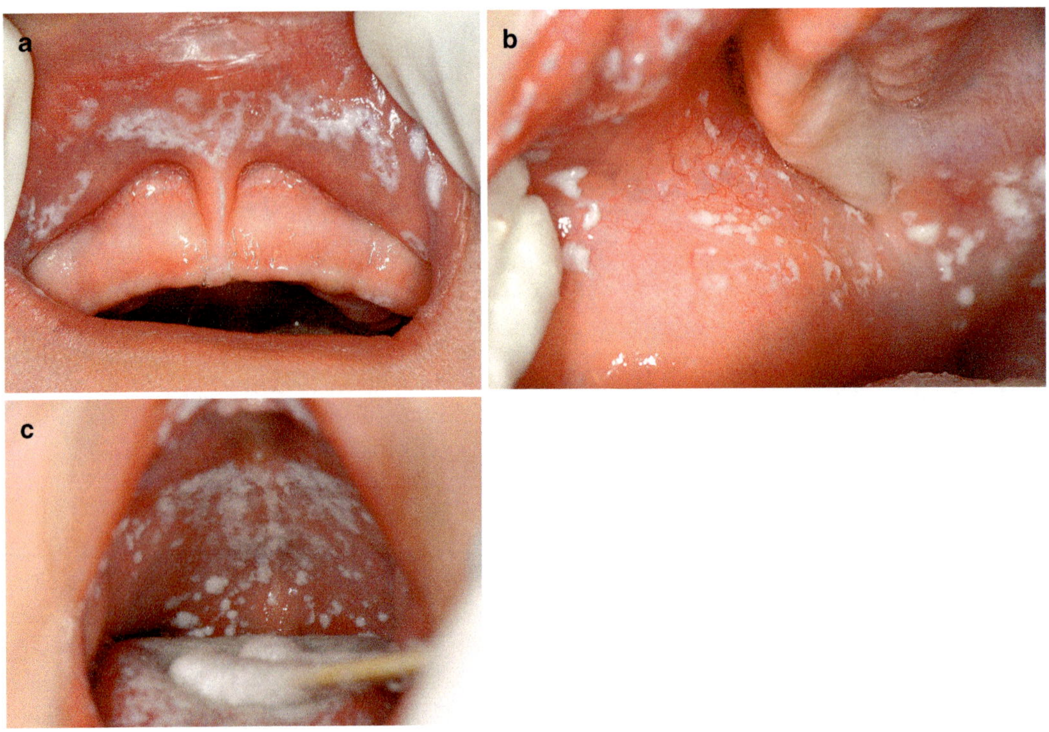

Fig. 1.11 (**a**) Widespread confluent white velvety plaques on the upper labium mucosa, which can be removed by gentle rubbing of the lesion. (**b**) White velvety plaques on the right buccal mucosa, which can be removed by gentle rubbing of the lesion. (**c**) Widespread confluent white velvety plaques on the palate, which can be removed by gentle rubbing of the lesion

Age: 3 months
Sex: male
Chief Complaints:
3-month-old boy with white patch for 4 days
History of Present Illness:
A 3-month-old boy presented to our clinic with oral white plaques for 4 days. No obvious discomfort was found. He had a fever 3 days ago, which had gone after unknown treatment.
Past Medical History: None.
Allergy: None.
Physical Examination:
Widespread confluent white velvety plaques were observed on the labium mucosa, dorsum of the tongue, palate, and buccal mucosa which can be removed by gentle rubbing of the lesion, leaving an erythematous surface (Fig. 1.11).
Diagnosis:
Pseudomembranous Candidosis

Diagnosis Basis:

1. The patient was an infant.
2. Oral lesions showed white velvety plaques which can be easily removed.

Management:

1. Medication
   Rp.: 1% sodium bicarbonate solution 250 ml × 4
   Sig.: topical use t.i.d. and soak the contact items
   Nystatin liniment 15 g × 2
   Sig.: topical use t.i.d.
2. Not only boil the contact items (such as bottles, spoon, cup, bowl and toys) following soaked with 1–2% sodium bicarbonate solution disinfectant, but also adhere to medication after the lesions regression for 10–14 days should be noted.

Case 12 Acute Erythematous Candidosis

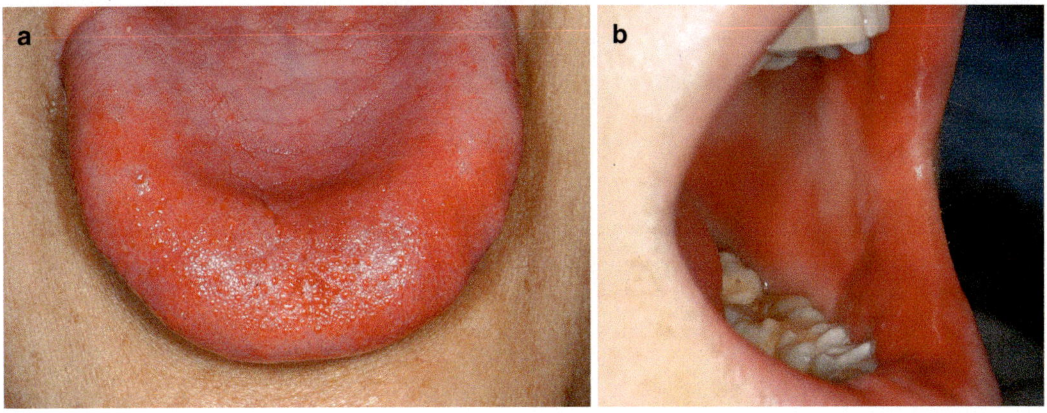

Fig. 1.12 (**a**) Disperse and irregular reddened lesions on the dorsum of the tongue. (**b**) Disperse hyperemia on the left buccal mucosa

Age: 51 years
Sex: female
Chief Complaints:
51-year-old woman with painful reddened mouth for 3 days
History of Present Illness:
A 51-year-old woman presented to our clinic complaining of multiple painful reddened lesions 3 days ago. It tends to develop after the receipt of broad-spectrum antibiotics for 1 week due to the cold he caught. Blood routine examination and blood sugar were normal.
Past Medical History: None.
Allergy: None.
Physical Examination:
Widespread reddened lesions with disperse and irregular appearance were noticed, with especially serious manifestations on the tongue and buccal

mucosa. Fungi were detected from samples taken from the buccal mucosa, dorsum of the tongue, and the palate by smear method (Fig. 1.12).

Diagnosis:

Acute Erythematous Candidosis

Diagnosis Basis:

1. History of antibiotics application to rule out anemia.
2. Oral reddened lesions with disperse appearance.
3. Fungi were detected by smear method.

Management:

1. Medication
   Rp.: Pidotimod 0.4 g × 18 tablets
   Sig.: 1 tablet p.o.
   Compound vitamin B 100 tablets
   Sig.: 2 tablets t.i.d. p.o.
   2% sodium bicarbonate solution 250 ml × 2
   Sig.: rinse t.i.d.
   Nystatin liniment 15 g × 2
   Sig.: topical use t.i.d.
2. Cessation of antibiotics abuse

Case 13 Chronic Erythematous Candidosis

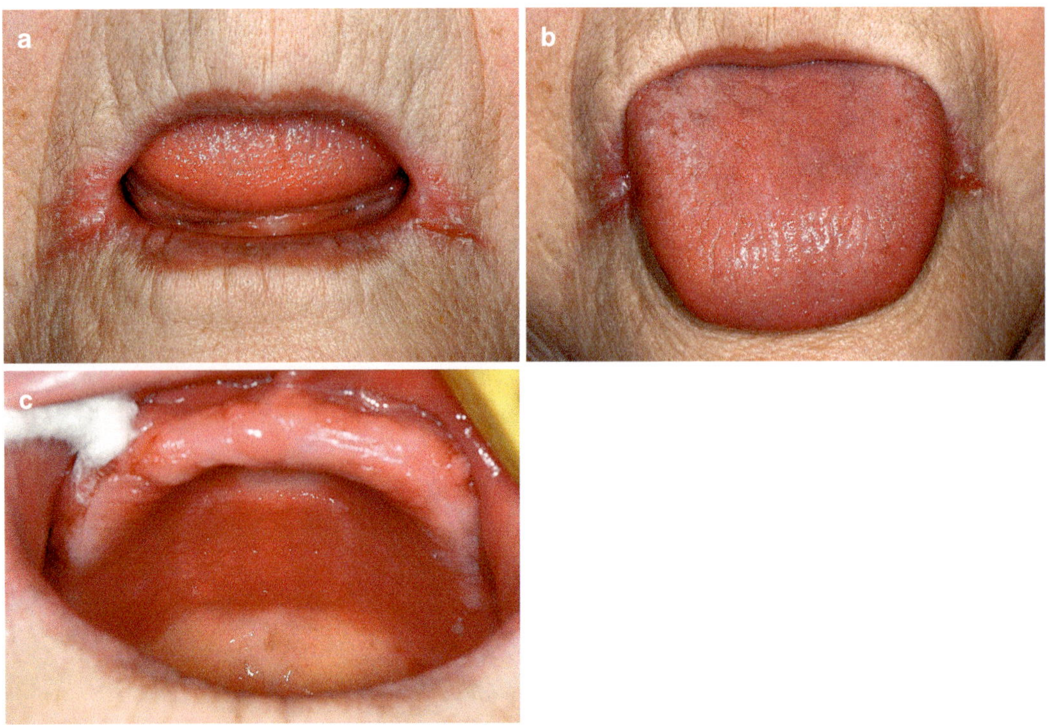

Fig. 1.13 (**a**) Fissures running in the corner of the mouth. (**b**) Atrophic dorsum of the tongue. (**c**) Widespread reddened lesions on the palate, with edema and papillary hyperplasia on the alveolar ridges and the palate

Age: 79 years

Sex: female

Chief Complaints:

79-year-old woman with painful reddened mouth for 4 years and fissure running in the corner of the mouth for 1 year

History of Present Illness:

A 79-year-old woman presented to our clinic complaining of painful reddened lesions with atrophic area on the dorsum of the tongue 4 years ago. Fissures running in the corner of the mouth occurred 1 year ago. Blood routine examination and blood sugar were normal.

Past Medical History: Hypertension.

Allergy: None.

Physical Examination:

Complete denture and low jaw spacing were observed. Widespread reddened lesions were noticed on the palate, with edema and papillary hyperplasia on the alveolar ridges. The dorsum of the tongue was atrophic, and fissures running in the corner of the mouth occurred. Fungi were detected from samples taken from the corner of the mouth, dorsum of the tongue, and the palate by smear method (Fig. 1.13).

Diagnosis:

Chronic Erythematous Candidosis; Candidal Angular Cheilitis

Diagnosis Basis:

1. The patient was an old lady with complete denture.
2. Widespread reddened lesions with edema and papillary hyperplasia were observed on the maxillary denture-supporting area.
3. Fungi were detected by smear method.

Management:

1. Medication
   Rp.: Pidotimod 0.4 g × 18 tablets
   Sig.: 1 tablet b.i.d. p.o.
   Compound vitamin B 100 tablets
   Sig.: 2 tablets t.i.d. p.o.
   2% sodium bicarbonate solution 250 ml × 4
   Sig.: rinse t.i.d.
   Nystatin liniment 15 g × 2
   Sig.: topical use t.i.d.
2. Attention to clean dentures followed by soaked with 2% sodium bicarbonate solution

Case 14 Chronic Hyperplastic Candidosis

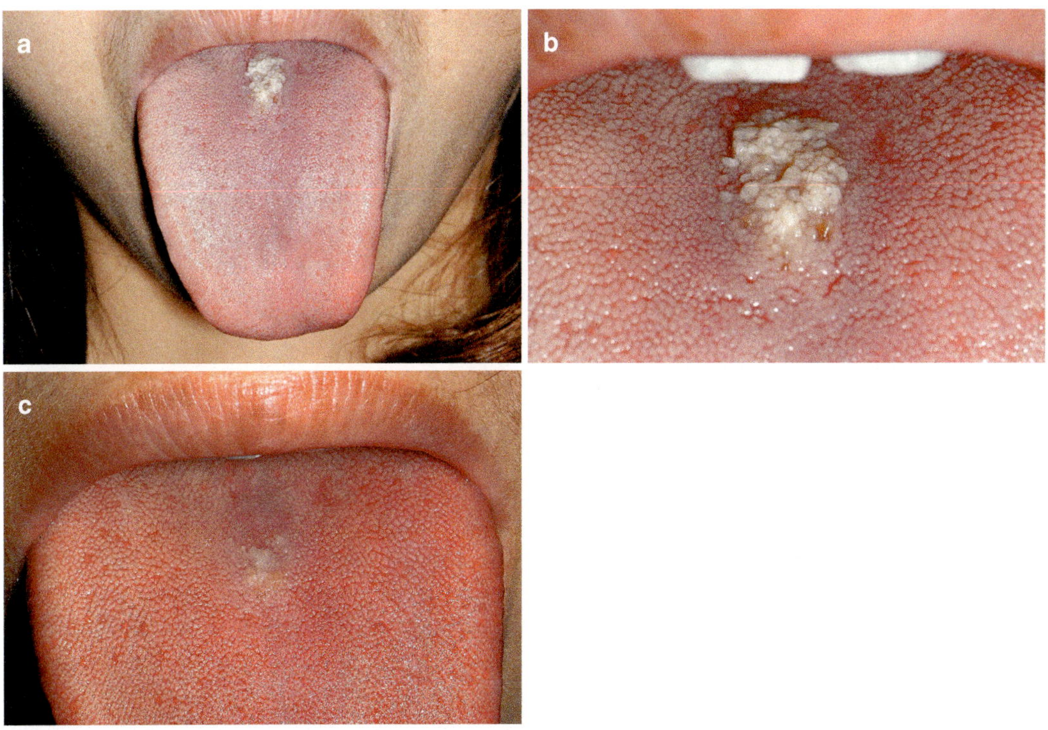

Fig. 1.14 (**a**) A 14 mm × 11 mm plaque on the posterior and middle dorsum of the tongue. (**b**) The plaque with white granular surface that protrudes from the mucosal surface. (**c**) The white lesion recessed mostly 1 week later

Age: 50 years
Sex: female
Chief Complaints:
White plaque on the dorsum of the tongue for 10 days

History of Present Illness:
The patient came across a painless white plaque on the posterior of the dorsum of the tongue with foreign body sensation. There was no obvious increase of this growth.

Past Medical History: None.
Allergy: None.
Physical Examination:
There was a 14 mm × 11 mm plaque on the posterior and middle dorsum of the tongue, with white granular surface. No local hyperemia or erosion was observed. It cannot be removed by gentle rubbing of the lesion. Smear method failed to detect fungi from the lesion (Fig. 1.14a, b).
Clinical Impression:
Chronic Hyperplastic Candidosis?
Management:

1. Medication
   Rp.: Pidotimod 0.4 g × 18 tablets
   Sig.: 1 tablet b.i.d. p.o.
   Compound vitamin B 100 tablets
   Sig.: 2 tablets t.i.d. p.o.
   2% sodium bicarbonate solution 250 ml × 4
   Sig.: rinse t.i.d.
   Nystatin liniment 15 g × 2
   Sig.: topical use t.i.d.
   Fluconazole 50 mg × 6 tablets
   Sig.: 50 mg b.i.d. suck
2. Subsequent visit 1 week later was suggested. Excision or biopsy would be considered if no remission occurred

Subsequent Treatment:
One week later, the white lesion recessed mostly (Fig. 1.14c); 2 weeks later, the lesions disappeared completely.
Diagnosis:
Chronic Hyperplastic Candidosis
Diagnosis Basis:

1. The dorsum of the tongue is a predilection site of chronic hyperplastic candidosis.
2. The plaque presented as white granular appearance.
3. Although definite diagnosis requires biopsy, complete recovery was achieved by antifungal therapy in this case.

[Review] Oral Candidosis
Oral candidosis is a fungal infection of *Candida* species on the mucous membranes of the mouth. In recent decades, the incidence of oral candidosis has markedly increased, mainly owing to the escalation of human immunodeficiency virus (HIV) infection, organ and bone marrow transplantation, and increasing use of immunosuppressive therapies as well as broad-spectrum antibiotics [33].

A change from the harmless commensal existence of *Candida* to a pathogenic state appears following alteration of the oral environment to one that favors the growth of *Candida*. The causes of such alterations are the so-called predisposing factors including host factors for *Candida* infection. With regard to the opportunistic pathogenic nature of *Candida*, candidiasis is often described as being "diseases of the diseased" [34]. *Candida albicans* is the most common in everyone, and mycological studies have revealed that *C. albicans* represents more than 80% of the specimen from all types of human candidosis [35]. It is noteworthy that the incidence of non-*C. albicans* species is increased in human candidosis. The reasons may partly relate to improved diagnostic methods. However, it could also reflect that more and more antifungal drug resistance was observed in some non-*Candida albicans* species compared with *C. albicans* [36]. The most predilection mucosa is superficial and moist, which is common in the vagina and oral cavity. Systemic infections are rare but are severe if they do develop, with mortality rates of up to 60% [37]. In the past 10 years, candidemia that has increased fivefold has been reported, with susceptible individuals suffering from leukemia or blood stem cell transplantation. In addition to candidosis, it has been considered that *Candida* species may be pathogenic factors in some oral disorders, including oral cancer, burning mouth syndrome, taste disorders, and endodontic disease, although the pathogenesis remains unclear [38–41].

C. albicans is heat-labile and is stable in acidic conditions. The pathogenic significance of being able to generate hyphae could associate with the greater enhanced adherence to host surfaces and invade epithelial layers resulting in tissue damage. Putative virulence factors have been identified, including adherence to host by cell surface hydrophobicity and expression of cell surface adhesins; through high-frequency phenotypic switching, hyphal generated, secreted aspartyl proteinase production, and complement binding to reduce phagocytosis, destruct secretory IgA and mask antigen; through hyphal development and hydrolytic enzyme production, to promote entry of oral mucosa, resulting in destruction of host cell and extracellular matrix [34].

A change from the harmless commensal existence to a pathogenic state relates to lots of predisposing factors. Local host factors include wearing denture, using steroid inhaler, declined salivary flow, high sugar diet, and smoking. Systemic host factors include extremes of age, diabetes, immunosuppression, receipt of broad-spectrum antibiotics, etc. [42].

Candidiasis is rare in immunocompetent populations; the incidence of fungal infection appears to increase in individuals presenting clinical features of acquired or primary immunodeficiencies. The HIV infection, immunosuppressive therapy, use of broad-spectrum antibiotics, and invasive surgical procedures such as solid organ or bone marrow transplantation are the main factors related to acquired immunodeficiencies. The primary immunodeficiency diseases are hereditary disorders involving one or multiple components of the immune system, which could lead to recurrent or persistent bacterial, fungal, and viral infections. Primary immunodeficiencies are usually diagnosed during early life, with more than 80% of cases diagnosed before the age of 20 years [43]. The diseases vary in the severity and spectrum of symptoms which need early diagnosis and treatment. There are many types of primary immunodeficiencies, such as familial/diffuse chronic mucocutaneous candidosis, candidosis-endocrinopathy syndrome, candidosis-thymoma syndrome, DiGeorge syndrome, chronic granulomatous disease, etc. Most of them manifest as chronic oral candida infections and other systemic symptoms, involving the oral mucosa, skin, and nail [44]. The initial skin lesions are usually erythema, verrucous proliferation, and scab formation, following marked hyperkeratosis and acanthosis, rarely, cutaneous horns.

Oral candidosis is mainly present as stomatitis, angular cheilitis, and cheilitis. Candida stomatitis includes two acute types, namely, pseudomembranous candidosis and acute erythematous candidosis, and two persistent forms, known as chronic erythematous candidosis and chronic hyperplastic candidosis.

Pseudomembranous candidosis is also known as the oral thrush and is mostly in neonates and 5–10% of the elderly. It is characterized by the painless confluent white velvety plaques that are easily removed by gentle rubbing of the lesion, leaving an erythematous surface which may easily bleed. The feature that plaques can be removed is a diagnostic point that differentiates pseudomembranous candidosis from other oral patch lesions. Histological inspections show fungal materials in the yeast and filamentous forms, together with food debris, leukocytes, and epithelial cells [45]. The adjacent oral mucosa is of normal color and texture. In the majority of immunocompromised patients, pseudomembranous candidosis often seems to be more extensive with thicker and widespread pseudomembranes, and the lesions will invariably relapse when treatment ceases.

Acute erythematous candidosis is often known as antibiotic sore mouth, as it tends to develop after the receipt of broad-spectrum antibiotics, resulting in a reduced bacterial level of the oral microflora [34]. It presents as a painful reddened lesion, the most common infection site is the dorsum of the tongue, and the palate or buccal mucosa may be involved. Cessation of antibiotic therapy results in the normal balance of the microflora, which subsequently resolves the candidosis without intervention. Inhaled corticosteroids are an additional factor.

Chronic erythematous candidosis is also known as *Candida*-associated denture stomatitis, which is almost exclusively encountered on palatal tissues beneath the fitting surface of a denture. It often presents as a reddened lesion, sometimes with papillary hyperplasia on the palate. The main host factors related to this disorder are poor oral hygiene, not removing dentures while sleeping, or bad denture fit. Up to 75% of denture wearers have clinical signs of this condition [46].

Chronic hyperplastic candidosis mainly manifests as a thickened white plaque, most commonly on the dorsum of the tongue. It has the potential of squamous cell carcinoma development at lesion locations, although the function of *Candida* in carcinogenesis remains unclear [47]. Several studies have shown that antifungal treatment may alter the clinical features of this lesion from a nonhomogeneous to a homogeneous leukoplakia, while others have demonstrated that part of the lesions completely disappears after antifungal therapy alone, thus confirming its fungal etiology [34].

Candidal angular cheilitis manifests as erythematous lesions at one or both of the angles of the mouth. The spectrum of microorganisms discovered from this disorder includes *Staphylococcus aureus*, streptococcal species, etc., other than *Candida*. As a result, the exact role of *Candida* in angular cheilitis remains uncertain [34].

Candidal cheilitis lacks the specific clinical features, which could manifest as erosions, crusting, or small granular lesions on the lips.

The diagnosis of oral candidosis is usually based on the clinical history and features; laboratory examinations are also needed [43]. The common tests include smear method, isolated culture, and histopathological examination. Generally, pseudomembranous and erythematous candidosis can be diagnosed without a biopsy.

A characteristic feature of chronic hyperplastic candidosis is hyperparakeratosis on the superficial mucosa with inflammatory cell infiltration and microabscesses formed. Epithelial cell edema, mild to moderate epithelium dysplasia, and a dense infiltration of lymphocytic cells into the mesenchyme of lamina propria were also found. The penetration of the oral mucosa by *C. albicans* hyphae, which are detected in biopsy sections following Periodic Acid-Schiff (PAS) or equivalent staining methods. Case 11 was diagnosed by the typical pseudomembranous lesions; Cases 12 and 13 were diagnosed by the typical history, clinical features, and smear method; and Case 14 was diagnosed by the clinical features and good response to antifungal therapy.

Management of oral candidosis requires identification and correction of the specific underlying predisposing factors in an individual patient, such as cessation of antibiotics and glucocorticoid abuse, cleaning the denture, and appropriate oral hygiene practices.

Local treatment has good effect on oral candidosis. Commonly used is 2–4% sodium bicarbonate solution and nystatin liniment. Nystatin liniment is a tetraene antibiotic, and 1 mg is equivalent to 2000 U. Aqueous suspensions of 0.05–0.1 million U/ml can be used for topical use, once every 2–3 h, and it can be swallowed after coated. For infants and young children with oral thrush, the lesions will regress after the application of the above drugs but are easy to relapse. Not only boiling the contact items (such as bottles, spoon, cup, bowl, and toys) followed by soaking with 1–2% sodium bicarbonate solution disinfectant but also adhering to the medication after the lesion regression for 10–14 days should be noted. In addition, if the child is still in the breastfeeding stage, the mother's nipple should also be cleaned with 1–2% sodium bicarbonate solution and coated with nystatin liniment or water suspension.

For patients with stubborn condition, combination of oral drugs that include antifungal agents, immunoenhancers, and vitamins can be effective. Oral antifungal drugs such as fluconazole tablets are suggested to be taken on the first day by 200 mg, followed by 50 mg, two times daily for 7–14 days, or itraconazole capsules, 100–200 mg orally, one time per day. However, it is critical to notice that the abovementioned oral antifungal drugs should not be used in infants and patients with serious systemic diseases. Immunoenhancers include pidotimod, 0.4–0.8 g each time, two times per day for 7–14 days; or thymopetidum enteric-coated tablets, 20 mg orally, two to three times daily, for 15–30 days; or transfer factor capsule, 6 mg each time, two to three times daily, for 15–30 days. Vitamin drugs include compound vitamin B, mecobalamin, folic acid, vitamin C, and so on.

1.6 Coccigenic Stomatitis (Membranous Stomatitis)

Case 15 Coccigenic Stomatitis (Membranous Stomatitis)

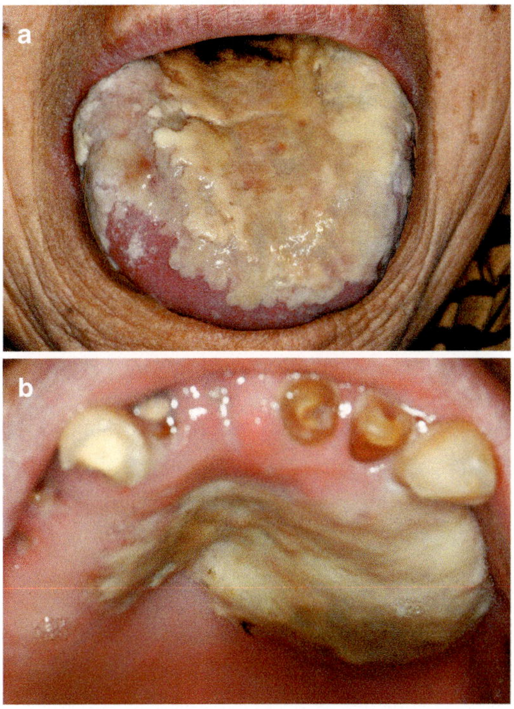

Fig. 1.15 (**a**) Widespread dense, smooth, thick, and yellowish-brown pseudomembrane on the dorsum of the tongue. (**b**) Widespread dense, smooth, thick, and yellowish-brown pseudomembrane on the palate

Age: 72 years
Sex: female
Chief Complaints:
72-year-old woman with an ulcerated tongue for 3 days
History of Present Illness:
A 72-year-old woman presented to our clinic with painful oral ulcers for 3 days, which impaired eating and speech. She had taken antibiotic drugs (unknown details) due to bronchitis 1 week ago in the local hospital.
Past Medical History: Bronchitis, hypertension.
Allergy: None.
Physical Examination:
Widespread dense, smooth, thick, and yellowish-brown pseudomembrane was observed on the dorsum of the tongue and palate, which can be removed by rubbing of the lesion. The floor of the mouth and ventral tongue were also involved (Fig. 1.15). White blood cell count was normal. The percentage of neutrophils increased slightly (75.84%), but the rate of lymphocytes decreased (11.74%).
Diagnosis:
Membranous Stomatitis
Diagnosis Basis:
Widespread dense, smooth, and thick pseudomembrane appeared on the oral mucosa.
Management:

1. Medication
   Rp.: Pidotimod 0.4 g × 12 tablets
   Sig.: 0.4 g b.i.d. p.o.
   Compound vitamin B 100 tablets
   Sig.: 2 tablets t.i.d. p.o.
   Compound chlorhexidine solution 300 ml × 1
   Sig.: rinse t.i.d.
   Dequalinium chloride buccal tablet 0.25 mg × 18 tablets
   Sig.: 0.25 mg 4–6 times/day suck
   2% sodium bicarbonate solution 250 ml × 2
   Sig.: rinse t.i.d.
   Nystatin liniment 15 g × 2
   Sig.: topical use t.i.d.

Subsequent Treatment:
One week later, the lesion was recession mostly, leaving superficial erosive surface. So the medications were adjusted to 2% sodium bicarbonate solution, oral rinse, three times daily; nystatin liniment, topical use, three times per day; and topical use of prednisolone acetate injection on the erosion to promote healing.

[Review] Coccigenic Stomatitis (Membranous Stomatitis)

The oral cavity is colonized by several hundred types of microorganisms. In healthy individuals, they are usually harmless and in balance. Oral microflora mainly consists of *Streptococci*,

Staphylococci, and *Diplococcus pneumonia*. The balance between the host and oral microflora breaking down relates to lots of predisposing factors, including cold and fever, acute infectious disease, radiotherapy and chemotherapy for malignancies, and long-term use of immunosuppressants, which could reduce the immune function, resulting in abnormal proliferation and virulence increase of bacteria responsible for coccigenic stomatitis. Advanced age, suffering from other oral mucosal disorders, dentures, and orthodontic materials may also be predisposing factors [48, 49].

Primary coccigenic stomatitis is uncommon, often occurred in weak patients with low resistance. Secondary coccigenic stomatitis is commonly seen in clinical practice occurring following other oral mucosal lesions, such as herpes simplex, allergies stomatitis, or erosive oral lichen planus. The anti-infectious treatment together with the treatment of primary lesions should be considered. Patient in Case 15 of this unit had medication history before oral erosion; therefore, drug allergic stomatitis initially, followed by secondary coccigenic stomatitis, was considered.

Coccigenic stomatitis can occur in any part of the oral mucosa, mainly for hyperemia and local erosions or ulcers. The ulcers and erosions are covered by a gray or yellowish-brown pseudomembrane, which is dense, smooth, and thick that are not easily removed by gentle rubbing of the lesion, leaving an erosive surface. So it is also called membranous stomatitis. The surrounding mucosal hyperemia and swelling could be observed, with obvious inflammatory reaction. The patients show significant pain and increased saliva, with bad breath, and lymphadenopathy may be accompanied by systemic symptoms such as fever. Coccigenic stomatitis may be the mixed infection that is caused by several kinds of *Coccus* coexistence. If necessary, smear or bacterial culture can be made to determine the main pathogens.

Increased permeability of the mucosal barrier because of mucositis may result in microbial dissemination into the bloodstream. Bacteremia poses a lethal threat to individuals with impaired immune mechanisms, leading to systemic infections, which should be noticed in clinical practices [50].

A patient accompanied by the systemic infection should be evaluated firstly. Targeted antibiotics should be chosen based on results of bacterial culture and drug sensitivity test, including penicillins, cephalosporins, and macrolides. The following drugs can be applied if without systemic infection: pidotimod, 0.4 g orally, twice a day for 1–2 weeks; compound vitamin B, two tablets orally, three times a day; 1% povidone iodine solution or compound chlorhexidine solution for oral rinse, three times a day; and topical use of compound ulcer paste. Lozenges can also be used, such as the cydiodine tablets, 1.5 mg suck, four to six times a day; lysozyme hydrochloride tablets, 20 mg suck, four to six times a day; and dequalinium chloride buccal tablet, 0.5 mg suck, four to six times a day. During the medication process, 2–4% sodium bicarbonate solution for oral rinse and topical use of nystatin liniment should be administrated to avoid fungal infection.

1.7 Oral Tuberculosis

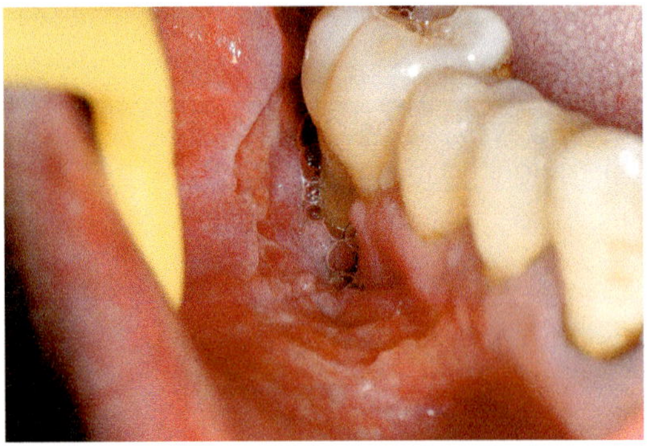

Fig. 1.16 A 20 mm × 10 mm ulcer with undermined edges, clear boundary, and a granulating floor on the right mandibular buccal gingival sulcus

Case 16 Tuberculosis Ulcer
Age: 46 years
Sex: male
Chief Complaints:
46-year-old man with ulcers on the right mandibular gingiva for 6 months

History of Present Illness:
A 46-year-old man complained of painless ulcers on the right mandibular gingiva, with weight loss for 6 months. He denied the history of hot flashes, night sweats, and tuberculosis.
Past Medical History: None.
Allergy: None.
Physical Examination:
There was a 20 mm × 10 mm ulcer on the right mandibular buccal gingival sulcus. It was stellate with undermined edges and clear boundary. After removing purulent exudates of the superficial ulceration, a granulating floor can be noticed (Fig. 1.16).
Clinical Impression:
Tuberculosis Ulcer?
Laboratories and Imaging Studies:

1. Routine blood test, blood glucose, and serological tests for syphilis and HIV were normal.
2. Tissue biopsy of the ulcer was performed. Histopathology exam showed chronic granulomatous inflammation with unstructured caseous material. The bacilli were identified by acid-fast stains, and *Mycobacterium tuberculosis* DNA was detected by DNA-qPCR. Tuberculosis ulcer was confirmed by pathological diagnosis.
3. Chest X-ray showed infectious disorder of bilateral lung.

Diagnosis:
Tuberculosis Ulcer
Diagnosis Basis:

1. The painless ulcer was stellate with undermined edges. A granulating floor can be noticed after removing purulent exudates of the superficial ulceration.
2. It was confirmed by histopathological examination.

Management:

1. He was advised to the department of infectious diseases for antituberculosis therapy.
2. Intralesional injection was adopted for oral tuberculosis ulcers: isoniazid 0.1 g, every other day, for ten times as the treatment course.
3. Topical use of compound chlorhexidine solution, oral rinse, three to four times daily.

[Review] Oral Tuberculosis
Oral tuberculosis (TB) is an infectious disease caused by *Mycobacterium tuberculosis*. It can be classified as primary and secondary oral TB. Primary oral TB was detected in 42% and secondary oral TB in 58% (of which 54% pulmonary, 4% extrapulmonary) of patients. The secondary oral lesion is more common in elder patients, whereas the primary type mainly affects the young. It has been reported that approximately 50% of patients with oral manifestation of TB has led to the diagnosis of a previously unknown systemic infection, which resulted in a timely and effective treatment [51].

Oral TB is rare and has been reported to occur in 0.05–5% of all TB infections, but it should be considered if particular oral ulcers encountered due to more drug-resistant TB and acquired immunodeficiency syndrome (AIDS) occur. Oral TB accounted for up to 1.33% of human immunodeficiency virus (HIV)-associated opportunistic infections, based on a cohort of 1345 patients [52].

Mycobacterium tuberculosis can survive in human adipocytes for a long time. Recent researches have indicated that radical cure for tuberculosis is difficult, for antituberculosis drugs are hard to get into the adipocytes directly. The mechanism of the oral *Mycobacterium tuberculosis* infection is not clear yet, but it is generally believed that oral mucous membrane presents a natural resistance to *Mycobacterium* invasion. This resistance has been attributed to the integrity and thickness of the oral epithelium, the cleansing action of saliva, and the presence of salivary enzymes and tissue antibodies. Any break or loss of this natural barrier, which may be a result of trauma, inflammation, tooth extraction, or poor oral hygiene, and preexisting lesions such as leukoplakias, periapical granulomas, periodontitis, etc., may provide an invasion route of *Mycobacterium*. Immunosuppression and nutritional deficiencies may also be the systemic predisposing factors [53, 54].

Mycobacterium tuberculosis infects all parts of the mouth. Oral tuberculous lesions include tuberculous chancre, tuberculosis ulcers, and lupus vulgaris, among which the most common symptoms are tuberculosis ulcers.

Tuberculous chancre (primary tuberculosis syndrome) is rare and more widely in children and adolescents [55]. The dorsal surface of the tongue is affected most commonly, followed by the buccal mucosa and lips. For those with negative tuberculin skin test, oral mucosa may be the first area invaded by *Mycobacterium tuberculosis*. Following an incubation period of 2–3 weeks, a nodule occurs at the entry part and develops into an intractable painless ulcer with surrounding induration, which is called tuberculous chancre. Enlarged cervical lymph nodes are common in primary infection.

Tuberculosis ulcer is the most common secondary tubercular lesion in the mouth. It tends to occur in the middle-aged and elderly, with the tongue and hard palate as the predilection sites. In addition, gums, floor of the mouth, lips, and buccal mucosa can also be involved. The typical oral lesions consist of a stellate ulcer with undermined edges and clear boundary. After removing purulent exudates of the superficial ulceration, a granulating floor can be noticed. There are yellowish-brown miliary nodules at the margin of the ulcers, which ruptured to form dark red mulberry-like granulomas, following the increased ulcers accordingly. Irregular appearance of tuberculosis ulcers is caused by variable locations of these nodules. The pain degree varies, but the lingual ulcers are obviously painful [54]. If the patients have poor resistibility, lesions can appear at the junction of the oral mucosa and skin. It is characteristic of superficial granulomatous ulcer initially, followed by widespread tissue damages and deformation tendency, which is called tuberculosis cutis ulcerosa with poor prognosis.

Lupus vulgaris are rare cutaneous tuberculosis skin lesions and appear mostly in adolescent or children with good immune function. It begins as painless reddish-brown nodules which is soft with clear boundaries. On diascopy, it shows characteristic "apple-jelly" color in the central area of the nodules, surrounded by pale normal skin. The term "lupus" may be derived from the rapacity and virulence of the disease. Tissue necrosis and defect resembling wolf bites can be observed if combined with secondary infection.

The differential diagnoses of oral tuberculous ulcers include recurrent aphthous ulcers, traumatic ulcers, squamous cell carcinoma, lymphoma, metastatic tumors, and so on [56].

The diagnosis of oral tuberculosis is mainly confirmed by the histopathological examination. The lesion is consisted of small tubercles, the center of which is unstructured caseous material, surrounded by multiple epithelioid cells and Langhans-type giant cells, with dense inflammatory cellular infiltration. Proliferation of fibroblasts among tubercles can be observed. For confirmation and differential diagnosis, the bacilli could be identified by acid-fast stains and culture. In addition, sputum culture, history of tuberculosis, tuberculin skin test, and chest X-ray would be beneficial in the diagnosis of oral tuberculosis [57].

Patients with oral tuberculosis should be advised to the department of infectious diseases for further inspection and antituberculosis therapy. Most oral lesions can be healed after receiving generalized anti-TB treatment. Intralesional injection can be adopted for oral tuberculosis ulcers simultaneously: streptomycin 0.5 g, once daily, or isoniazid 0.1 g, once daily or every other day, for ten times as a treatment course. Topical therapeutic options are mainly symptomatic treatment, including compound chlorhexidine solution, oral rinse, three to four times daily. The patients still need to finish the course of anti-TB treatment in the department of infectious diseases, although oral lesions are healed.

References

1. Arduino PG, Porter SR. Herpes simplex virus type 1 infection: overview on relevant clinico-pathological features. J Oral Pathol Med. 2008;37(2):107–21.
2. Siegel MA. Diagnosis and management of recurrent herpes simplex infections. J Am Dent Assoc. 2002;133(9):1245–9.
3. Gilmour TK, Meyer PA, Rytina E, et al. Antiepiligrin (laminin 5) cicatricial pemphigoid complicated and exacerbated by herpes simplex virus type 2 infection. Australas J Dermatol. 2001;42(4):271–4.

4. Itin PH, Lautenschlager S. Viral lesions of the mouth in HIV-infected patients. Dermatology. 1997;194(1):1–7.
5. Cataldo F, Violante M, Maltese I, et al. Herpetic gingivostomatitis in children: the clinico-epidemiological aspects and findings with acyclovir treatment. A report of the cases of 162 patients. Pediatr Med Chir. 1993;15(2):193–5.
6. Wutzler P, Doerr HW, Farber I, et al. Seroprevalence of herpes simplex virus type 1 and type 2 in selected German populations-relevance for the incidence of genital herpes. J Med Virol. 2000;61(2):201–7.
7. Amir J. Clinical aspects and antiviral therapy in primary herpetic gingivostomatitis. Paediatr Drugs. 2001;3(8):593–7.
8. Kiderman A, Furst AL, Miller T, et al. How successfully do general practitioners diagnose herpetic gingivo-stomatitis clinically. Br J Gen Pract. 2002;52(479):481–2.
9. Arduino PG, Porter SR. Oral and perioral herpes simplex virus type 1 (HSV-1) infection: review of its management. Oral Dis. 2006;12(3):254–70.
10. World Health Organization. WHO model formulary for children. Geneva: WHO Press; 2010.
11. Wilson JF. Herpes zoster. Ann Intern Med. 2011;154(5):ITC31-15; quiz ITC316.
12. Schmader KE, Dworkin RH. Natural history and treatment of herpes zoster. J Pain. 2008;9(Suppl 1):S3–9.
13. Weinberg A, Levin MJ. VZV T cell-mediated immunity. Curr Top Microbiol Immunol. 2010;342:341–57.
14. Levy O, Orange JS, Hibberd P, et al. Disseminated varicella infection due to the vaccine strain of varicella-zoster virus, in a patient with a novel deficiency in natural killer T cells. J Infect Dis. 2003;188(7):948–53.
15. Arvin AM. Varicella-zoster virus. Clin Microbiol Rev. 1996;9(3):361–81.
16. Pereira FP, Guskuma MH, Luvizuto ER, et al. Unilateral facial paralysis caused by Ramsay hunt syndrome. J Craniofac Surg. 2011;22(5):1961–3.
17. Harpaz R, Ortega-Sanchez IR, Seward JF. Prevention of herpes zoster: recommendations of the advisory committee on immunization practices (ACIP). MMWR Recomm Rep. 2008;57(RR-5):1–30; quiz CE2-4.
18. Oxman MN, Levin MJ, Johnson GR, et al. A vaccine to prevent herpes zoster and postherpetic neuralgia in older adults. N Engl J Med. 2005;352(22):2271–84.
19. Kuter BJ, Weibel RE, Guess HA, et al. Oka/Merck varicella vaccine in healthy children: final report of a 2-year efficacy study and 7-year follow-up studies. Vaccine. 1991;9(9):643–7.
20. Muppa R, Bhupatiraju P, Duddu M, et al. Hand, foot and mouth disease. J Indian Soc Pedod Prev Dent. 2011;29(2):165–7.
21. Chang ZR, Zhang J, Sun JL, et al. Epidemiological features of hand, foot and mouth disease in China, 2008–2009. Zhonghua Liu Xing Bing Xue Za Zhi. 2011;32(7):676–80.
22. McMinn P, Stratov I, Nagarajan L, et al. Neurological manifestations of enterovirus 71 infection in children during an outbreak of hand, foot, and mouth disease in Western Australia. Clin Infect Dis. 2001;32(2):236–42.
23. Chan KP, Goh KT, Chong CY, et al. Epidemic hand, foot and mouth disease caused by human enterovirus 71, Singapore. Emerg Infect Dis. 2003;9(1):78–85.
24. Lin TY, Twu SJ, Ho MS, et al. Enterovirus 71 outbreaks, Taiwan: occurrence and recognition. Emerg Infect Dis. 2003;9(3):291–3.
25. Chan LG, Parashar UD, Lye MS, et al. Deaths of children during an outbreak of hand, foot, and mouth disease in Sarawak, Malaysia: clinical and pathological characteristics of the disease. For the Outbreak Study Group. Clin Infect Dis. 2000;31(3):678–83.
26. Puenpa J, Theamboonlers A, Korkong S, et al. Molecular characterization and complete genome analysis of human enterovirus 71 and coxsackievirus A16 from children with hand, foot and mouth disease in Thailand during 2008–2011. Arch Virol. 2011;156(11):2007.
27. Frydenberg A, Starr M. Hand, foot and mouth disease. Aust Fam Physician. 2003;32(8):594–5.
28. Bryant PA, Tingay D, Dargaville PA, et al. Neonatal coxsackie B virus infection—a treatable disease. Eur J Pediatr. 2004;163(4–5):223–8.
29. Huang YC, Chu YH, Yen TY, et al. Clinical features and phylogenetic analysis of Coxsackievirus A9 in northern Taiwan in 2011. BMC Infect Dis. 2013;13:33.
30. Chen YJ, Chang SC, Tsao KC, et al. Comparative genomic analysis of coxsackievirus A6 strains of different clinical disease entities. PLoS One. 2012;7(12):e52432.
31. Park K, Lee B, Baek K, et al. Enteroviruses isolated from herpangina and hand-foot-and-mouth disease in Korean children. Virol J. 2012;9:205.
32. Yamashita T, Ito M, Taniguchi A, et al. Prevalence of coxsackievirus A5, A6, and A10 in patients with herpangina in Aichi Prefecture, 2005. Jpn J Infect Dis. 2005;58(6):390–1.
33. Reichart PA, Samaranayake LP, Philipsen HP. Pathology and clinical correlates in oral candidiasis and its variants: a review. Oral Dis. 2000;6(2):85–91.
34. Williams DW, Kuriyama T, Silva S, Malic S, Lewis MA. Candida biofilms and oral candidosis: treatment and prevention. Periodontol 2000. 2011;55(1):250–65.
35. Pfaller MA, Diekema DJ. Epidemiology of invasive candidiasis: a persistent public health problem. Clin Microbiol Rev. 2007;20(1):133–63.
36. González GM, Elizondo M, Ayala J. Trends in species distribution and susceptibility of bloodstream isolates of Candida collected in Monterrey, Mexico, to seven antifungal agents: results of a 3-year (2004 to 2007) surveillance study. J Clin Microbiol. 2008;46(9):2902–5.

37. Leroy O, Gangneux JP, Montravers P, et al. Epidemiology, management, and risk factors for death of invasive Candida infections in critical care: a multicenter, prospective, observational study in France (2005–2006). Crit Care Med. 2009;37(5):1612–8.
38. Sitheeque MA, Samaranayake LP. Chronic hyperplastic candidosis/candidiasis (candidal leukoplakia). Crit Rev Oral Biol Med. 2003;14(4):253–67.
39. Samaranayake LP, Lamb AB, Lamey PJ, MacFarlane TW. Oral carriage of Candida species and coliforms in patients with burning mouth syndrome. J Oral Pathol Med. 1989;18(4):233–5.
40. Sakashita S, Takayama K, Nishioka K, Katoh T. Taste disorders in healthy "carriers" and "non-carriers" of *Candida albicans* and in patients with candidosis of the tongue. J Dermatol. 2004;31(11):890–7.
41. Nair PN, Sjögren U, Krey G, Kahnberg KE, Sundqvist G. Intraradicular bacteria and fungi in root-filled, asymptomatic human teeth with therapy-resistant periapical lesions: a long-term light and electron microscopic follow-up study. J Endod. 1990;16(12):580–8.
42. Williams D, Lewis M. Pathogenesis and treatment of oral candidosis. J Oral Microbiol. 2011;3:5771.
43. Antachopoulos C, Walsh TJ, Roilides E. Fungal infections in primary immunodeficiencies. Eur J Pediatr. 2007;166(11):1099–117.
44. Report of a WHO Scientific Group. Primary immunodeficiency diseases. Clin Exp Immunol. 1995;99(Suppl 1):1–24.
45. Kennedy MJ, Rogers AL, Hanselmen LR, Soll DR, Yancey RJ. Variation in adhesion and cell surface hydrophobicity in *Candida albicans* white and opaque phenotypes. Mycopathologia. 1988;102(3):149–56.
46. Barbeau J, Séguin J, Goulet JP, et al. Reassessing the presence of Candida albicans in denture-related stomatitis. Oral Surg Oral Med Oral Pathol Oral Radiol Endod. 2003;95(1):51–9.
47. Williams DW, Potts AJ, Wilson MJ, Matthews JB, Lewis MA. Characterisation of the inflammatory cell infiltrate in chronic hyperplastic candidosis of the oral mucosa. J Oral Pathol Med. 1997;26(2):83–9.
48. Dahlen G. Bacterial infections of the oral mucosa. Periodontol. 2009;49:13–38.
49. Aas JA, Paster BJ, Stokes LN, et al. Defining the normal bacterial flora of the oral cavity. J Clin Microbiol. 2005;43(11):5721–32.
50. Olczak-Kowalczyk D, Daszkiewicz M, Krasuska-Slawinska, et al. Bacteria and Candida yeasts in inflammations of the oral mucosa in children with secondary immunodeficiency. J Oral Pathol Med. 2012;41(7):568–76.
51. Kakisi OK, Kechagia AS, Kakisis IK, Rafailidis PI, Falagas ME. Tuberculosis of the oral cavity: a systematic review. Eur J Oral Sci. 2010;118(2):103–9.
52. Miziara ID. Tuberculosis affecting the oral cavity in Brazilian HIV-infected patients. Oral Surg Oral Med Oral Pathol Oral Radiol Endod. 2005;100(2):179–82.
53. Ito FA, de Andrade CR, Vargas PA, Jorge J, Lopes MA. Primary tuberculosis of the oral cavity. Oral Dis. 2005;11(1):50–3.
54. Kumar V, Singh AP, Meher R, Raj A. Primary tuberculosis of oral cavity: a rare entity revisited. Indian J Pediatr. 2011;78(3):354–6.
55. Sezer B, Zeytinoglu M, Tuncay U, Unal T. Oral mucosal ulceration: a manifestation of previously undiagnosed pulmonary tuberculosis. J Am Dent Assoc. 2004;135(3):336–40.
56. Von Arx DP, Husain A. Oral tuberculosis. Br Dent J. 2001;190(8):420–2.
57. Kamala R, Sinha A, Srivastava A, Srivastava S. Primary tuberculosis of the oral cavity. Indian J Dent Res. 2011;22(6):835–8.

2 Oral Hypersensitive Reactive Diseases

Yu Zhou, Xin Jin, and Qianming Chen

Keywords
Hypersensitivity · Erythema multiforme · Angioneurotic edema · Erosion · Bulla

Y. Zhou
State Key Laboratory of Oral Diseases, National Clinical Research Center for Oral Diseases, Department of Oral Medicine, West China Hospital of Stomatology, Sichuan University, Chengdu, Sichuan, China

X. Jin
College of Stomatology, Chongqing Medical University, Chongqing Key Laboratory of Oral Diseases and Biomedical Sciences, Chongqing, China

Q. Chen (✉)
Changjiang Scholars Program, Ministry of Education, Beijing, China

State Key Laboratory of Oral Diseases, National Clinical Research Center for Oral Diseases, Department of Oral Medicine, West China Hospital of Stomatology, Sichuan University, Chengdu, Sichuan, China
e-mail: qmchen@scu.edu.cn

Q. Chen, X. Zeng (eds.), *Case Based Oral Mucosal Diseases*,
https://doi.org/10.1007/978-981-13-0286-2_2

2.1 Allergic Medicamentosus Stomatitis

Case 17 Allergic Medicamentosus Stomatitis

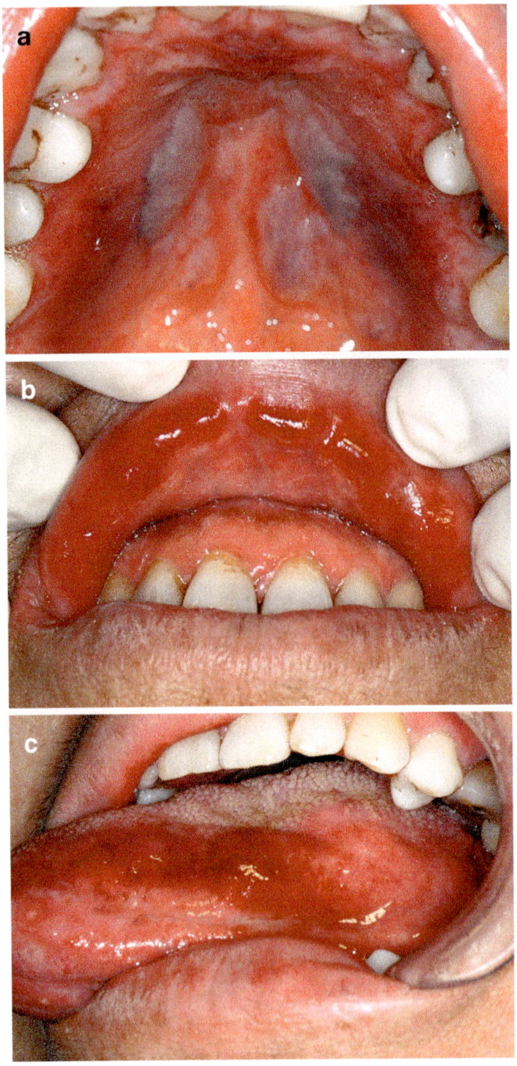

Fig. 2.1 (**a**) Multiple sizes of blisters on hard palate surrounding with hyperemia. (**b**) Diffuse hyperemia, edema, and blister seen on the inside of the upper lip. (**c**) Hyperemia swelling on the left side of tongue abdomen with blood blister and small dot erosion

Age: 46 years
Sex: Male
Chief Complaints:
46-year-old man with hyperemia and blister in oral cavity for one day

History of Present Illness:
A 46-year-old man presented to our clinic with ulcers on the surface of tongue abdomen for 2 days. He had used the propolis sticker 1 day ago. 3 hours after that, he felt his lips numb and swell, and then hyperemia and blister appeared on his hard palate and lips.
Past Medical History: Hypertension
Allergy: Alcohol and iodine
Physical Examination:
Diffuse hyperemia and edema were seen on the lips, tongue, and hard palate. Three blisters about 1.8 cm × 1 cm were seen on hard palate, surrounding with a number of small blood blister and blister (Fig. 2.1).
Diagnosis:
Allergic medicamentosus stomatitis
Diagnosis Basis:

1. Acute onset and local drug history before erosion.
2. Diffuse hyperemia, edema, and blood blisters with different sizes were seen on the oral mucosa.

Management:

1. Medication
   Rp.: Prednisone acetate 5 mg × 35
   Sig.: 25 mg p.o. q.m.
   Loratadine 10 mg × 6
   Sig.: 10 mg p.o. q.d.
   Vitamin C 0.1 g × 100
   Sig.: 0.2 g p.o. t.i.d.
   Compound chlorhexidine solution 300 ml × 1
   Sig.: rinse t.i.d.
   Dexamethasome paste 15 g × 2
   Sig.: topical use t.i.d.
2. Aerosol therapy
   Rp.: Dexamethasone sodium phosphate injection 1 ml × 1
   Gentamycin sulfate injection 2 ml × 1
   Vitamin B12 injection 1 ml × 1
   Vitamin C injection 2.5 ml × 1
   Sig.: Aerosol therapy b.i.d.
3. Drink more water and avoid using the sensitization sticker.

Case 18 Allergic Stomatitis

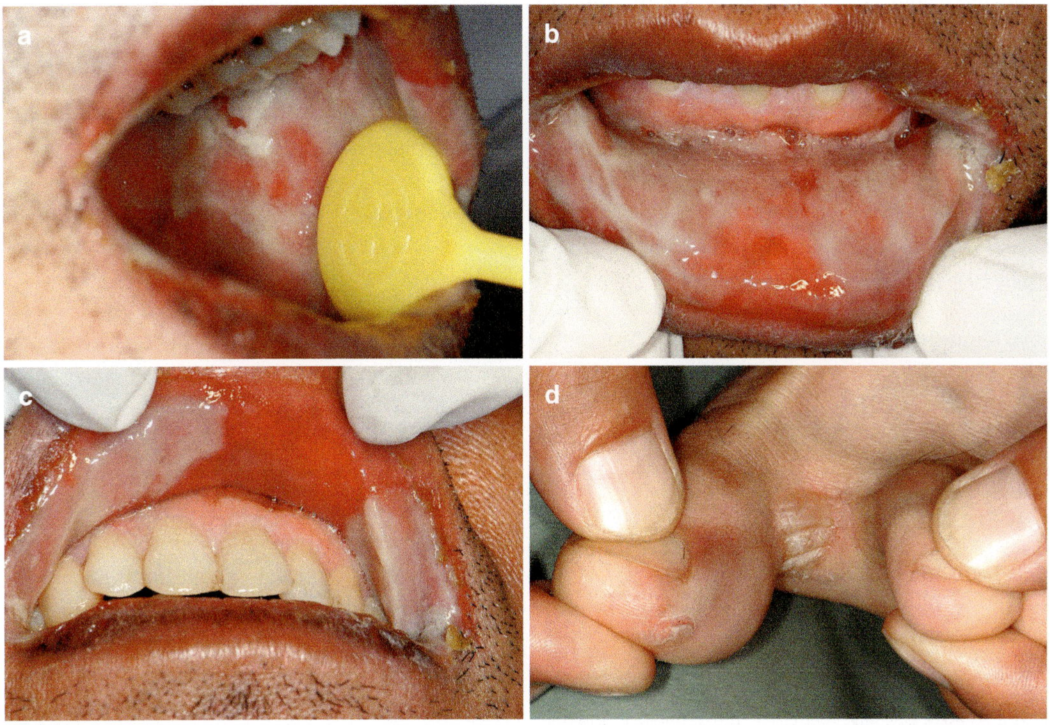

Fig. 2.2 (**a**) Extensively erosion seen on the left buccal mucosa, covering with yellow membrane. (**b**) Extensively erosion seen on the lower lip, covering with yellow membrane. (**c**) Extensively irregular erosion seen on the inside of the upper lip, surrounding with hyperemia. (**d**) Multiple sizes of blisters on left toe, parts of which busted

Age: 53 years
Sex: Male
Chief Complaints:
53-year-old man with ulcer in oral cavity for 5 days
History of Present Illness:
A 53-year-old man presented to our clinic with ulcer in cavity for 5 days. He felt pain. Anti-inflammatory and antiviral treatment in local hospitals is invalid. Multiple sizes of blisters appeared on left toe 2 days ago (Fig. 2.2).
Past Medical History: None
Allergies: None
Physical Examination:
Extensive irregular erosions were revealed in the cavity, covering with yellow membrane, surrounding with hyperemia, tenderness obviously. Four 3–5 mm^2 of blisters been seen on left toe.
Diagnosis:
Allergic stomatitis

Diagnosis Basis:

1. Acute onset and short duration
2. Extensive irregular erosions, covered with yellow membrane

Management:

1. Medication
   Rp.: Prednisone acetate 5 mg × 35
   Sig.: 25 mg p.o. q.m.
   Loratadine 10 mg × 6
   Sig.: 10 mg p.o. q.d.
   Vitamin C 0.1 g × 100
   Sig.: 0.2 g p.o. t.i.d.
   Compound chlorhexidine solution 300 ml × 1
   Sig.: rinse t.i.d.
   Dexamethasone paste 15 g × 2
   Sig.: topical use t.i.d.

2. Aerosol therapy
   Rp.: Dexamethasone sodium phosphate injection 1 ml × 1
   Gentamycin sulfate injection 2 ml × 1
   Vitamin B12 injection 1 ml × 1
   Vitamin C injection 2.5 ml × 1
   Sig.: Aerosol therapy b.i.d.
3. Drink more water and pay attention to finding allergen.

Case 19 Fixed Drug Eruption

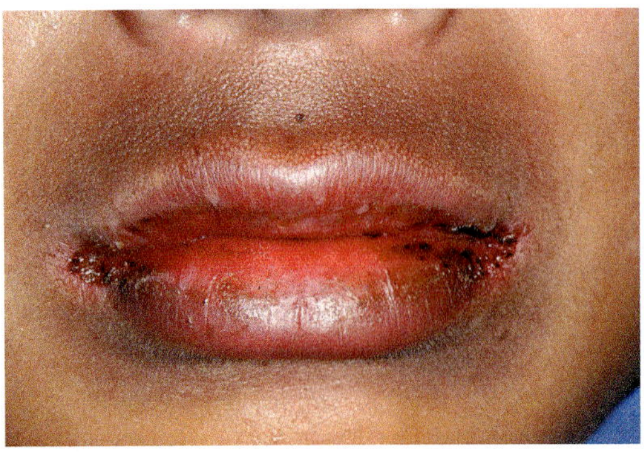

Fig. 2.3 Erosions and scabs on the corner of mouth, black pigmentation surrounding the lips

Age: 12 years
Sex: Male
Chief Complaints:
12-year-old boy with black pigmentation surrounding the lips for 1 year, aggravating for 4 days
History of Present Illness:
A 12-year-old boy presented to our clinic with recurrent dull red "particles" after taking certain cold medicine for almost 1 year. Since then, it occurred three times, each happened after taking this cold medicine. It kept about 10 days healing, but the dull red on lips didn't cure completely. Four days ago, the boy caught a cold and has taken the same medicine as before. Then the erosion on the lips happened again, and it became blacker.
Past Medical History: None
Allergies: None
Physical Examination:
The lips were congestive. Erosions and scabs were seen on the corner of mouth, with black pigmentation around the lips (Fig. 2.3).

Diagnosis:
Fixed drug eruption
Diagnosis Basis:

1. Pigmentation rounding mouth
2. Taken the same medicine, recurrent on the same place and same sample

Management:

1. Medication
   Rp.: Loratadine 10 mg × 6
   Sig.: 10 mg p.o. q.d.
   Vitamin C 0.1 g × 100
   Sig.: 0.2 g p.o. t.i.d.
   Compound chlorhexidine solution 300 ml × 1
   Sig.: rinse t.i.d.
   Dexamethasone paste 15 g × 2
   Sig.: topical use t.i.d.
2. Drink more water, pay attention to find allergen, and avoid contacting.

[Review] Allergic Medicamentosus Stomatitis
Drug can been used to prevent, diagnose, and treat the disease; however, it could also have a harmful and un-therapeutic effect, which is called adverse drug reaction. Drug eruption, a kind of adverse drug reaction, appears multiple skin symptoms, such as measles, urticaria, erythema appearance, pustules or bulla, purpura, lichenoid lesions, or itchy skin with normal appearance. It also can be called allergic medicamentosa stomatitis when swellings, blisters, erosions, and ulcers occur in oral mucosa. It is also normal to see nails change to green-purple or pigmentation. It is mild in most patients and can disappear after drug withdrawal. It can be diagnosed according to medical history and clinical examination; however, it is easy to misdiagnosis and delayed diagnosis for diversiform [1].

Allergic medicamentosa stomatitis defined as drugs taken by different ways, such as mouth, injection, suction, patches or local inunction, and wash into allergic constitution and cause mucous membrane and skin hypersensitivity disease. Severe cases can also cause the disease of other systems. Sometimes patients denied medication history. Allergen can be substances such as food, pollen, spices, medicinal liquor, and so on. But if it is similar to the onset and damage of allergic medicamentosa stomatitis, then it also can be diagnosed as allergic medicamentosa stomatitis (or allergic stomatitis). The patient of case 18 in this unit denied taking drugs or special food, which can cause such symptoms, but according to its characteristics of acute damage process and the onset of clinical disease, it also can be diagnosed as allergic stomatitis.

Lots of drugs can cause allergic medicamentosa stomatitis, among which antipyretic analgesics, sleeping sedatives, sulfa drugs, and antibiotic medicine are common to see. Some so-called "safe" drugs such as vitamins and herbs may also have allergenic. Corticosteroid drugs could also be allergen. Most of allergic medicamentosa stomatitis is type I allergy. The performance of allergic medicamentosa stomatitis is acute. Lesions can be seen in any part of oral cavity. Sometimes at the beginning of the disease, a larger blister can be found on the mucous membrane. It often appears as large and irregular edema, congestion, and erosion in the lip buccal, tongue, and palate with a large number of effusions. It is covered with yellowish-white coating membrane in oral cavity, with thick yellow-black scab shells on lips. Sometimes patients feel discomfort and pain. Thus it is difficult to feed.

Allergic medicamentosa stomatitis may be accompanied with the skin and other parts of mucosal lesions. It is common to see the lesions at the hand and foot, characterized by erythema, papule, bulla, and so on, among which circular erythema is the most common. It is often accompanied with itching but is painful.

If the pathogenic damage caused by allergic medicamentosa stomatitis happens in the same position and form repeatedly, it is called fixed drug eruption (FDE). Avoid using sensitized drugs and treating process; it is often cured within 10 days, but pigmentation is observed [2, 3]. The lips and perioral skin are its predilection site. Allergic medicamentosa stomatitis is typical delayed-type hypersensitivity (DTH) induced by $CD8^+$ T lymphocytes. Once $CD8^+$ T lymphocytes within the skin have been activated, it will not only kill the keratinocytes surrounding but also release cytokines such as IFN-γ and cytotoxic granules, recruit $CD4^+$ T lymphocytes and neutrophil, and cause the damage location [4]. It has been reported that lymphocyte transformation test (LTT) can be successfully used to identify drug allergens [5].

Lyell syndrome, also called toxic epidermal necrolysis, is a severe allergic medicamentosa stomatitis. Bulla is widely distributed to the whole body and orifices such as the eyes, the nose, the vagina, the urethra, the anus, and the internal organs.

The first thing to treat allergic medicamentosa stomatitis is to find suspicious allergen and avoid it immediately. Common drugs include cortin (prednisone acetate 15–30 mg, q.m.), antihistamine (Loratadine 10 mg p.o. q.d.), and vitamin C (100–200 mg t.i.d. p.o.). The course of treatment is about 1 week. Local drugs include 0.05% compound chlorhexidine solution or 0.01% dexamethasone solution (rinse t.i.d.) hydropathical compress on lips or mouthwash, 0.1% triamcinolone acetonide oral ointment, 0.1% dexamethasone ointment, prednisone acetate injection, or triamcinolone acetonide injection (1:5 dilution, topical use t.i.d.). Analgesic agents include compound chamomile, lidocaine hydrochloride gel, and compound benzocaine gel. Otherwise, cooperating with excessive atomization treatment is another choice, including prednisone acetate injection, vitamin C injection, and vitamin B12 injection.

2.2 Erythema Multiforme

Case 20 Erythema Multiforme

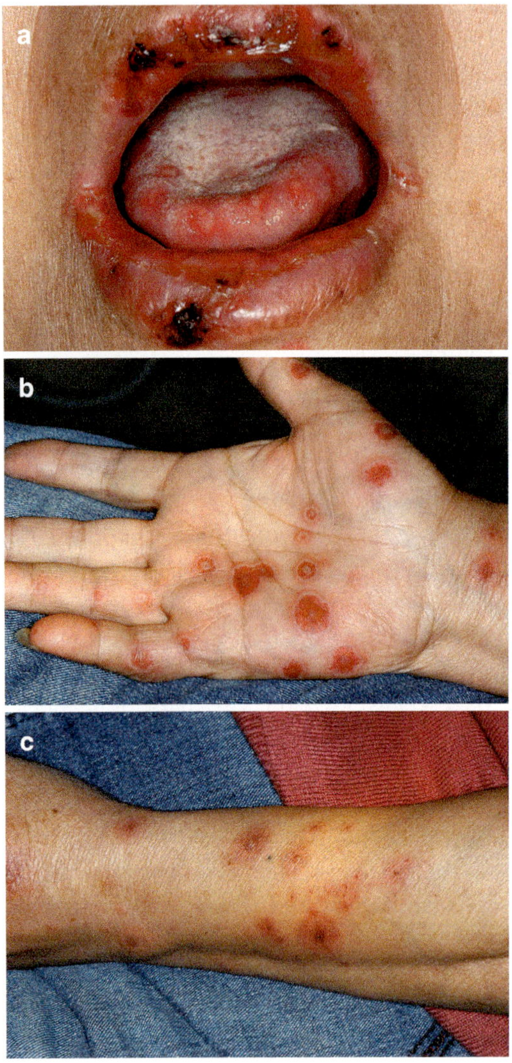

Fig. 2.4 (**a**) Erosions and crusts appeared on the lips and corner of the mouth, multiple irregular erosions appeared on the front of the dorsum. (**b**) Multiple target lesions of erythema on palms. (**c**) Target lesions appeared on upper limbs

Age: 68 years
Sex: Female
Chief Complaints:
Oral erosive lesions for 7 days

History of Present Illness:
Seven days ago, with no clear etiology, patient developed oral erosions and pain, accompanied by skin erythema and itching. A similar condition occurred a year ago. Two days ago patient underwent for blood routine examination and blood glucose test in the local hospital with no obvious abnormalities.
Past Medical History: None
Allergy: None
Physical Examination:
Erosion and bloody encrustations were observed in the upper and lower lip area, with multiple irregular oral mucosa erosions covered by yellow-white pseudomembrane. Multiple target lesions of erythema were observed on upper limbs and palms with occasional blistering in the center (Fig. 2.4).
Diagnosis:
Erythema multiforme
Diagnosis Basis:

1. Sudden onset without specific cause
2. Typical target lesion and blistering erythema on the skin
3. Irregular oral erosive lesions with bloody encrustations on lips

Management:

1. Medication
   Rp.: Prednisone acetate 5 mg × 35
   Sig.: 25 mg p.o. q.m.
   Loratadine 10 mg × 6
   Sig.: 10 mg p.o. q.d.
   Vitamin C 0.1 g × 100
   Sig.: 0.2 g p.o. t.i.d.
   Compound chlorhexidine solution 300 ml × 1
   Sig.: rinse t.i.d.
   Dexamethasone paste 15 g × 2
   Sig.: topical use t.i.d.
2. Aerosol therapy
   Rp.: Dexamethasone sodium phosphate injection 1 ml × 1
   Gentamycin sulfate injection 2 ml × 1
   Vitamin B12 injection 1 ml × 1
   Vitamin C injection 2.5 ml × 1
   Sig.: aerosol therapy q.d.-b.i.d. for 3 days
3. Drink more water.

[Review] Erythema Multiforme

Erythema multiforme (EM) is a rare acute disorder of the skin and mucosal membranes manifesting in the skin as erythematous lesions and blisters, and the oral cavity as erosive lesions and blisters. The skin lesions are of a characteristic bull's-eye or target morphology, comprising a central vesicle with peripheral rounded and symmetrical erythematous papules or maculae [6]. It is accepted that it can be categorized as EM minor and major, as well as Stevens-Johnson syndrome (SJS), and toxic epidermal necrolysis (TEN) based on the severity of the disease [7]. However some researchers suggest that SJS and TEN are distinct conditions because of their variations in clinical manifestations, although some are the same, and also different etiology; thus, TEN should not be considered a type of EM [8]. Other researchers classified EMM and SJS as the same category.

These diseases do not yet have clear classification criteria and are mainly distinguished based on clinical symptoms and the size and extent of skin and mucosal lesions. EM is self-limiting.

Currently it is believed that EM is associated with HSV infection. It was reported that 71% of EM patients have HSV infection, and most are herpes labialis lesions [9]. HSV-DNA can also be detected on the surface of residual pigmented skin after healing for several weeks [10]. HSV is considered to be the most common individual cause of EM. EM can occur after 10–14 days after the onset of HSV infection symptoms. HSV-related EM results from attacks by T cells against HSV antigen-positive cells that contain the HSV DNA, which is engulfed by CD34+ cells, resulting in epidermal cell damage [11, 12]. Immunological and genetic factors are also important in pathogenesis EM. Human leukocyte antigen HLA-DQ3 is closely related with HSV-related EM [13]. Other viral, bacterial, and fungal infections may also cause EM.

EM may also be caused by drugs. Fifty-nine percent of cases have medication history. Due to the use of cephalosporins, the incidence of EM greatly increased [14]. Cases induced by phenytoin and radiation therapy of the craniofacial area are not uncommon. EM is believed to result from a T cell-mediated immune reaction to the precipitating agent, which leads to a cytotoxic immunological attack on keratinocytes that express nonself antigens, with subsequent subepithelial and intraepithelial vesiculation; this leads to widespread blistering and erosions [15]. SJS and TEN are predominantly drug-related [16].

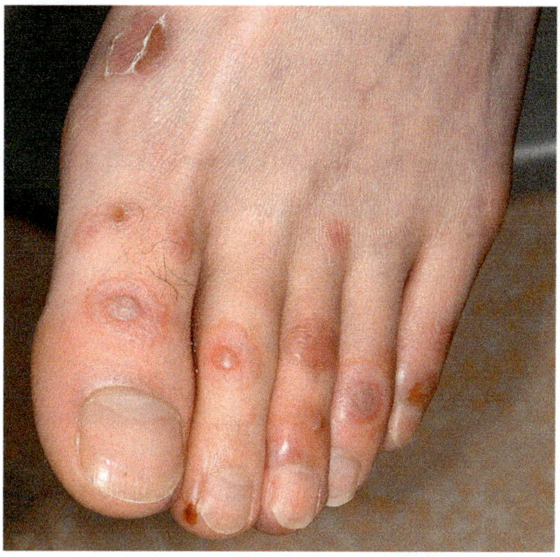

Fig. 2.5 Target lesion and blister erythema appeared on the plantar skin

Erythema multiforme minor is an acute, self-limiting disease that may be episodic or recurrent, sometimes showing a seasonal pattern. Erythema multiforme minor tends to arise in the third and fourth decades of life, although it can also affect children and adolescents, and rarely affects individuals under the age of 3 or older than 50.The cutaneous lesions of erythema multiforme comprise typical targets, which are concentric rings that look like iris, and occasionally accompanied by blisters, called blister erythema (Fig. 2.5). Other types of lesions include raised atypical targets, flat atypical targets, and macules with or without blisters. The cutaneous lesions affect less than 10% of the body surface area. The lesion often symmetric distributed, with a predilection for the extensor surfaces of the extremities. Itching and discomfort, but not pain, are the main symptoms of cutaneous lesions. Lesions last for 1–3 weeks and heal without scarring. Mucosa lesions are not very severe. The oral mucosa is the most commonly involved mucosal surface. The oral lesions initially manifest with edema, erythema, and erythematous macules, followed by the development of multiple vesicles and bullae that quickly rupture and result in pseudomembrane formation. The lips tend to become swollen and show diagnostically distinctive bloody encrustations. Prodromal symptoms are usually absent in most instances of the EM minor, but some patients may experience mild systemic symptoms such as fever or chills [13].

Erythema multiforme major spans a wide range of clinical presentations that include mucocutaneous involvement. Some authors have suggested that EMM differs from EMm by the involvement of at least two different mucosal sites. The oral mucosa is the most commonly involved mucosal surface, but any mucosal site can be affected in the course of EMM, including the epithelium of the trachea, bronchi, or gastrointestinal tract. The involvement of conjunctival and nasal mucosa is quite common too. In EMM oral lesions are larger than that of EMm, and in more than 50% of cases, patients have ulceration of all oral mucosal surfaces, which are manifested by superficial irregular erosions with red margins and are usually covered by a yellow fibrinous pseudomembrane. The oral lesions often occur on the tongue, buccal mucosa, and lips, with difficulties in mouth opening. After healing, the lesions don't leave scars. The cutaneous involvement of EMM is usually less than 10% of the body surface but is generally more severe and lasts 1–6 weeks [6, 13].

Stevens-Johnson syndrome is characterized by sudden onset of erosions of the mucous membranes (predominantly the oral mucosa, lips, and conjunctivae) together with widespread blistering of the skin. Stevens-Johnson affects up to 10% of the body surface and has mucosal involvement of two or more sites. SJS lesions extend to involve the nasal cavity, pharynx, larynx, and esophagus. The oral lesions sometimes precede skin involvement by several days. The skin lesions of SJS are primarily atypical flat target lesions and macules rather than classic target lesions, are more widespread (rather than involving only the acral areas), and can lead to significant percutaneous loss of fluid and electrolytes. Nikolsky's sign is positive. One third of affected individuals have a prodromal symptom that includes fever, pharyngitis, headache, and arthralgias/myalgias, and rarely pneumonia, nephritis, or myocarditis. There is a risk of scarring of mucosal lesions, which may lead to synechiae formation of the conjunctiva or laryngeal and/or vaginal strictures [13, 15].

Toxic epidermal necrolysis occurs in patients after receiving suspected stimulation: develop fever, sore throat, and other precursor symptoms, followed by the development of blistering in 1–16 days. Extensive blisters cover the body, with epidermal detachment of >30% of the body surface which is similar to second-degree burns. More mucosa lesions are involved including oral mucosa, oropharynx, esophagus, conjunctiva, genitals, and so on. The overall mortality rate of TEN is approximately 30–40% with poor prognosis [17].

A retrospective study of patients with recurrent erythema multiforme showed that most patients did not have a clear onset for recurrent EM. HSV infection rate is not high and not statistically significant. Moreover, the effect for continuous antiviral and immunosuppressive therapy is not clear [18].

The diagnosis of erythema multiforme is mainly based on the onset and recurrence, oral mucosal lesions, and characteristic multiform skin lesions. There is no specific diagnostic method, and the significance of pathological diagnosis mainly serves to different EM from bullous disease.

First step for treating erythema multiforme should be stopping suspicious drugs or allergens. Use of medication should be with caution. Avoid using drugs unless urgently needed ones to prevent exposure to new allergens and aggravate allergic reactions. Treatment of mild erythema multiforme is the same with drug-allergic stomatitis. Systemic medication includes glucocorticoid, such as prednisone 15–30 mg/d, q.m. for 5–7 days; antihistamines such as oral administration of loratadine 10 mg, 1 time/day, for 6 days; and oral administration of vitamin C tablets, 0.2 g for 3 times/day. Topical use medications include compound chlorhexidine solution or 0.01% dexamethasone solution for hydropathic compress and rinse, three times/day; 0.1% triamcinolone acetonide dental paste, 0.1% dexamethasone ointment, prednisolone acetate injection, and intralesional triamcinolone acetonide (TA) injection (1:5 dilution); and hydropathic compress on the affected area three times/day; analgesic preparations include the use of compound chamomile and lidocaine hydrochloride gel or compound benzocaine gel. In addition, these treatments can be accompanied by aerosol therapy using dexamethasone sodium phosphate injection and vitamin C injection. Because of eating difficulties exhibited by patients, extra supportive care should be given to patients.

Due to the seriousness of these conditions, severe erythema multiforme, SJS, and TEN patients should be promptly transferred to dermatology department of hospital for treatment.

2.3 Contact Stomatitis

Case 21 Primary Contact Stomatitis (Drinking Pesticides by Accident)

Age: 80 years

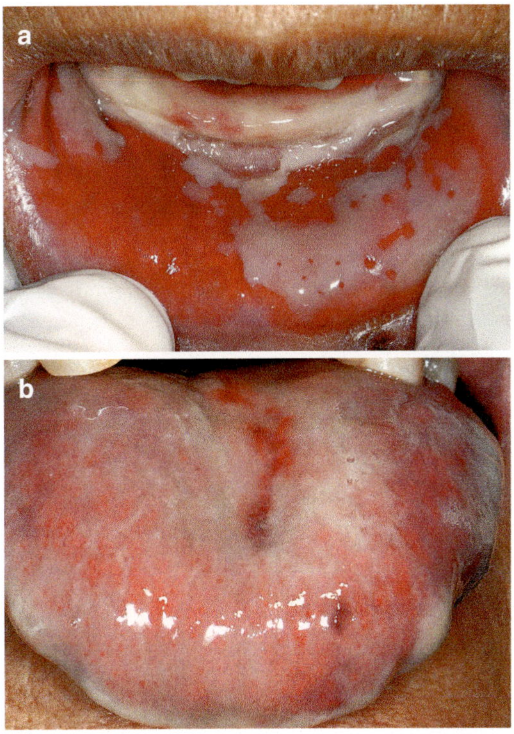

Fig. 2.6 (**a**) Widespread congestion and irregular erosions on the lower lip, with white pseudomembrane and plenty of inflammatory exudate. (**b**) Widespread erosions on the dorsum of the tongue, with white pseudomembrane and plenty of inflammatory exudate

Sex: Female

Chief Complaints:

80-year-old woman with oral erosion for 5 days

History of Present Illness:

A 80-year-old woman presented to our clinic with oral erosion for 5 days after drinking pesticides (paraquat) by accident and spitting it out immediately. But at once her oral mucosa became erosion and too painful to eat.

Past Medical History: None

Allergy: None

Physical Examination:

Widespread congestion and irregular erosions were detected on the lips, tongue, and both sides of buccal mucosa covered by white pseudomembrane. There lies plenty of inflammatory exudate (Fig. 2.6).

Diagnosis:

Primary contact stomatitis

Diagnosis Basis:

1. Paraquat is one of pesticides with extreme toxicity, and contacting with it can injure skins and mucosa.
2. The oral mucosa contacting with paraquat will grow congestion and erosion immediately.

Management:

1. Medication
   Rp.: Prednisone acetate 5 mg × 35
   Sig.: 25 mg p.o. q.m.
   Vitamin C 0.1 g × 100
   Sig.: 0.2 g p.o. t.i.d.
   Compound chlorhexidine solution 300 ml × 1
   Sig.: rinse t.i.d.
   Dexamethasone paste15 g × 2
   Sig.: topical use t.i.d.
2. Aerosol therapy
   Rp.: Dexamethasone sodium phosphate injection 1 ml × 1
   Gentamycin sulfate injection 2 ml × 1
   Vitamin B12 injection 1 ml × 1
   Vitamin C injection 2.5 ml × 1
   Sig.: aerosol therapy q.d.-b.i.d. for 3 days
3. Transferring the patient to the internal medicine department in a general hospital immediately to exclude the possibility of toxication.

Case 22 Primary Contact Stomatitis (Rinsing White Spirit)

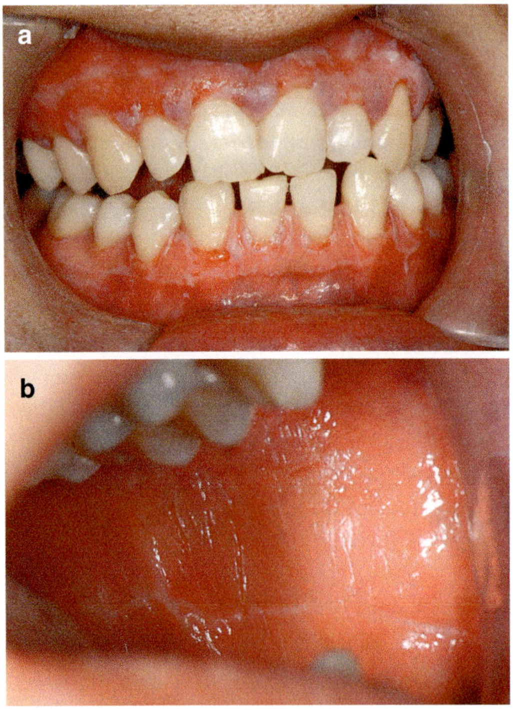

Fig. 2.7 (**a**) Congestion and erosions covered with white pseudomembrane on the buccal gingival margin. (**b**) White lesions with fine wrinkles appeared on the left buccal mucosa

Age: 35 years
Sex: Female
Chief Complaints:
Gingival erosion for 3 days
History of Present Illness:
Three days ago, her tongue appeared to have "mung bean"-sized ulcers with pain, which is rinsed with white spirit to treat it, contributing to white lesion in the whole oral cavity and too much pain when eating.
Past Medical History: None
Allergy: None
Physical Examination:
The buccal gingival margin in the oral cavity developed congestion and erosion covered with white pseudomembrane that can be wiped. White lesions with fine wrinkles were observed on the left buccal mucosa (Fig. 2.7).

Diagnosis:
Primary contact stomatitis (alcohol burn)
Diagnosis Basis:

1. The history of rinsing white spirit.
2. The oral mucosa contacting with white spirit will grow congestion and erosion.

Management:

1. Medication
   Rp.: Zhongtong'an capsules 0.28 g × 48
      Sig.: 0.56 g p.o. t.i.d.
      Dexamethasone sodium phosphate injection 1 ml × 5
      Sig.: 50-fold dilution rinse t.i.d.
      Compound chlorhexidine solution 300 ml × 1
      Sig.: rinse t.i.d.
      Dexamethasone paste 15 g × 2
      Sig.: topical use t.i.d.
2. Aerosol therapy
   Rp.: Dexamethasone sodium phosphate injection 1 ml × 1
      Gentamycin sulfate injection 2 ml × 1
      Vitamin B12 injection 1 ml × 1
      Vitamin C injection 2.5 ml × 1
      Sig.: aerosol therapy q.d.-b.i.d. for 3 days

Case 23 Allergic Contact Cheilitis

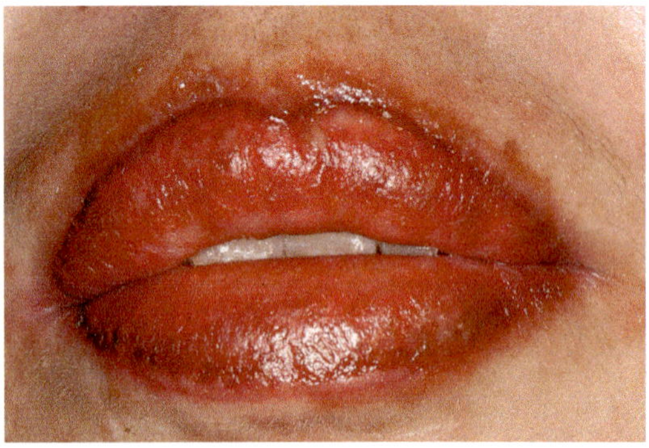

Fig. 2.8 Swelling and congestion with fine erosions and thin crusts on the lips

Age: 42 years
Sex: Female
Chief Complaints:
Lips swelling for 1 week after tattooing on them

History of Present Illness:
One week ago, her lips became swollen after tattooing; sometimes "yellow liquid" exuded and had burning or itching sensation. In recent days, the symptoms aggravated. She used acyclovir gel to hydropathic compress, but there was no remission.
Past Medical History: None
Allergy: None
Physical Examination:
Swelling and congestion with fine erosions and thin crusts were detected on the lips (Fig. 2.8).
Diagnosis:
Allergic contact stomatitis
Diagnosis Basis:

1. The history of contacting allergen.
2. The contacting part of oral mucosa exposed to the antigen became congestion and erosion.

Management:

1. Medication
   Rp.: Prednisone acetate 5 mg × 35
   Sig.: 25 mg p.o. q.m.
   Loratadine 10 mg × 6
   Sig.: 10 mg p.o. q.d.
   Vitamin C 0.1 g × 100
   Sig.: 0.2 g p.o. t.i.d.
   Compound chlorhexidine solution 300 ml × 1
   Sig.: rinse t.i.d.
   Dexamethasone paste 15 g × 2
   Sig.: topical use t.i.d.
2. Aerosol therapy
   Rp.: Dexamethasone sodium phosphate injection 1 ml × 1
   Gentamycin sulfate injection 2 ml × 1
   Vitamin B12 injection 1 ml × 1
   Vitamin C injection 2.5 ml × 1
   Sig.: aerosol therapy q.d.-b.i.d. for 3 days

[Review] Contact Stomatitis
Contact stomatitis (CS) could be divided into two types. One is primary contact stomatitis associated with severely irritant substance, and everyone would have this reaction after contacting, for instance, strong acid, strong base, or food within irritation and high temperatures. The other type called allergic contact stomatitis is that when allergic constitution's local oral cavity is exposed to exogenous materials, inflammatory response will be caused. The materials exist no irritation, and only individuals who have previously been sensitized to the allergen are affected [19]. Common allergens contain silver amalgam fillings and methyl methacrylate, self-curing plastic in the denture materials, and certain composition of food, flavor, candy, toothpaste, lipstick, and ointment. Allergic contact stomatitis is a hypersensitivity reaction (type IV) [20]. Antigen with low molecular weight passing through the susceptible population's skin and mucosa combines with epithelial protein into hapten. Epithelial Langerhans cells take the hapten to regional lymph nodes submitting and activating T lymphocytes. Upon second contact recognition of the antigen, lesions typically develop at sites of direct exposure to allergen. Contact allergies are common in the skin but rare in the mouth due to the protective role of saliva against the accumulation of allergens, the high concentration of blood vessels in oral epithelium that prevents the long-term maintenance of allergens in contact with the mucosa by absorption and removal, and the reduced activation of cellular immunity as less antigen-presenting cells are found in the oral mucosa in comparison to skin. When confronted with allergic diseases in clinical practice, usually anaphylaxis isn't single anaphylaxis, but hybrid and certain type plays a main role.

Lesions appear at local oral mucosa of direct exposure to allergen, and sometimes they extend to the nearby. The clinical features of CS are multiple, for instance, erythema, erosions, and lichenoid reaction, and patients complain of burning sensation. Until 2–3 days after exposure to the antigen, the contacting part of oral mucosa becomes congestion and edema and can grow blisters, erosion, and ulcer covered with pseudomembrane.

One special kind of allergic contact stomatitis is plasma cell gingivitis, appearing as generalized erythema and edema of the attached gingiva, occasionally accompanied by cheilitis or glossitis (Fig. 2.9). The histopathologic aspect of allergic contact stomatitis shows plenty of plasma cells

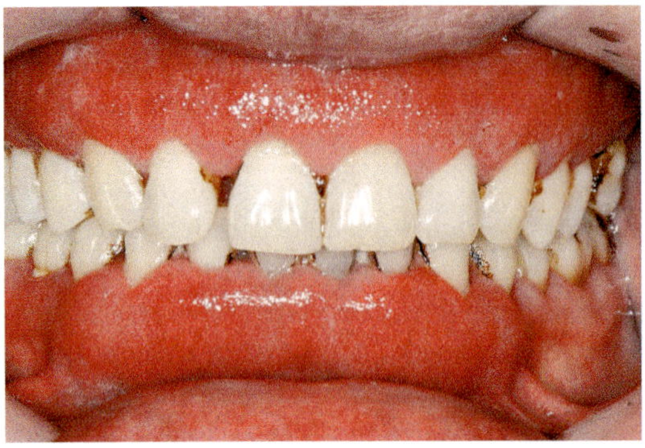

Fig. 2.9 Generalized erythema and edema of the attached gingiva

replace normal connective tissue. In the some of the reported cases, the oral mucosal lesions were associated with the use of toothpaste, chewing gum, and candies containing allergen. As to others, the pathogenesis is still unknown even after the allergen examination. The differential diagnosis is with malignant plasmacyte disease, such as plasmacytoma and multiple myeloma [21].

The clinical manifestation of primary contact stomatitis resembles to allergic contact stomatitis. The causes for it consist of suiciding by pesticides, drinking pesticides or hot water carelessly, rinsing white spirit for oral diseases, or pasting aspirin and vitamin C for toothache.

The diagnosis of CS is generally based on typical contact history and clinical manifestation.

Severe primary contact stomatitis could take prednisone (Sig.: 15–30 mg q.m. p.o.; a treatment course is 5–7 days) to control inflammation, but don't need to take loratadine. Primary contact stomatitis can also use Zhongtong'an capsules (Sig. 0.56 g t.i.d. p.o.).

The treatment of allergic contact stomatitis is similar to allergic medicamentosa stomatitis. Preventing exposure to the allergenic drugs and allergen could lead to resolution of the condition. Reduce systematic therapy to avoid new anaphylaxis. Common medicines contain cortin, like prednisone (Sig.: 15–30 mg q.m. p.o.); antihistamine, like loratadine (Sig.: 10 mg q.d. p.o.); and vitamin C (Sig.: 100–200 mg t.i.d. p.o.), and its treatment course is 5–7 days.

The topical medication of primary and allergic contact stomatitis includes compound chlorhexidine solution or 0.01% dexamethasone sodium phosphate injection used as hydropathic compressing on lips and rinsing, t.i.d.; 0.1% triamcinolone acetonide dental paste, 0.1% dexamethasone ointment, prednisolone acetate injection or triamcinolone acetonide injection (6-fold dilution), hydropathic compress, t.i.d.; and compound chamomile and lidocaine hydrochloride gel and compound benzocaine gel regarded as anodyne. Moreover, it can cooperate with aerosol therapy by dexamethasone sodium phosphate injection, gentamycin sulfate injection, vitamin C injection, and vitamin B12 injection.

2.4 Angioneurotic Edema

Case 24 Angioneurotic Edema

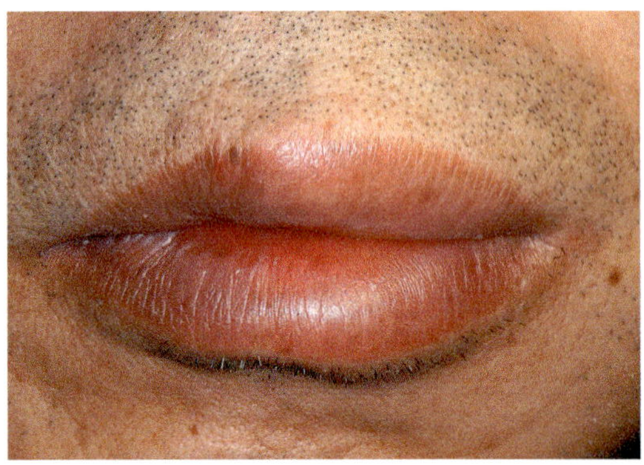

Fig. 2.10 Obvious swelling observed on the left lips

Age: 58 years
Sex: Male
Chief Complaints:
A 58-year-old male with 6-hour history of swelling lips
History of Present Illness:
A 58-year-old male presented with 6-hour history of suddenly swelling double lips and lower left cheek, painless.
Past Medical History: Myocardial infarction
Allergy: None

Physical Examination:
Obvious tough swelling was observed on the left lips and lower left cheek, without tenderness (Fig. 2.10).

Diagnosis:
Angioneurotic edema

Diagnosis Basis:

1. Acute onset
2. Painless swelling on lip mucosa, without tenderness

Management:

1. Medication
   Rp.: Prednisone Acetate 5 mg × 15
   Sig.: 15 mg p.o. q.m.
   Loratadine 10 mg × 6
   Sig.: 10 mg p.o. q.d.
   Vitamin C 0.1 g × 100
   Sig.: 0.2 g p.o. t.i.d.
2. Drink plenty of water.
3. Trace allergens.

[Review] Angioneurotic Edema

Angioneurotic edema is a disease of dermal mucosa characterized by edema of the deep dermal and subcutaneous tissues.

It can be categorized into hereditary angioedema, acquired angioedema, and allergic angioedema according to different incentives [22]. Hereditary angioedema is a common autosomal dominant disease caused by a deficiency of complement factor 1 inhibitor, leading to the activation of complement classic pathway and an increase in bradykinin [23]. Acquired angioedema is considered to be an autoimmune disease that often appears in patients with lymphoproliferative disorders.

In general cases angioneurotic edema is an allergic disease. It is an IgE-mediated I type reaction in which drugs or their metabolites enter the body and induce IgE production. IgE then attaches to the surface of mast cells, causing the production of vasoactive substances such as histamine, leukotriene, prostaglandins, and bradykinin. The process in turn provokes vasodilatation and increases vascular permeability and therefore leads to swelling in tissues [24].

Current studies on angioneurotic edema are mostly found in the form of case report in which the symptom is often caused by drugs, e.g., recombinant tissue plasminogen activator (rt-PA) used in thrombolysis [25], angiotensin-converting enzyme inhibitors (ACEI) in hypertension treatment, antipsychotics, insulin, aspirin, NSAID (nonsteroidal anti-inflammatory drugs), β-lactam antibiotics, sulfonamides, etc. [26]. There have been reports indicating a link between the disease and drug dosage, and low-dose treatment is recommended in the absence of alternative drugs [22].

Most patients with angioneurotic edema experience acute onset with sudden symptoms that typically disappear within hours to days without long-term sequelae and can be recurrent. Acute angioneurotic edema, however, can become chronic when the dissipation of symptoms slows down or stops due to the recurrence. Clinical symptoms involve limited tough elastic swellings with no pain, itch, depression, tenderness, or wave-like motion. Angioneurotic edema occurs on the face, tongue, extremities, genitals, and especially loose tissues in cephalic region such as the lips (Figs. 2.11 and 2.12), and serious symptoms can lead to laryngeal edema, airway obstruction, and even death [27].

The first step of treatment for angioneurotic edema involves the diagnosis and prevention of allergies; meanwhile oral medication can be applied (the same as the oral medication for drug-allergic stomatitis). Though localized angioneurotic edema usually does not need specific treatment, for patients with symptom recurrence

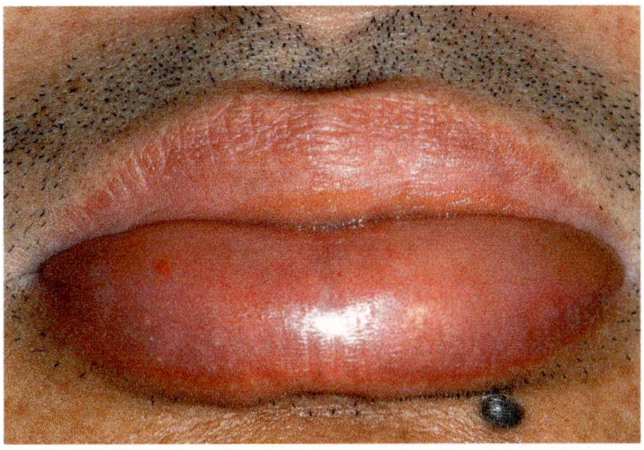

Fig. 2.11 Obvious swelling on the lower lip

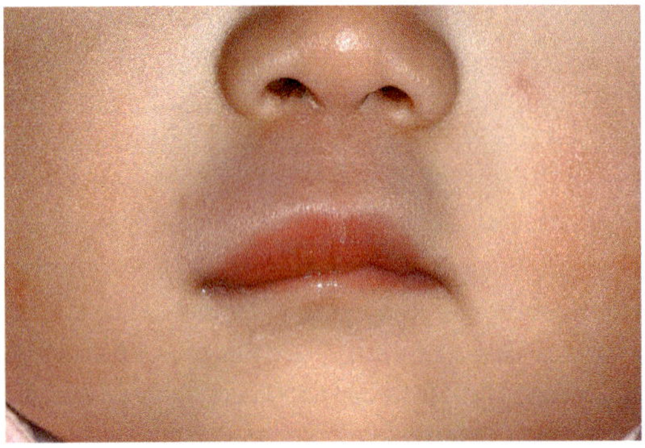

Fig. 2.12 Obvious swelling on the right upper lip

that prevents the swelling from dissipating completely, we recommend low-dose, multi-point injection into the swelling with mixture of 1 ml of triamcinolone acetonide and equal volume of sterile water, once per week or every 2 weeks. For patients with laryngeal edema and anhelation, careful observation and hospitalization are necessary.

References

1. Khan DA. Cutaneous drug reactions. J Allergy Clin Immunol. 2012;130(5):1225–e6.
2. Shiohara T. Fixed drug eruption: pathogenesis and diagnostic tests. Curr Opin Allergy Clin Immunol. 2009;9(4):316–21.
3. Ozkaya E. Oral mucosal fixed drug eruption: characteristics and differential diagnosis. J Am Acad Dermatol. 2013;69(2):e51–8.
4. Marya CM, Sharma G, Parashar VP, Dahiya V. Mucosal fixed drug eruption in a patient treated with ornidazole. J Dermatol Case Rep. 2012;6(1):21–4.
5. Kim MH, Shim EJ, Jung JW, Sohn SW, Kang HR. A case of allopurinol-induced fixed drug eruption confirmed with a lymphocyte transformation test. Allergy Asthma Immunol Res. 2012;4(5):309–10.
6. Sanchis JM, Bagan JV, Gavalda C, et al. Erythema multiforme: diagnosis, clinical manifestations and treatment in a retrospective study of 22 patients. J Oral Pathol Med. 2010;39(10):747–52.
7. Katz J, Livneh A, Shemer J, et al. Herpes simplex-associated erythema multiforme (HAEM): a clinical therapeutic dilemma. Pediatr Dent. 1999;21(6):359–62.
8. Watanabe R, Watanabe H, Sotozono C, et al. Critical factors differentiating erythema multiforme majus from Stevens-Johnson syndrome (SJS)/toxic epidermal necrolysis (TEN). Eur J Dermatol. 2011;21(6):889–94.
9. Schofield JK, Tatnall FM, Leigh IM. Recurrent erythema multiforme: clinical features and treatment in a large series of patients. Br J Dermatol. 1993;128(5):542–5.
10. Imafuku S, Kokuba H, Aurelian L, et al. Expression of herpes simplex virus DNA fragments located in epidermal keratinocytes and germinative cells is associated with the development of erythema multiforme lesions. J Invest Dermatol. 1997;109(4):550–6.
11. Ono F, Sharma BK, Smith CC, et al. CD34+ cells in the peripheral blood transport herpes simplex virus DNA fragments to the skin of patients with erythema multiforme (HAEM). J Invest Dermatol. 2005;124(6):1215–24.
12. Kokuba H, Imafuku S, Huang S, et al. Erythema multiforme lesions are associated with expression of a herpes simplex virus (HSV) gene and qualitative alterations in the HSV-specific T-cell response. Br J Dermatol. 1998;138(6):952–64.
13. Al-Johani KA, Fedele S, Porter SR. Erythema multiforme and related disorders. Oral Surg Oral Med Oral Pathol Oral Radiol Endod. 2007;103(5):642–54.
14. Stewart MG, Duncan NO 3rd, Franklin DJ, et al. Head and neck manifestations of erythema multiforme in children. Otolaryngol Head Neck Surg. 1994;111(3 Pt 1):236–42.
15. Scully C, Bagan J. Oral mucosal diseases: erythema multiforme. Br J Oral Maxillofac Surg. 2008;46(2):90–5.
16. Auquier-Dunant A, Mockenhaupt M, Naldi L, et al. Correlations between clinical patterns and causes of erythema multiforme majus, Stevens-Johnson syndrome, and toxic epidermal necrolysis: results of an international prospective study. Arch Dermatol. 2002;138(8):1019–24.
17. Schwartz RA. Toxic epidermal necrolysis. Cutis. 1997;59(3):123–8.
18. Wetter DA, Davis MD. Recurrent erythema multiforme: clinical characteristics, etiologic associations, and treatment in a series of 48 patients at Mayo Clinic, 2000 to 2007. J Am Acad Dermatol. 2010;62(1):45–53.
19. Chen Q. Oral medicine. 4th ed. Beijing: People's Medical Publishing House; 2013.
20. Ozkaya E, Babuna G. Two cases with nickel-induced oral mucosal hyperplasia: a rare clinical form of allergic contact stomatitis. Dermatol Online J. 2011; 17(3):12.
21. Greenberg MS, Glick M, Ship JA. Burket's oral medicine: diagnosis & treatment. 11th ed. Hamilton: BC Decker Inc; 2008.
22. Soumya RN, Grover S, Dutt A, et al. Angioneurotic edema with risperidone: a case report and review of literature. Gen Hosp Psychiatry. 2010;32(6):646.e1–3.
23. Velasco-Medina AA, Cortes-Morales G, Barreto-Sosa A, et al. Pathophysiology and advances in the

treatment of hereditary angioedema. Rev Alerg Mex. 2011;58(2):112–9.
24. Warnock JK, Knesevich JW. Adverse cutaneous reactions to antidepressants. Am J Psychiatry. 1988; 145(4):425–30.
25. Ekmekci P, Bengisun ZK, Kazbek BK, et al. Oropharyngeal angioneurotic edema due to recombinant tissue plasminogen activator following massive pulmonary thromboembolism. Int Immunopharmacol. 2011;11(9):1384–5.
26. Mishra B, Sahoo S, Sarkar S, et al. Clozapine-induced angioneurotic edema. Gen Hosp Psychiatry. 2007;29(1):78–80.
27. Akkaya C, Sarandol A, Aydogan K, et al. Urticaria and angio-oedema due to ziprasidone. J Psychopharmacol. 2007;21(5):550–2.

Ulcerative Lesions of the Oral Mucosa

3

Yu Zhou, Xiaoying Li, Xin Jin, and Qianming Chen

Keywords
Recurrent aphthous ulcer · Behcet's disease · Radiation stomatitis · Traumatic mucosal hematotoma · Traumatic ulceration · Necrotizing sialometaplasia

Y. Zhou
State Key Laboratory of Oral Diseases, National Clinical Research Center for Oral Diseases, Department of Oral Medicine, West China Hospital of Stomatology, Sichuan University, Chengdu, Sichuan, China

X. Li
State Key Laboratory of Oral Diseases, National Clinical Research Center for Oral Diseases, Department of Oral Medicine, West China Hospital of Stomatology, Sichuan University, Chengdu, Sichuan, China

X. Jin
College of Stomatology, Chongqing Medical University, Chongqing Key Laboratory of Oral Diseases and Biomedical Sciences, Chongqing, China

Q. Chen (✉)
Changjiang Scholars Program, Ministry of Education, Beijing, China

State Key Laboratory of Oral Diseases, National Clinical Research Center for Oral Diseases, Department of Oral Medicine, West China Hospital of Stomatology, Sichuan University, Chengdu, Sichuan, China
e-mail: qmchen@scu.edu.cn

3.1 Recurrent Aphthous Ulcer

Case 25 Minor Aphthous Ulcer

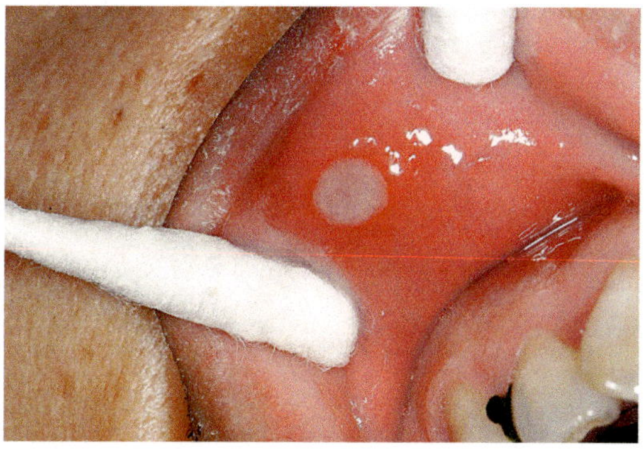

Fig. 3.1 A rounded ulcer appeared on the inner side mucosa of the upper lip, with the characteristics of "red, yellow, concave, tenderness"

Age: 46 years
Sex: Male
Chief Complaints:
Recurrent oral ulcer for 6 years, aggravation 6 months, recurrence 3 days
History of Present Illness:
The patient was recurring oral ulcers for 6 years. The oral ulcer always recurs once a month with one ulcer at a time, lasting 5–6 days. For the last 6 months, the oral ulcer recurred in every 2 weeks, 1–2 ulcers every time, and lasted for 1 week. Three days ago, there was an ulcer recurring in the inner side mucosa of the upper

Q. Chen, X. Zeng (eds.), *Case Based Oral Mucosal Diseases*,
https://doi.org/10.1007/978-981-13-0286-2_3

lip. He didn't have any medical history of ocular disease and genital ulcers. He usually catches a cold.

Past Medical History: None

Allergy: None

Physical Examination:

An ulcer with about 5 mm in diameter appeared on the inner side mucosa of the upper lip, with the characteristics of "red, yellow, concave, tenderness (Fig. 3.1)."

Diagnosis:

Minor aphthous ulcer

Diagnosis Basis:

1. History of recurrence.
2. The ulcer had the characteristics of "red, yellow, concave, tenderness."

Management:

1. Medication

   Rp.: Thymopeptide enteric-coated tablets 20 mg × 30

   Sig.: 20 mg p.o. b.i.d.

   Multivitamin formula with mineral tablets 30 tablets

   Sig.: 1 tablet p.o. q.d.

   Dexamethasone paste 15 g × 1

   Sig.: topical use t.i.d.

Follow-Up Management:

If the medication is effective, continue taking the above drugs for 1–2 months. If not, switching to immunomodulatory drugs is considered.

Case 26 Herpetiform Aphthous Ulcer

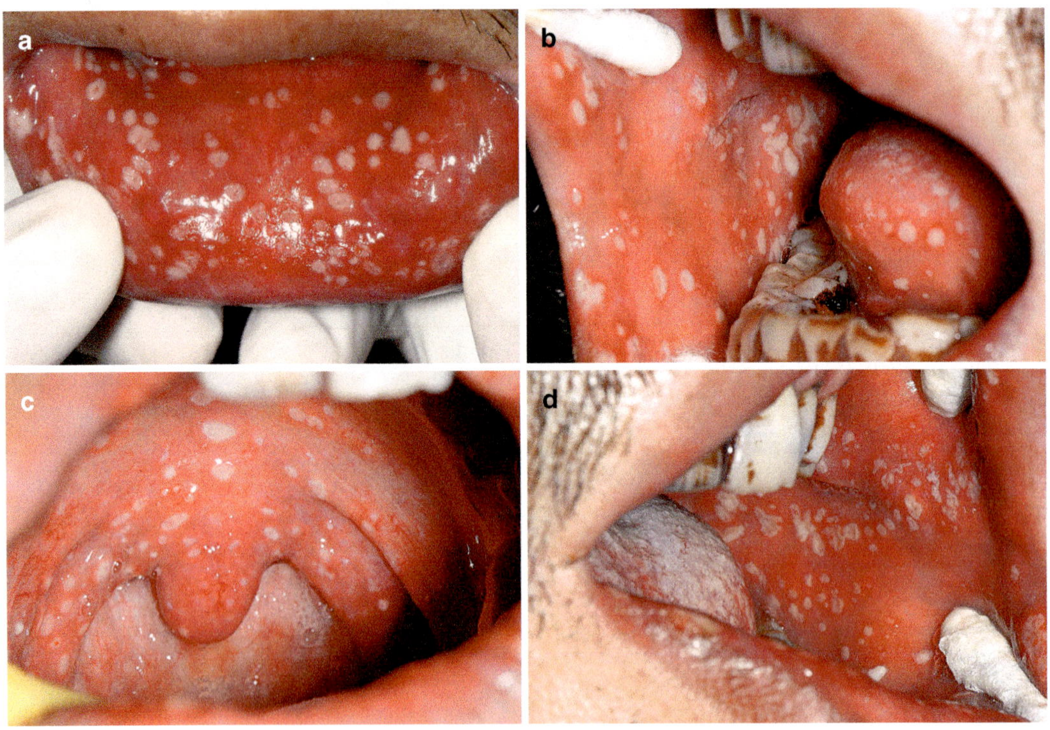

Fig. 3.2 (**a**) Dozens of small rounded ulcers appeared on the inner side mucosa of the lower lip, presenting like stars in the sky. (**b**) Dozens of small rounded ulcers appeared on the right buccal mucosa and right tongue. (**c**) Dozens of small rounded ulcers appeared on the soft palate. (**d**) Dozens of small rounded ulcers appeared on the left buccal mucosa

Age: 48 years
Sex: Male
Chief Complaints:
Recurrent oral ulcer for 2 years, reappear 5 days
History of Present Illness:
The patient was recurring oral ulcers for 2 years. Usually 3–6 ulcers appeared at one time with the intermission of 1–2 months. Five days ago, without obvious causes, ten ulcers recurred in his oral cavity, with a severe pain. He didn't have any medical history of ocular disease and genital ulcers.
Past Medical History: None
Allergy: None
Physical Examination:
There were dozens of small (about 2–3 mm in diameter) ulcers on the lips, anterior tongue, buccal mucosa, and soft palate, presenting as stars in the sky (Fig. 3.2).
Diagnosis:
Herpetiform aphthous ulcer
Diagnosis Basis:

1. History of recurrence
2. Dozens of small ulcers presenting like stars in the sky

Management:

1. Medication
   Rp.: Prednisone acetate 5 mg × 25 tablets
   Sig.: 25 mg p.o. q.m.
   Zhongtong'an capsules 0.28 g × 48 tablets
   Sig.: 0.56 g p.o. q.d.
   Compound vitamin B 100 tablets
   Sig.: two tablets p.o. t.i.d.
   Dexamethasone sodium phosphate injection 1 ml × 5
   Sig.: 1:50 dilution rinse t.i.d.
   Compound chlorhexidine solution 300 ml × 1
   Sig.: rinse t.i.d.
   Dexamethasone paste 15 g × 1
   Sig.: topical use t.i.d.
2. Aerosol therapy
   Rp.: Dexamethasone sodium phosphate injection 1 ml × 1
   Gentamicin sulfate injection 2 ml × 1
   Vitamin B12 injection 1 ml × 1
   Vitamin C injection 2.5 ml × 1
   Sig.: aerosol therapy b.i.d.

Follow-Up Treatment:
It will be switched to the same treatment plan as minor aphthous ulcer until the disease is controlled.

Case 27 Major Aphthous Ulcer

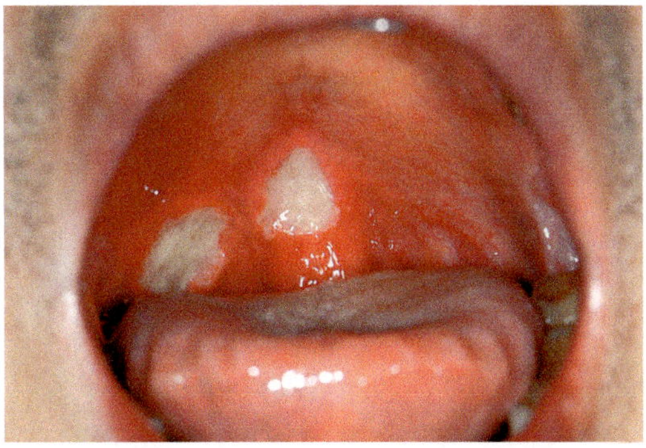

Fig. 3.3 Two large and deep ulcers on the left soft palate, with the characteristics of "red, yellow, concave, tenderness"

Age: 42 years
Sex: Male
Chief Complaints:
Recurrent oral ulcer for 6 years, aggravation for 1 year
History of Present Illness:
The patient was recurring oral ulcers for 6 years. The oral ulcer always recurred one at a time occasionally, lasting 2–3 days. For the last 1 year, the oral ulcer recurred frequently, 2–3 times in every month, 2–3 ulcers every time, and lasted for 10–20 days, with the intermission of 2–3 days. Twenty days ago, the oral ulcer recurred and had yet to heal. He didn't have any medical history of ocular disease and genital ulcers.
Past Medical History: None
Allergy: None
Physical Examination:

There were two large and deep ulcers on the left soft palate, about 10 mm in diameter, covering with yellowish-white pseudomembrane (Fig. 3.3).

Diagnosis:

Major aphthous ulcer

Diagnosis Basis:

1. History of recurrent ulcers
2. Single ulcer with the characteristics of "red, yellow, concave, tenderness"
3. Major ulcer with long-lasting ulcer stage

Management:

1. Medication

   Rp.: Prednisone acetate 5 mg × 25 tablets
   - Sig.: 20 mg p.o. q.m. (first 5 days)
   - Thalidomide 25 mg × 20 tablets
   - Sig.: 50 mg p.o. q.n. (from the sixth day)
   - Zhongtong'an capsules 0.28 g × 48 tablets
   - Compound vitamin B 100 tablets
   - Sig.: two tablets p.o. t.i.d.
   - Dexamethasone sodium phosphate injection 1 ml × 5
   - Sig.: 1:50 dilution rinse t.i.d.
   - Recombinant human epidermal growth factor spray 15 ml × 1
   - Sig.: topical use t.i.d.

Follow-Up Management:

After the disease control, we suggest the injection of *Bacillus* Calmette-Guerin polysaccharide nucleic acid (BCG-PSN) for 18 times (sig.: 1 ml i.m. q.o.d.). If the disease is poorly controlled, we recommend to add the dose of thalidomide to 75–100 mg, q.d., 2 weeks as a course; or change to tripterygium hypoglaucum tablet (sig.: 2 g p.o. t.i.d.), 1 month as a course; or change to tripterygium glycoside tablet (sig.: 1–1.5 mg/(kg.d) p.o. t.i.d.), 1 month as a course.

Case 28 Teenage Periglandular Aphtha

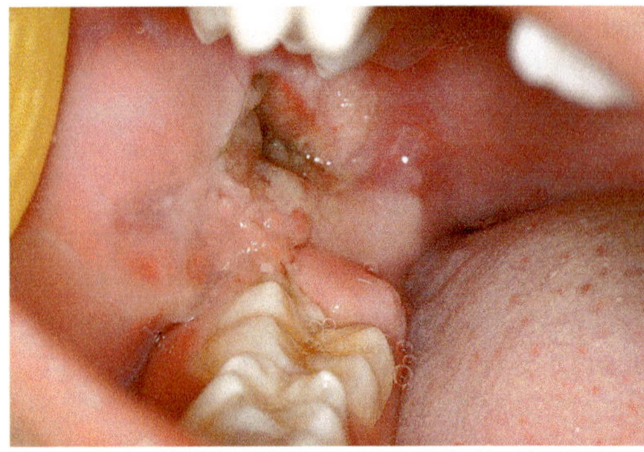

Fig. 3.4 Large and deep ulcer appeared on the right retromolar region, surrounding with gray mucosa

Age: 8 years

Sex: Male

Weight: 25 kg

Chief Complaints:

One ulcer appeared on the right buccal mucosa for 1 week

History of Present Illness:

One week ago, there was an ulcer recurring on the right buccal mucosa, with pain. The similar lesion had appeared for three times at the same position, lasting for 10 days in every time. He usually catches a cold, and didn't like to eat vegetables.

Past Medical History: None

Allergy: None

Physical Examination:

There was one obvious large and deep ulcer on the right retromolar region with about 12 mm in diameter, covered with yellowish-white pseudomembrane, without obvious red and swollen (Fig. 3.4).

Diagnosis:

Teenage periglandular aphtha

Diagnosis Basis:

1. History of recurrent ulcer.
2. The ulcer was deep, large, crater-like, and appearing in teenagers.

Management:

1. Medication
   Rp.: Pidotimod 0.4 g × 18 tablets
   Sig.: 0.4 g p.o. q.d.
   Junior multivitamin formula with mineral tablets 30 tablets
   Sig.: one tablet p.o. q.d.
   Compound chlorhexidine solution 300 ml × 1
   Sig.: rinse t.i.d.
   Recombinant human epidermal growth factor spray 15 ml × 1
   Sig.: spray t.i.d.
   Dexamethasone paste 15 g × 1
   Sig.: topical use t.i.d.

Follow-Up Management:
If the disease has no obvious remission, we suggest multiple-point injection of small dose at the base of the ulcer with triamcinolone acetonide injection plus equal water for injection or 2% lidocaine. *Bacillus* Calmette-Guerin polysaccharide nucleic acid (BCG-PSN), 0.5 ml i.m. q.o.d., is also suggested. If necessary, prednisone acetate (15 mg, p.o. q.m, for 3–5 days) could be applied.

[Review] Recurrent Aphthous Ulcer
Recurrent aphthous ulcer (RAU), also called as recurrent oral ulcer (ROU), has the characteristics of recrudescence, self-healing, and burning sensation. It is the most common ulcerative disease affecting the oral mucosa, with the incidence varies from 5% to 60% depending on the ethnic and socioeconomic groups studied [1]. RAU results in considerable pain and distress and may lead to difficulty in speaking, eating, and swallowing and thus may negatively affect patients' quality of life [2].

The etiology and pathogenesis of RAU are still unknown, existing individual differences. Most scholars believe that RAU is a result from the comprehensive effect of many factors including immunologic, genetic, and systemic diseases, infection, and so forth.

It is generally accepted that the immune pathogenesis plays an important role but without exact theories about immunological etiology. Cell-mediated and immune complex mechanisms are probably involved in RAS pathogenesis. An increase in γδ T cells further suggests a role for antibody-dependent cell-mediated cytotoxicity in RAU pathogenesis. These T cells produce tumor necrosis factor-a (TNF-a), a major inflammatory mediator responsible for initiation of the inflammatory process by its effects on endothelial cell adhesion, neutrophil chemotaxis, a vascular obstruction, and activation of lysosomal enzymes, resulting in the appearance of ulcer lesion [3]. Different inflammatory mediators have been found in the lesions of RAU. A markedly increased plasma IL-2 has been recorded in the active stage of RAU. IL-10 usually stimulates epithelial proliferation in a healing process. Salivary prostaglandin E2 and epidermal growth factor may potentially aid mucosal healing. Both are reduced in the early stages of RAS ulcer and then rise in the healing phase [4]. Besides cellular immunity, the production of immune complex also relates to RAU. Immune deposits occur in lesional biopsy specimens, especially in the stratum spinosum. Immune mechanisms appear to play an important role in the etiology of RAU; a positive family history is seen in one-third of RAU patients. A genetic predisposition is suggested by the presence of an increased frequency of human leukocyte antigen types A2, A11, B12, and DR2.

A positive family history is seen in one-third of RAU patients. A genetic predisposition is suggested by the presence of an increased frequency of human leukocyte antigen types A2, A11, B12, and DR2, as well as the inheritance of either an allele of interleukin-1 (IL-1β-51) or an allele of IL-6 (IL-6174) [5].

Many systemic diseases relate to RAU. However, the evidence, system disease-related ulcer is the real RAU or just like RAU, still need to be studied. These include celiac disease, iron-deficiency anemia, human immunodeficiency virus (HIV) infection, neutropenia, and vitamin B12, folic acid, and zinc deficiencies. These patients need to actively improve the systemic factors. However, neither iron nor vitamin supplementation has been shown to enhance the resolution of ulcers [5, 6].

Microbial infection is the incidence of RAU or secondary infection and is still controversial. There are studies to indicate that RAU may be a T-cell-mediated response to antigens of *Streptococcus sanguis*, which cross-react with the mitochondrial heat shock protein and induce oral mucosal damage [4]. The evidence that various bacteria and viruses can cause ulcers is not very reliable.

Anxiety and stress have been associated with the onset and recurrence of RAU. There are reports that by avoiding allergic food (e.g., chocolate, wheat flour, tomato, strawberry, and peanut), the clinical symptoms of RAU can be improved. Because nicotine may promote keratinized mucosa, thus smoking can induce RAU. Hormonal changes related to the menstrual cycle may also be related to RAU, but the clinical evidence is scarce. What's more, RAU development is related to several chemical compounds and medications. These include nonsteroidal anti-inflammatory agents, nicorandil, beta-blockers, angiotensin-converting enzyme inhibitors, antiarrhythmic drugs, and sodium lauryl sulfate (a detergent in some oral healthcare products) [5, 6].

RAU present, as well as demarcated, oval or round recurrent oral ulcers with a white or yellow pseudomembrane and a surrounding erythematous halo. They may rarely appear initially as red macules or papules but quickly form the classic ulcer. Especially for longer-lasting ulcers, a gray membrane may replace the central yellow pseudomembrane. The ulcers are painful and interfere with eating and speaking. A prodromal burning or tingling sensation may occur. Aphthous ulcers have a predilection for lining mucosa and specialized mucosa, like the labial mucosa, buccal mucosa, floor of the mouth, soft palate, ventral and lateral tongue, and oropharynx [7]. Generally ulcers do not occur on the masticatory mucosa like the hard palate and gingiva.

RAU are conventionally classified, based on their size, duration, and presence or absence of scarring after healing into minor, major, and herpetiform ulcers [8]. Minor aphthae comprise about 75–85% of RAU and present as one to five painful ulcers each less than 1.0 cm in diameter that last for 10–14 days and heal spontaneously without scarring. Regional lymphadenopathy may rarely be present depending on the severity and number of lesions. The process is self-limited but recurs with high variability. In some patients, ulcer activity is almost continuous with new ulcers developing as old ones heal.

Major aphthae (periadenitis mucosa necrotica recurrens) comprise about 10–15% of cases. Ulcers are greater than 1.0 cm in diameter, deeper, and more painful and may take up to weeks or longer to heal. Dysphagia and fever are common. Scarring is common (Fig. 3.5). Ulcers occur on the posterior oral cavity where they may interfere with eating. Ulcers may be secondarily infected with bacteria or fungi. When it appears in teenagers, it is known as juvenile periglandular aphtha, characterized by great and deep ulcer. The inflammation of mucosa surrounding the ulcer is not obvious. And the ulcer always recurs on the tip of buccal pad and lateral and tip of the tongue in the boys. Patients often bite the cheek or tongue due to the symptom of itchiness.

Herpetiform ulcers are seen in 5–10% of cases and present as crops (as many as 100) of 1–3 mm ulcers that heal within 10–14 days without scarring. They may appear anywhere throughout the

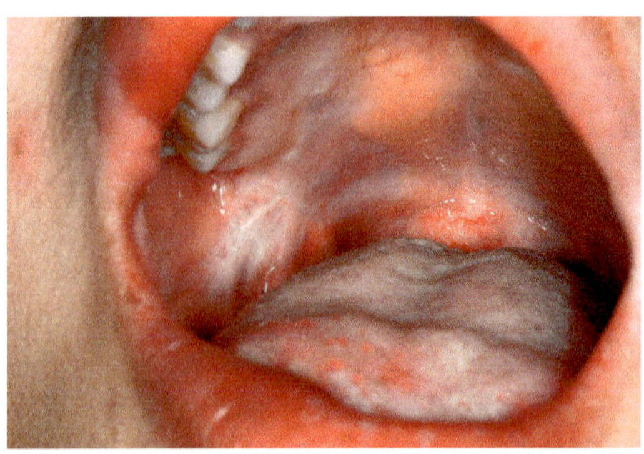

Fig. 3.5 The white mucosa on the right soft palate is MaRAU scar after healing

oral cavity except masticatory mucosa. Women are more frequently affected.

The diagnosis of RAU is based on the characteristics of recurrence, periodicity, and self-healing and the features of "painful round hollow ulcers with white or yellow pseudomembrane and a surrounding erythematous halo." RAU is not cancerous ulcer and also has no malignant potential. However, for the deep, large, long course and different with the past of the ulcer, we should be vigilant. Conduct a biopsy to rule out cancerous ulcer or other diseases when necessary. Cancerous ulcer (Fig. 3.6) occurs in elderly patients, characterized by uneven depth and edge, infiltration and hard in quality of surrounding tissue, and cauliflower-like of the bottom, without recurrence and self-healing. These characteristics are different from the characteristics of RAU.

It is noteworthy that RAU is also available for the extraintestinal manifestations of inflammatory bowel disease (Figs. 3.7 and 3.8). The inflammatory bowel disease refers to ulcerative colitis and Crohn's disease. The investigation should be carried out in inflammatory bowel disease, if the RAU patients have persistent or recurrent diarrhea, purulent stools accompanied by abdominal pain and tenesmus.

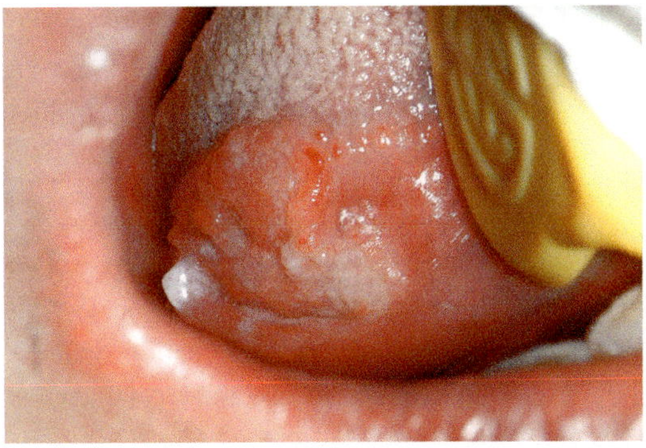

Fig. 3.6 Ulcer with unclear border and cauliflower-like surface on the right root of the tongue

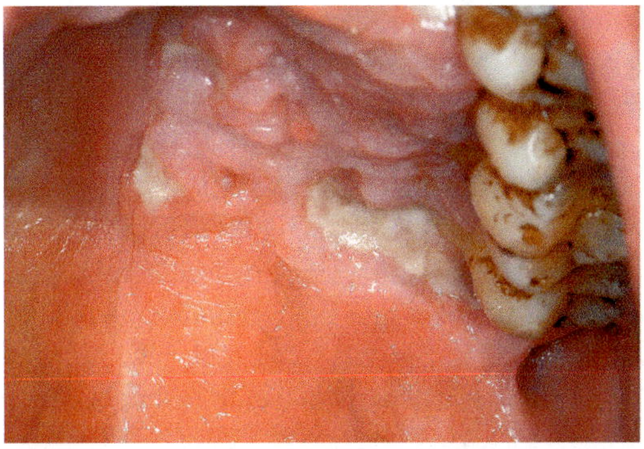

Fig. 3.7 Deep ulcer with 1cm in diameter on the left posterior maxillary palatal gingiva, surrounding with small ulcers

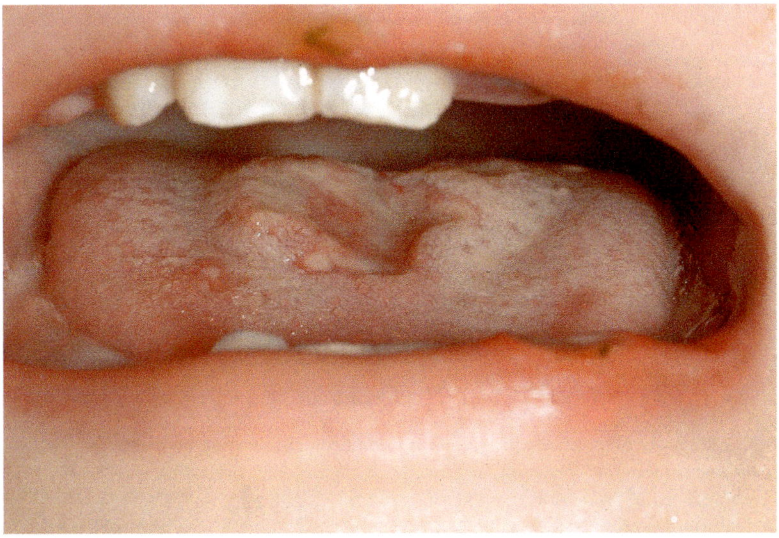

Fig. 3.8 Ulcer with 1 cm in diameter on the dorsum of the tongue, covered with yellow pseudomembrane

Because of the multiple and complex factors of RAU, it still has no definitive treatment [5]. The goals of therapy are to decrease frequency of recurrence, prolong the interval, decrease pain, and promote healing.

Commonly used systemic agents for the treatment of RAU include glucocorticoid (like prednisone), immunosuppressant (like thalidomide), Chinese patent medicine with immunosuppressive effect (like tripterygium glycoside tablet, tripterygium hypoglaucum tablet), and immunomodulator (like thymosin, transfer factor, licorzine granules). Commonly used topical agents include gargle (chlorhexidine solution, dexamethasone solution), paste (like amlexanox paste, dexamethasone paste, triamcinolone acetonide dental paste, dexamethasone ointment), spray (like recombinant human epidermal growth factor spray, recombinant bovine basic fibroblast growth factor spray), lozenge (like penicillin V potassium lozenge), patch (amlexanox patch, dexamethasone patch), gelatin (like compound chamomile and lidocaine hydrochloride gel, compound benzocaine gel, recombinant bovine basic fibroblast growth factor gel, recombinant human epidermal growth factor hydrogel), and injections (like triamcinolone acetonide injection, compound betamethasone injection).

For patients with minor RAU, who had only a few days or no significant intermittent periods, and with a major RAU or a herpetiform ulcer, they can take prednisone (sig.: 15–30 mg p.o. q.m), 1–2 weeks as a course, or thalidomide (Sig.: 50 mg p.o. q.n.), 10–14 days as a course, together with vitamins, trace elements, and topical agents. For the patients with deep and prolonged unhealed ulcers, cancer was excluded, eliminating malignant lesion; we suggest patients take multiple-point injection of small dose at the base of the ulcer with triamcinolone acetonide injection plus equal water for injection or 2% lidocaine.

For patients with poor constitution, reduced immune function, and minor RAU, they can choose thymopeptide enteric-coated tablets (Sig.: 20 mg p.o. q.d. or b.i.d), 1–2 months as a course; or transfer factor capsules (Sig.: 6 mg p.o. b.i.d. or t.i.d), 1–2 months as a course; or use *Bacillus* Calmette-Guerin polysaccharide nucleic acid (Sig.: 1 ml i.m. q.o.d.), 18 times as a course. The above drugs can be used in combination with the use of vitamins, trace elements, and topical agents.

3.2 Behcet's Disease

Case 29 Behcet's Disease

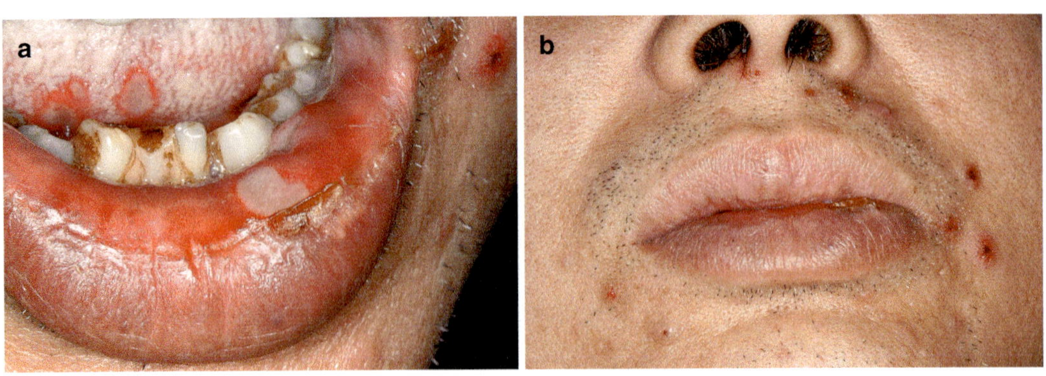

Fig. 3.9 (**a**) Dozens of rounded ulcer appeared on the inner side mucosa of lower lip and tongue tip, with the characteristics of "red, yellow, concave, tenderness". (**b**) Acneiform lesions appeared on the perioral skin. (**c**) The acupuncture point in the hand emerged red and swollen after needling. (**d**) Round and small ulcers appeared on the genitalia, with the characteristic of "red, yellow, concave, tenderness". (**e**) Round and small ulcers appeared on the perianal region, with the characteristic of "red, yellow, concave, tenderness"

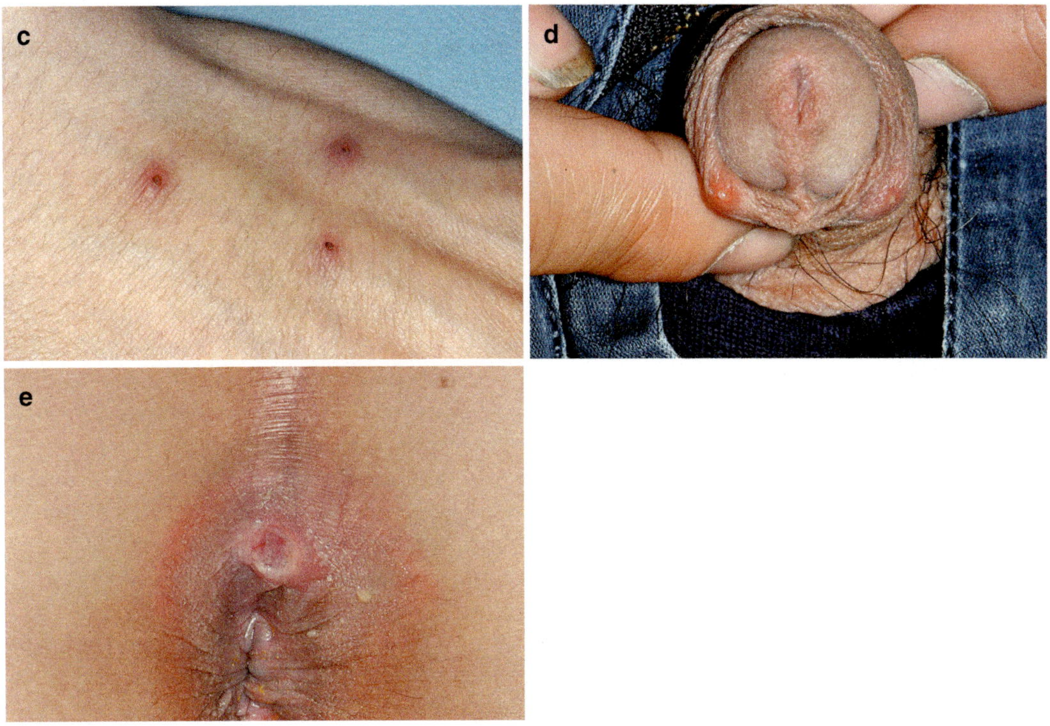

Fig. 3.9 (continued)

Age: 42 years
Sex: Male
Chief Complaints:
A 42-year-old male with recurrent oral ulcers for 3 years and recurrent genital ulcers for 1 year
History of Present Illness:
A 42-year-old male presented to our clinic with recurrent oral ulcers for 3 years. He had a number of ulcers every time with obvious pain, often accompanied by perioral skin pustules. Every time he self-medicated with two tablets of dexamethasone, p.o. twice a day, 2–3 days to ease the pain. The intermittent period was 7–8 days. In addition to oral ulcers, he also presented to our clinic with recurrent genital ulcers for 1 year. The attack frequency seemed to oral ulcers, but not necessarily attacked at the same time. Four days before relapse, the lesions appeared as multiple ulcers in oral and also occurred perianal ulcer with infusion invalid.
Past Medical History: None
Allergy: None
Physical Examination:
More than ten small red papules on the perioral skin with brown scab shell covered on the top. There were several 2–8-mm-diameter ulcers on the lower buccal mucosa, right mouth angular inside, tip of the tongue, and ventral tongue. The ulcers were covered with a yellow pseudomembrane on the surface, periphery with a red band and central depression, obviously painful. There were redness and swelling around the infusion needle point on the back of the hand. There was a 5-mm-diameter ulcer on the perianal mucosa, and there were two 2-mm-diameter ulcers on the wrapper. All of the three were in line with the features, which were covered with a yellow pseudomembrane on the surface, periphery with a red band and central depression, obviously painful (Fig. 3.9).
Diagnosis:
Behcet's disease
Diagnosis Basis:

1. Recurrent oral ulcers and history of genital ulcers
2. Acnes on the facial skin and redness and swelling around the skin acupuncture points

Management:

1. Medication
   Rp.: Thalidomide 25 mg × 40 tablets
   Sig.: 75 mg p.o. q.n.
   Zhongtong'an capsules 0.28 g × 48 tablets
   Sig.: 0.56 g p.o. q.d.
   Compound vitamin B 100 tablets
   Sig.: two tablets p.o. t.i.d.
   Dexamethasone paste 15 g × 1
   Sig.: topical use t.i.d.

Subsequent Management:
After disease is controlled, *Bacillus* Calmette-Guerin polysaccharide nucleic acid (BCG-PSN), intramuscular injection, 1 ml each time, every other day can be used. If the disease is poorly controlled, increase dose of thalidomide as appropriate to 100 mg each time; or replacement with tripterygium hypoglaucum tablet, 2 g each time, three times a day; or replacement with tripterygium glycoside tablet could be considered.

[Review] Behcet's Disease
Behcet's disease is a systemic disease caused by an unknown etiology, with vasculitis as the pathological basis, with the features of chronic progressive, recurrent, system damage and so on [9].

The etiology of Behcet's disease and the performance of oral ulcers are similar to recurrent aphthous ulcers, but most scholars still believe that the two are different independent diseases. The specific etiology of Behcet's disease is also not clear; some scholars believe that it is a systemic vasculitis with an unknown etiology affecting the small and large vessels of the venous and arterial systems [10]. Behcet's disease has a genetic basis; the most consistent genetic association has been with HLA-B51, which explains only about 20% of the disease heritability [11]. It is also in vogue to group BD with autoinflammatory disease [12]. Our current understanding is that an exogenous trigger(s) modulating the immune system in a genetically susceptible host lead to disease expression in BD [13]. The exogenous trigger(s) include viruses, bacteria, and heat shock proteins [14]. BD's regional differences are obvious and often occur in Asia and the Middle East; many of the local patients with recurrent aphthous ulcers well develop to BD and often involve multi-systems with severe symptoms. However, in Western Europe and North America, many patients have RAU, but very few of patients have BD; the symptoms are mild, and the prognosis is well [6].

BD's clinical manifestations include common signs and rare signs of two categories. Common signs include oral, genital, skin, eye, and other symptoms. Rare symptoms include joint, cardiovascular, nervous, digestive, urinary, and other systemic diseases.

Oral ulcerations are seen in almost all patients of BD, mostly minor, or herpetiform RAU also can be major.

The incidence of genital ulcers accounts for about 75% of patients with BD. It is also often recurrent but with fewer occurrences and fewer numbers. The ulcers are often seen in the labia, penis, glans, and scrotum and can also be found in the perianal, etc. [15].

The incidence of skin lesions in patients with BD is second only to oral ulcers, including:

1. Erythema nodosums are frequently seen at the lower limbs in the form of several 1–2-cm-diameter erythema lesions and are of moderate hardness and painful when touched. The erythema lesions usually spend 1 month to self-heal, and the new erythema lesions would emerge.
2. Folliculitis-like lesions are mainly seen at the head, the face, the upper chest, and the upper back and present as papulopustular lesions with wide flush around.
3. Skin prick reaction is a nonspecific hyperreactivity of the peripheral vessel to trauma and is a BD's characteristic performance having a diagnostic value and accounting for about 65%.

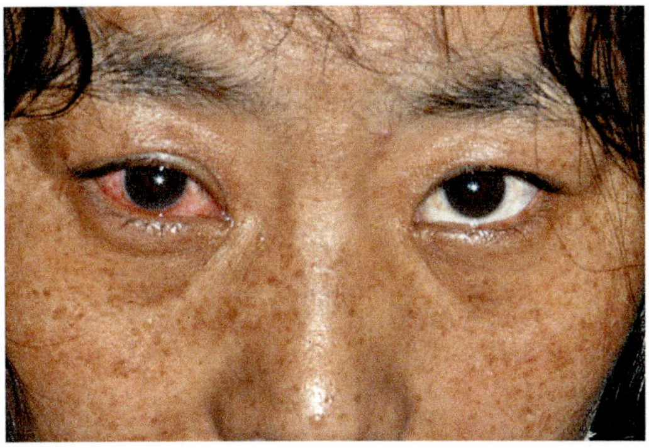

Fig. 3.10 Congestion appeared on the conjunctiva of the right eye

It refers to that after patients receiving intramuscular injection, the needle could present as a papule or pustule, or after patients receiving intravenous injection, the patients could appear with thrombophlebitis and dissipate in 3–7 days. The clinical trial method of skin prick reaction is that after 75% ethanol disinfection of the skin, prick the forearm skin with a sterile needle directly or pin containing 0.1 ml saline, and observe the needle point 24–48 h later. If it presents as a papule or pustule, it means positive of the skin prick reaction. Other skin lesions include acne-like lesions and so on.

Eye involvements generally appear later, which mainly present as iridocyclitis, hypopyon, conjunctivitis, and keratitis (Fig. 3.10). Severe patients can present choroiditis, neuropapillitis, optic atrophy, and vitreous diseases, which can lead to cataracts, glaucoma, and blindness [16].

Rare lesions include arthritis and cardiovascular system, central nervous system, digestive system, and other system damage [9].

Fifty percent of patients with Behcet's disease can present with arthritis or joint pain. The knee is the most easy to be affected, followed by the ankle, wrist, and elbow. It rarely leads to joint deformity; X-ray examination has generally no abnormal findings.

Vascular involvement is more common in male BS patients than in female patients. One-third of cases have thrombophlebitis of the deep or superficial veins, usually of the lower extremities. Thromboembolism is rare, probably due to the high adherence of thrombi to the diseased veins. Arterial disease is occurring in <5% of cases, but the serious cases can present as aneurysm, which would lead to death if it breaks. Cardiac lesion, such as myocarditis, valve involvement, pericarditis, etc., is even rarer.

Five to ten percent of patients can present with central nervous system involvement, which is one of the most serious damages of BD, and may lead to death. Eighty percent of patients with CNS disease features have parenchymal brain involvement. This mainly affects the brainstem and is manifested by pyramidal sign and cerebellar sign. Non-parenchymal disease, which is seen as intracranial hypertension due to dural sinus thrombosis, is manifested by headaches and papilloedema.

Gastrointestinal involvement disease is common among patients from Japan. Symptoms include anorexia, vomiting, dyspepsia, diarrhea, and abdominal pain. Gastrointestinal mucosal ulceration is most commonly seen in the ileum, followed by the cecum and other parts of the colon. Ileocecal ulcers have a distinct tendency to perforate. It can be difficult to distinguish inflammatory bowel disease from BD histologically.

Renal involvement is usually mild and characterized by glomerulonephritis. Renal amyloidosis (type AA) is more likely to occur in patients with vascular involvement of BD and affects its prognosis [13].

The common diagnosis of BD consists of the presence of recurrent oral ulceration in addition to two of the following features: recurrent genital ulcers, skin lesions, eye lesions, and positive skin prick reaction.

Treatment of BS is based largely on literature reports, including glucocorticoids, colchicine, azathioprine, cyclosporine, tumor necrosis factor (TNF)-a inhibitors (such as infliximab, etanercept), interferon-a, cyclophosphamide, etc. [13]. If the clinical manifestations of patients are limited to oral ulcers, genital ulcers, and skin lesions, the way of treatment is similar to the treatment of major recurrent aphthous ulcers. But it requires paying close attention to the patient's general condition; if associated with the eye, joint, and other system organ damage, the patient should be transferred to the appropriate sections for further examination and treatment.

3.3 Radiation Stomatitis

Case 30 Radiation Stomatitis

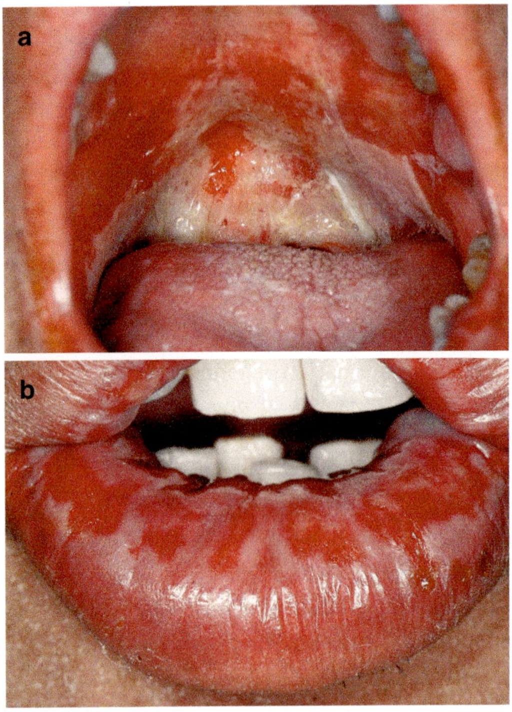

Fig. 3.11 (**a**) Widespread irregular hyperemia and erosions appeared on the palate, covered with yellow-white pseudomembrane. (**b**) Irregular hyperemia and erosions appeared on the lower lip, covered with yellow-white pseudomembrane

Age: 42 years
Sex: Male
Chief Complaints:
A 42-year-old man with oral canker for 14 days
History of Present Illness:
Twenty days ago, he had begun to receive radiotherapy due to nasopharyngeal carcinoma. Four days ago, he presented oral canker with obvious pain.
Past Medical History: Nasopharyngeal carcinoma, cholecystitis, hepatic adipose infiltration, gastric ulcer, and denied other medical history.
Allergy: None
Physical Examination:
Widespread irregular hyperemia and erosions were observed on the tongue, palate, labial, and buccal mucosa, covered with yellow-white pseudomembrane. There was much secretion of inflammation in the oral cavity (Fig. 3.11).
Diagnosis:
Radiation stomatitis
Diagnosis Basis:

1. History of radiotherapy
2. Widespread irregular hyperemia and erosion on oral mucosa

Management:

1. Medication
   Rp.: Compound chlorhexidine solution 300 ml × 1
      Sig.: rinse t.i.d.
      2% sodium bicarbonate solution 250 ml × 1
      Sig.: rinse t.i.d.
      Dexamethasone paste 15 g × 2
      Sig.: topical use t.i.d.
      Recombinant human epidermal growth factor hydrogel 20 g × 1
      Sig.: topical use q.d.
      2. Aerosol therapy
   Rp.: Dexamethasone sodium phosphate injection 1 ml × 1
      Gentamicin sulfate injection 2 ml × 1
      Vitamin B12 injection 1 ml × 1
      Vitamin C injection 2.5 ml × 1
      Sig.: aerosol therapy b.i.d.

[Review] Radiation Stomatitis
Radiation stomatitis or radiation oral mucositis is a radiation-induced damage in the oral mucosa, is generally seen in patients with head and neck cancer receiving radiotherapy, and is a common side effect of radiotherapy [17].

Radiotherapy is one of the common treatments of head and neck cancer. In 90–100% of patients whose irradiation fields include the oral cavity, some degree of oral complication will develop as a result. Radiotherapy affects not only the oral mucosa but also the adjacent salivary glands, bone, dentition, and masticatory musculature and apparatus, leading to mucositis, dry mouth, bacterial or fungal infection, dental caries, perversion or loss of taste, osteoradionecrosis, etc. The radiation dose needed for cancer treatment is based on the location and type of malignant disease and whether or not radiotherapy will be used on its own or in combination with other treatment options. The severity of oral complications is related to the daily and total cumulative dose of radiation, the volume of irradiated tissue, and use of concurrent radiation-sensitizing drugs [18–20].

Radiation stomatitis has a clear etiology and is associated with radiation. Its specific mechanisms still have different views. High-energy radiation can induce the damage and necrosis of basal keratinocytes, resulting in the gradual decrease of the number of epithelial cells. As radiotherapy continues, a temporary steady state between death and regeneration of mucosal cells could occur because surviving cells are produced at an increased rate. However, cell regeneration often cannot keep up with the rate of cell death, resulting in some or complete denudation of the mucosa, presenting a variety of clinical manifestations [21]. In addition to the abovementioned direct tissue injury, the oral microbial flora is also contributed to radiotherapy-induced mucositis. Some scholars believe that endotoxins produced by gram-negative bacilli are potent mediators of the inflammatory process. Resident bacteria on ulcerated surfaces can amplify inflammatory response and enhance local injury. Mucosal barrier injury associated with mucositis promotes adherence and invasion by oral organisms [17, 22].

According to the course of the disease, radiation stomatitis can be divided into acute and chronic. Acute lesions occur early in the course of radiotherapy, lasting up to 2–3 weeks after radiotherapy. Chronic or advanced symptoms can occur at any time after radiotherapy, ranging from weeks to years. Clinical symptoms of radiation-induced mucositis include oral intense pain, odynophagia, dysphagia, anorexia, and difficulty speaking. Signs of radiation-induced mucositis might include oral mucosa hyperemia, erosion and ulceration formation, pseudomembrane covered, easy bleeding, and obvious tenderness. These complications often seriously affect the quality of life and the radiotherapy effect of patients and sometimes can be forced to change the treatment or termination of radiotherapy because it is difficult to tolerate [23, 24].

The treatment of radiation stomatitis is mainly through local therapy to promote erosion healing and anti-infection and relieve pain and dry mouth. Local therapies include aerosol therapy, gargarism rinse, and topical use or hydropathic compress. Medications include: 0.05% compound chlorhexi-dine solution or 0.01% dexamethasone solution, soak or mouthwash, three times a day; 0.1% triamcinolone acetonide dental paste or 0.1% dexamethasone ointment, coat, three times a day; recombinant human epidermal growth factor hydrogel (or spray), recombinant bovine basic fibroblast growth factor gel, or recombinant human acidic fibroblast growth factor spray, once or twice a day; analgesic can chose compound chamomile and lidocaine hydrochloride gel and compound benzocaine gel, or chose 2% lidocaine to rinse after diluting with water. In addition, ultrasonic aerosol therapy is also suggested, medications include dexamethasone sodium phosphate injection, gentamicin sulfate injection, vitamin C injection, and vitamin B12 injection, twice a day. If the aerosol therapy lasts for more than 3 days, it needs to combine with 2–4% sodium bicarbonate solution to rinse and nystatin liniment to topical use, to prevent secondary fungal infection.

3.4 Traumatic Mucosal Hematoma and Traumatic Ulceration

Case 31 Traumatic Mucosal Hematoma

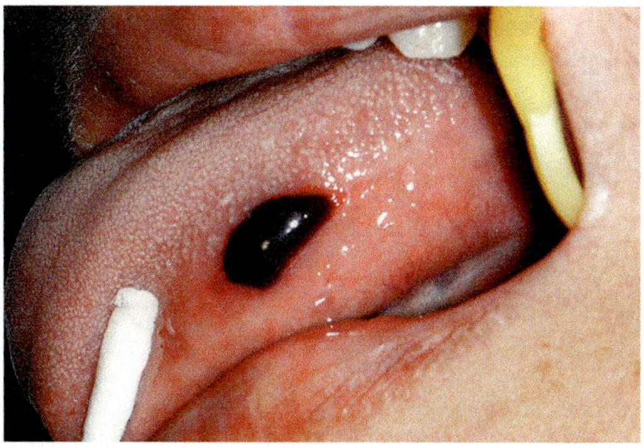

Fig. 3.12 Mucosal hematoma on the left lateral part of the tongue

Age: 66 years
Sex: Female
Chief Complaints:
A 66-year-old woman with a hematoma on the left lateral part of the tongue for 1 day
History of Present Illness:
A 66-year-old woman presented to our clinic with a hematoma on the left lateral part of the tongue for 1 day. One day before, the hematoma soon occurred just after she accidentally bit her left lateral part of tongue when she was eating. The hematoma caused pain, and its size was like a broad bean. The patient suffered from hypothyroidism, hypertension, hyperlipidemia, and hypercholesterolemia (Fig. 3.12).
Past Medical History: None
Allergy: None
Physical Examination:
A dark purple hematoma was on the left lateral part of the tongue. The size was about 3 mm × 10 mm. The lingual margins of D5, D6, and D7 were sharp.
Laboratories and Imaging Studies:
Normal blood routine and coagulation function
Diagnosis:
Traumatic mucosal hematoma
Diagnosis Basis:

1. The history of bite.
2. The lingual margins of nearby teeth were sharp.

Management:

1. Grinding lingual margins of D3, D4, and D5
2. Medication
   Rp.: Compound chlorhexidine solution 300 ml × 1
   Sig.: rinse t.i.d.
   Zhongtong'an capsules 0.28 g × 48
   Sig.: 0.56 g p.o. t.i.d.
   Dexamethasone paste 15 g × 1
   Sig.: topical use after rupture of the hematoma t.i.d.

Case 32 Traumatic Ulcer (After Rupture of the Hematoma)

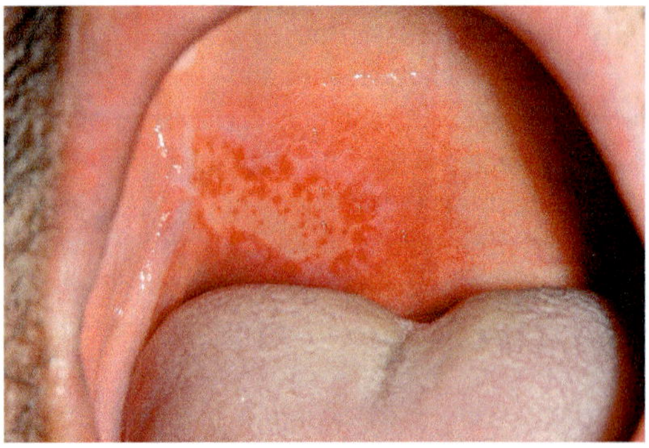

Fig. 3.13 Localized erosion on the posterior right soft palate covered with yellowish-white pseudomembrane and margined by a few white striae

Age: 64 years
Sex: Male
Chief Complaints:
A 64-year-old man with an ulcer on the soft palate for 5 days
History of Present Illness:
A 64-year-old man presented to our clinic with an ulcer on the soft palate for 5 days. Five days ago, a hematoma occurred on the soft palate when he was eating hot food. After that, the hematoma soon ruptured, and an ulcer formed accompanied by acute pain. He checked his blood routine in the local hospital, and it turned out normal. He went on intravenous infusion with unknown drugs for 2 days. After that, he took an unknown anti-inflammatory drug and metronidazole by himself. The infusion treatment and the drugs both failed to relieve the symptom.
Past Medical History: None
Allergy: None
Physical Examination:
A large area of erosion on the soft palate was detected with irregular shape covered with yellowish-white pseudomembrane and margined by a few white striae (Fig. 3.13).

Diagnosis:
Traumatic ulcer (after rupture of the hematoma)
Diagnosis Basis:

1. The history of scald.
2. After the scald on the soft palate, a hematoma occurred.

Management:

1. Medication
   Rp.: Compound chlorhexidine solution 300 ml × 1
   Sig.: rinse t.i.d.
   Zhongtong'an capsules 0.28 g × 48
   Sig.: 0.56 g p.o. t.i.d.
   Dexamethasone paste 15 g × 1
   Sig.: topical use t.i.d.
   Recombinant human epidermal growth factor spray 15 ml × 1
   Sig.: topical use t.i.d.
2. Aerosol therapy
   Rp.: Dexamethasone sodium phosphate injection 1 ml × 1
   Gentamicin sulfate injection 2 ml × 1
   Vitamin B12 injection 1 ml × 1
   Vitamin C injection 2.5 ml × 1
   Sig.: aerosol therapy b.i.d.

Case 33 Traumatic Ulcer (Decubital Ulcer)

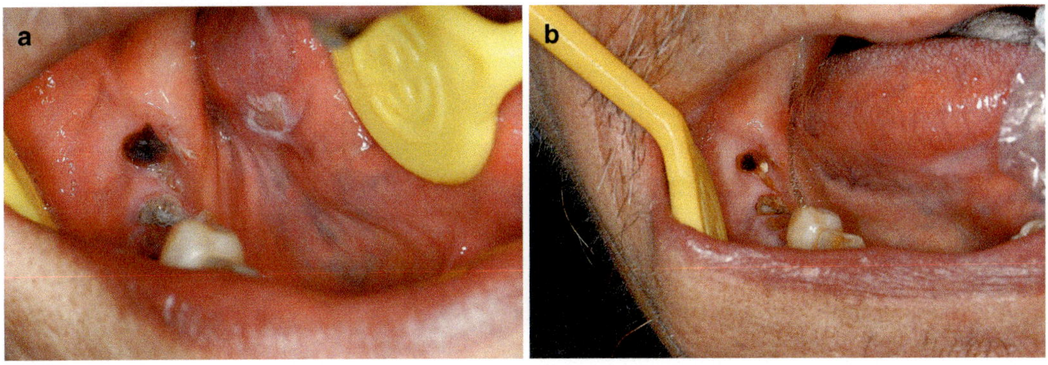

Fig. 3.14 (**a**) Residual roots of C5, C6, and C7 with sharp edges. An ulcer on nearby ventrum of the tongue with white margins. (**b**) Sharp edges of residual roots were removed, and after a week, the patient returned with the ulcer healed

Age: 68 years
Sex: Male
Chief Complaints:
A 68-year-old man with an ulcer on the tongue for 20 days
History of Present Illness:
A 68-year-old man presented to our clinic with an ulcer on the tongue for 20 days. Twenty days ago, an ulcer occurred on the right part of the tongue. The ulcer caused severe pain, and different kinds of unknown drugs which are applied by the patient were useless.
Past Medical History: None
Allergy: None
Physical Examination:
An ulcer with 4 mm × 5 mm in size was observed on the posterior ventrum of the tongue covered with white pseudomembrane. The ulcer is tough when touched. The edges of the residual roots of C5, C6, and C7 were sharp (Fig. 3.14).
Diagnosis:
Traumatic ulcer (decubital ulcer)
Diagnosis Basis:

1. The ulcer occurs in the elderly.
2. The residual roots near the ulcer had sharp edges.

Management:

1. Extract the residual roots of C5, C6, and C7 as soon as possible. (If the teeth cannot be extracted immediately, the teeth can be grinded to remove the sharp edges.) The patient chose to grind the teeth first.

2. Medication
   Rp.: Compound chlorhexidine solution 300 ml × 1
   Sig.: rinse t.i.d.
   Dexamethasone paste 15 g × 1
   Sig.: topical use t.i.d.
3. The patient is advised to return to clinic after a week, and excision biopsy is needed if necessary.

Case 34 Traumatic Ulcer (Bednar Ulcer)

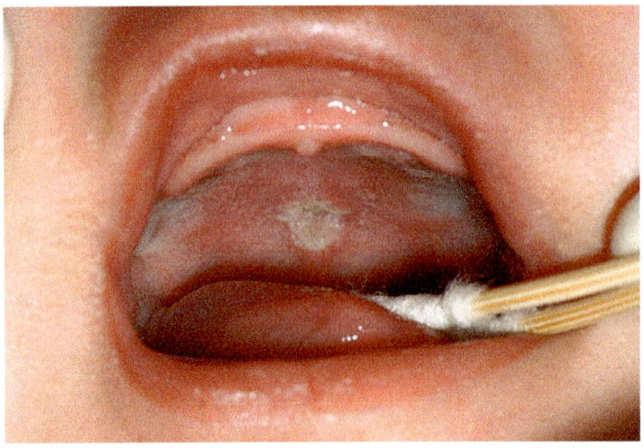

Fig. 3.15 An ulcer on the posterior palate, covered with white pseudomembrane

Age: 70 days
Sex: Male
Chief Complaints:
A 70-day-old boy with an ulcer on the hard palate for 2 weeks
History of Present Illness:
A 70-day-old boy presented to our clinic with an ulcer on the hard palate for 2 weeks. Two weeks ago, his parents found an ulcer on his hard palate which became larger gradually. The boy cried a lot and was bottle-fed.
Past Medical History: None
Allergy: None
Physical Examination:
A 5 mm × 10 mm ulcer was detected on the medial posterior hard palate, covered with white pseudomembrane (Fig. 3.15).
Diagnosis:
Traumatic ulcer (Bednar ulcer)
Diagnosis Basis:

1. The ulcer happened to a baby on his palate.
2. His feeding pattern was bottle-feeding.

Management:

1. Medication
   Rp.: Compound ulcer paste 15 g × 1
   Sig.: topical use t.i.d.
   Recombinant human epidermal growth factor hydrogel 20 g × 1
   Sig.: topical use q.d.
2. His parents were advised to use a softer pacifier and adjust their posture when feeding.

Case 35 Traumatic Ulcer (Rida-Fede Ulcer)

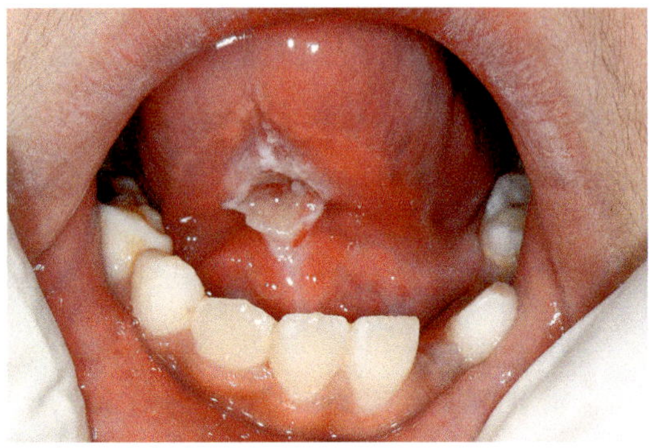

Fig. 3.16 A deep ulcer on the lingual frenum with whitish margin

Age: 8 years
Sex: Male
Chief Complaints:
An 8-year-old boy with an ulcer under the tongue for 20 days
History of Present Illness:
An 8-year-old boy presented to our clinic with an ulcer under the tongue for 20 days. Twenty days ago, an ulcer occurred under his tongue under no obvious predisposing causes. It became larger and deeper gradually and caused a lot of pain.
Past Medical History: None
Allergy: None
Physical Examination:
A deep ulcer was seen on the lingual frenum and ventrum of the tongue whose size was 7 mm × 5 mm. It was sunken and coated with white pseudomembrane. The ulcer is tough when touched. No obvious congestion was seen on the surrounding soft tissue. The incisal ridge of man-

dibular bilateral central incisors was sharp, and the lingual frenum was short (Fig. 3.16).

Diagnosis:

Traumatic ulcer (Riga-Fede ulcer)

Diagnosis Basis:

1. The ulcer happened to a child on his lingual frenum.
2. The lingual frenum was short, and the incisal ridge of the opposite newly erupted incisors was sharp.

Management:

1. Grind C1 and D1 to remove the sharp edges.
2. Medication

   Rp.: Compound chlorhexidine solution 300 ml × 1

   Sig.: topical rinse t.i.d.

   Dexamethasone paste 15 g × 1

   Sig.: topical use t.i.d.

   Recombinant human epidermal growth factor hydrogel 20 g × 1

   Sig.: topical use q.d.

Case 36 Traumatic Ulcer (Factitial Ulcer)

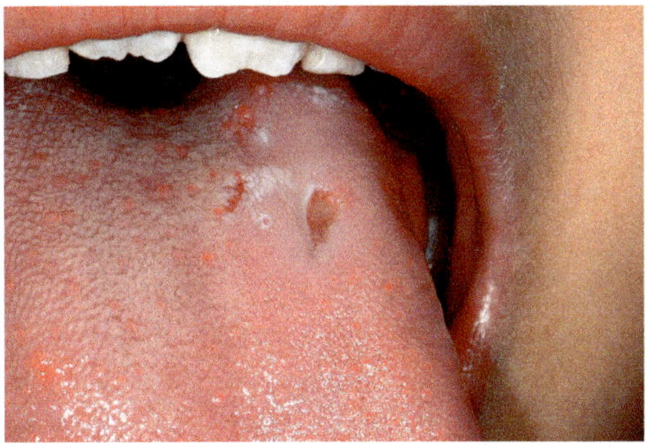

Fig. 3.17 An ulcer on the posterior left dorsum of the tongue with nearby mucosa whitened

Age: 8 years

Sex: Male

Chief Complaints:

An 8-year-old boy with a sore tongue for 20 days

History of Present Illness:

An 8-year-old boy presented to our clinic with a sore tongue for 20 days. Twenty days ago, the boy scratched the dorsum of his tongue repeatedly because of the itchy tongue. After that his tongue began to ache. Medication from other hospital which was unknown was ineffective.

Past Medical History: None

Allergy: None

Physical Examination:

A 3 mm × 5 mm ulcer was seen on the left dorsum of the tongue. It was sunken and coated with yellow pseudomembrane. The ulcer is tough when touched, and its nearby mucosa was whitened (Fig. 3.17).

Diagnosis:

Traumatic ulcer (factitial ulcer)

Diagnosis Basis:

1. The ulcer occurred in an active little boy.
2. The history of self-injury where matched up with the location of the ulcer.

Management:

1. Medication

   Rp.: Dexamethasone paste 15 g × 1

   Sig.: topical use t.i.d.

   Recombinant human epidermal growth factor hydrogel 20 g × 1

   Sig.: topical use q.d.
2. The patient was advised not to scratch his tongue.

[Review] Traumatic Mucosal Hematoma and Traumatic Ulceration

Traumatic mucosal hematoma refers to hematoma which occurs on oral mucosa when eating hot food, masticating large dry or solid food, swallowing too fast, or biting oneself. It is also called mucosal hematoma.

Hematomas caused by swallowing too fast usually happen on the border of hard palate and soft palate. The hematoma soon becomes larger, leading to foreign body sensation. The pain is not obvious. At first the fluid is scarlet. Soon after, it turns into dark purple. The wall of hematoma is thin and tends to rupture. After the hematoma ruptures, a scarlet wound surface is left, forming erosion or ulceration. The pain of the ulcer is obvious, which affects swallowing.

Hematomas caused by bites often happen on the buccal mucosa near the corner of the mouth and occlusion line. They also tend to happen on the lateral part of the tongue. The edges of corresponding teeth are usually sharp. After the hematoma ruptures, an erosion or ulcer forms, and it will soon heal.

Traumatic mucosal hematoma should be distinguished from mucosal hematoma caused by idiopathic thrombocytopenic purpura. Hematoma caused by ITP is usually multiple. Patients with hematomas caused by ITP do not have obvious history of eating too fast. Blood routine often shows extremely low level of blood platelet, and coagulation function test is often abnormal [2]. Besides ITP, traumatic mucosal hematoma should be distinguished from mucosal hematoma caused by blood system diseases like hemophilia.

Under the premise of ruling out blood system diseases, for large unruptured hematomas, we could use sterilized syringes to suck out blood or cut the wall of hematoma to let out blood. For small ones, no treatment is required. For those ruptured hematomas, we could use sterilized surgical scissors to trim the residual wall of the hematoma and then proceed to topical treatment of ulcer. 0.05% chlorhexidine solution or 0.01% dexamethasone solution can be used to rinse the ulcer three times a day. Recombinant human epidermal growth factor hydrogel or spray can also be applied to the ulcer once a day. 0.1% triamcinolone acetonide oral paste or 0.1% dexamethasone ointment is suggested three times a day. To relieve pain, compound chamomile and lidocaine hydrochloride gel are recommended. Besides, if the wound surface is quite large after the hematoma ruptures, aerosol therapy is advised which includes dexamethasone sodium phosphate injection, gentamicin sulfate injection, vitamin C injection, and vitamin B12 injection (one each).

Traumatic ulceration is a series of mucosal lesions which are caused by physical, mechanical, or chemical stimulus. According to different traumatic stimulus, traumatic ulceration is divided into these types:

1. **Decubital Ulcer:** Decubital ulcer usually happens to the elderly. It is caused by chronic stimulation by residual root or crown and the bad prosthesis. It can also be caused by chronic stimulation by massive calculus on the lingual side of mandibular anterior teeth. The ulcer usually reaches submucosal layer. The margin of the ulcer is slightly swollen, and the color is pale. It is often accompanied by pain [25].
2. **Bednar Ulcer:** Bednar ulcer which is caused by sucking thumbs or hard pacifiers often happens to infants. It usually occurs on the hard palate or mucosa near pterygoid hamulus. If it happens bilaterally, the lesion often is symmetrically distributed. The ulcer is superficial. The infant usually cries a lot and refuses to eat.
3. **Riga-Fede Ulcer:** Riga-Fede ulcer refers to ulcers which happen to children on the lingual frenum. It is caused by longtime friction between short lingual frenum and sharp newly erupted central incisors. Congestion, swelling, and ulceration can be seen on the lingual frenum. The longtime unhealed ulcer tends to transform into granulomatous ulcer, which often toughens when touched [26] (Fig. 3.18).
4. **Factitial Ulcer:** Factitial ulcer refers to the ulcer which is caused by bad habits including biting lips or buccal mucosa and using sharp objects like pencils or chopsticks to stab buccal mucosa. It appears mostly in active children or children suffering from attention

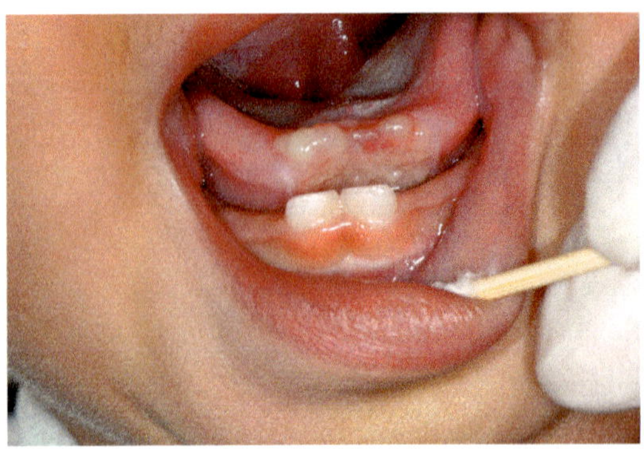

Fig. 3.18 Riga-Fede ulcer on the child's ventral tongue

deficit hyperactivity disorder. The ulcer is usually deep. The longtime unhealed ones have slightly tough base or granulation tissue. The pain is often not obvious, and sometimes, it is accompanied by itchiness.

5. **Chemically Burnt Ulcer:** It is usually caused by chemical stimulus including taking strong acid or alkali by mistake, iodophenol overflowing into the mouth during dental treatment, taking aspirin or alcohol, and applying propolis due to toothache. On the surface of the ulcer, there are usually pieces of fragile membrane. The ulcer is often superficial, and the pain is obvious.
6. **Thermally Burnt Ulcer:** It is usually caused by drinking hot water or drinks. It mostly manifests as large scale of erosion or superficial ulceration with sharp pain.

Ulcers caused by chemical or thermal burns of wide range can also be diagnosed as primary contact stomatitis.

Traumatic ulceration is easily diagnosed according to definite cause and history of disease. Usually the location and the shape of ulcer correspond to the stimulating factor. And there is no recurrent history. After removing the stimulus, the ulcer will soon improve or heal.

The priority of the treatment of traumatic ulceration is removing the stimulus, which includes extracting the residual root or crown, grinding or using composite resin to cover the sharp cusp or marginal ridge, modifying the bad prosthesis, as well as correcting bad habits like biting lips or buccal mucosa. For Bednar ulcer, the feeding pattern of the infant should be changed. Softer pacifiers, little spoon instead of bottle-feeding, and pacifiers with larger holes will all help improve the ulcer. For Riga-Fede ulcer, besides changing feeding pattern into spoon-feeding, ankylotomy is another option to correct short lingual frenulum. When the lesion is quite severe and the conventional treatment is ineffective, extraction of the incisors or excision of the ulcer could be used.

After removing the stimulating factor, there are several drugs as alternatives for topical treatment. 0.05% chlorhexidine solution or 0.01% dexamethasone solution can be used to rinse the ulcer three times a day. Compound ulcer paste could be applied, three times per day. Recombinant human epidermal growth factor hydrogel or spray can also be applied to the ulcer once a day. (If the ulcer tends to cancerate, it must be used with caution.) 0.1% triamcinolone acetonide oral paste and 0.1% dexamethasone ointment or prednisolone acetate injection and triamcinolone acetonide injection (in 1:5 dilution level) are suggested three times a day. Steroid preparations must be used with caution when treating children below the age of 6. But if the condition of the patient is rather severe, steroid preparations can be topically used as appropriate. To relieve pain, compound chamomile and lidocaine hydrochloride gel or compound benzocaine gel is recommended. After a series of therapies mentioned above, if the ulcer is deep and large and longtime unhealed, especially those that happened to the elderly, biopsy should be taken into consideration to rule out the possibility of cancerization.

3.5 Necrotizing Sialometaplasia

Case 37 Necrotizing Sialometaplasia

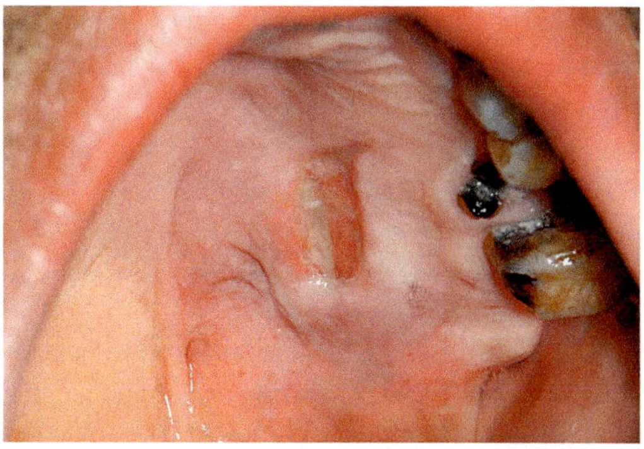

Fig. 3.19 Oral ulcer on the left side of the hard palate with well-defined borders and raised margins

Age: 70 years
Sex: Male
Chief Complaint:
A burning sensation on the palate for 10 days

History of Present Illness:
A 70-year-old male presented to our hospital with a burning sensation on the palate of 10 days' duration, accompanied by numbness and slightly pain when eating. An ulcer was discovered by self-checking. Blood test performed at a local hospital was normal. Taking amoxicillin and metronidazole did not work. He complained of fever and sweating at night.
Past Medical History: None
Allergy: None
Physical Examination:
A 1 cm × 0.5 cm oral ulcer was located on the left side of the hard palate with distinct borders and raised margins. Adjacent mucosa manifested no congestion. The base of ulcer was flat covered with a little yellow pseudomembrane (Fig. 3.19).
Clinical Impression: Ulcer of palate to be diagnosed
Management and Further Examination:

1. Medication
   Rp.: Dexamethasone paste 15 g × 1
   Sig.: topical use t.i.d.
2. Chest X-ray: No obvious anomalies.
3. After 1 week of treatment, the condition was not significantly improved. A biopsy was performed, and results showed necrotizing sialometaplasia.

Diagnosis:
Necrotizing sialometaplasia
Diagnosis Basis:

1. Ulcer on the palate.
2. The diagnosis was confirmed by biopsy.

Management:
NSM is self-limiting and usually requires only supportive treatment, including oral hygiene control and local antiseptics. The palatal ulcer healed spontaneously 4 weeks without complications after the biopsy. A 12-month follow-up of the patient demonstrated no recurrence.

[Review] Necrotizing Sialometaplasia
Necrotizing sialometaplasia (NSM) is a benign, self-healing lesion of salivary glands. The proposed pathological changes of NSM are ischemic circulation of the minor salivary gland and adjacent tissues by a necrotizing inflammatory response [27].

The most commonly proposed and generally accepted etiology for NSM relates to ischemia. It is caused mainly by traumatic injuries, such as accidental injury of maxillary teeth extraction, trachea after intubation, denture wear, injecting a local anesthetic, alcohol and tobacco use, and cocaine abuse. Respiratory infections and secondary atheromatous embolization have been implicated as potential predisposing factors [27, 28]. An emerging associated etiology is that seen in the setting of bulimia, which mainly affects young adult females. Bulimia is characterized by recurrent episodes of binge eating, followed by compensatory behaviors, including self-induced vomiting by a mechanical gag reflex, excessive exercise, and misuse of laxatives and enemas. Bulimic patients will often use their fingers to mechanically induce vomiting. Therefore, there may be a combination of mechanical and chemical factors affecting these patients. The low pH of the gastric contents contacting the oral mucosa is suggested as a major etiologic factor. The clinical scenario of normal body weight or lighter weight in an adolescent or young adult patient with clinical signs of bulimia should greatly increase suspicion for NS [29, 30].

The incidence appears higher in male patients [30], with a male-to-female ratio of approximately 2:1 [31], and particularly is increased in men older than 40 years. The lesion can be found in salivary glands and at other sites that contain salivary glands. It commonly occurs as a deep single ulcer on the unilateral posterior hard palate or at the junction of the hard and soft palates. The lesion also can be found at other sites such as the tongue, nasal cavity, larynx, maxillary sinus, and tonsil [32, 33]. The disease manifests as a deep-seated ulcer, measuring on average 1–3 cm in its major diameter. The ulcer borders are often erythematous and may be raised. Bony involvement is not generally described or to be expected in NSM. Pain and rapid progression are almost universal features, with pain often described as sharp, and it often precedes mucosal changes. Necrotizing sialometaplasia resolves spontaneously, and the lesion heals by secondary intention within 3–12 weeks [33]. However, a number of cases manifested as a fluctuant mass on the palate. A biopsy was performed, and the diagnosis of NSM was rendered; no further treatment was performed, and the lesion healed completely [34, 35].

Histopathological examination is necessary for the diagnosis of necrotizing sialometaplasia, because the clinical features of this condition can mimic other malignant diseases, particularly squamous cell carcinoma. Histopathological features of NSM include pseudoepitheliomatous hyperplasia of the overlying epithelium; the squamous metaplasia of minor salivary gland ducts and acini may contain apoptotic cells and areas of inflammation as well as mucin spillage. The preservation of the normal lobular architecture of the salivary glands is a key feature [27]. While there is no definitive immunophenotype, a properly oriented HE section remains the gold standard for diagnosis. But a study shows Ki-67, p53 down-expression [36], and calponin overexpression [37] in NSM compared with squamous cell carcinoma. It has been suggested that using the pattern of cytokeratin expression, p53, calponin may aid in the differentiation of NS from its mimics. The patient of case 37 underwent fever and sweating at night, so in symptomatic treatment to observe the curative effect of 1 week suggest that patients with chest X-ray, to eliminate TB.

NSM is self-limiting and usually requires only supportive treatment, including pain control and local antiseptics. Necrotizing sialometaplasia does not usually recur. Overtreatment such as surgical excision is avoided. Although there is usually no need for surgery in treatment of NSM, rare cases may reach significantly large sizes. In these cases, surgical debridement should be considered as a viable treatment option, providing better conditions for healing as well as decreasing the risk of sepsis [33]. But when NSM and malignant neoplasm (e.g., adenoid cystic carcinoma) coexist, the situation is more complicated [38]. To confirm the range of biopsy and accepting parts become extremely critical. The doctors should choose standard biopsy site and prevent misdiagnosis of malignant lesions and excessive treatment such as the expanded resection of NSM lesions at the same time. Rely mainly on intraoperative frozen section examination at this moment, and pay attention to regular follow-up observation.

References

1. Akintoye SO, Greenberg MS. Recurrent aphthous stomatitis. Dent Clin North Am. 2015;49(1):31–47, vii-vii.
2. Sawair FA. Recurrent aphthous stomatitis: do we know what patients are using to treat the ulcers. J Altern Complement Med. 2010;16(6):651–5.
3. Lewkowicz N, Lewkowicz P, Banasik M, et al. Predominance of type 1 cytokines and decreased number of CD4+CD25+ high T regulatory cells in peripheral blood of patients with recurrent aphthous ulcerations. Immunol Lett. 2005;99(1):57–62.
4. Femiano F, Lanza A, Buonaiuto C, et al. Guidelines for diagnosis and management of aphthous stomatitis. Pediatr Infect Dis J. 2007;26(8):728–32.
5. Messadi DV, Younai F. Aphthous ulcers. Dermatol Ther. 2010;23(3):281–90.
6. Baccaglini L, Lalla R, Bruce A, et al. Urban legends series: recurrent aphthous stomatitis. Oral Dis. 2011;17(8):755–70.
7. Chattopadhyay A, Chatterjee S. Risk indicators for recurrent aphthous ulcers among adults in the US. Community Dent Oral Epidemiol. 2007;35(2):152–9.
8. Rogers RS 3rd. Recurrent aphthous stomatitis: clinical characteristics and associated systemic disorders. Semin Cutan Med Surg. 1997;16(4):278–83.
9. Yazici Y, Yurdakul S, Yazici H. Behcet's syndrome. Curr Rheumatol Rep. 2010;12(6):429–35.
10. Yurdakul S, Hamuryudan V, Fresko I, et al. Behcet's syndrome. In: Hochberg MC, Silman AJ, Smolen YS, et al., editors. Rheumatology. 4th ed. Philadelphia, PA: Mosby Elsevier; 2008. p. 1561–5.
11. Verity DH, Marr JE, Ohno S, et al. Behcet's disease, the Silk Road and HLA-B51: historical and geographical perspectives. Tissue Antigens. 1999;54(3):213–20.
12. Gul A. Behcet's disease as an autoinflammatory disorder. Curr Drug Targets Inflamm Allergy. 2005;4(1):81–3.
13. Dalvi SR, Yildirim R, Yazici Y. Behcet's syndrome. Drugs. 2012;72(17):2223–41.
14. Gul A. Behcet's disease: an update on the pathogenesis. Clin Exp Rheumatol. 2001;19(5 Suppl 24):S6–12.
15. Mat MC, Goksugur N, Engin B, et al. The frequency of scarring after genital ulcers in Behcet's syndrome: a prospective study. Int J Dermatol. 2006;45(5):554–6.
16. Tugal-Tutkun I, Onal S, Altan-Yaycioglu R, et al. Uveitis in Behcet disease: an analysis of 880 patients. Am J Ophthalmol. 2004;138(3):373–80.

17. Feller L, Essop R, Wood NH, et al. Chemotherapy- and radiotherapy-induced oral mucositis: pathobiology, epidemiology and management. SADJ. 2010;65(8):372–4.
18. Herrestedt J. Prevention and management of mucositis in patients with cancer. Int J Antimicrob Agents. 2000;16(2):161–3.
19. Raber-Durlacher JE, Elad S, Barasch A. Oral mucositis. Oral Oncol. 2010;46(6):452–6.
20. Scardina GA, Pisano T, Messina P. Oral mucositis. Review of literature. N Y State Dent J. 2010;76(1):34–8.
21. Sciubba JJ, Glodenberg D. Oral complications of radiotherapy. Lancer Oncol. 2006;7(2):175–83.
22. Scully C, Epstein J, Sonis S. Oral mucositis. Head Neck. 2003;25(12):1057–70.
23. Napenas JJ, Shetty KV, Streckfus CF. Oral mucositis: review of pathogenesis, diagnosis, prevention, and management. Gen Dent. 2007;55(4):335–44; quiz 345-346, 376.
24. Wong PC, Dodd MJ, Miaskowski C, et al. Mucositis pain induced by radiation therapy: prevalence, severity, and use of self-care behaviors. J Pain Symptom Manage. 2006;32(1):27–37.
25. Santangelo A, Testai M, Ossino MC, et al. Management and treatment of decubital ulcers of an elderly population in the assisted sanitary residence of Futura-Viagrande (Catania, Sicily, Italy). Arch Gerontol Geriatr. 2009;48(3):332–4.
26. van der Meij EH, de Vries TW, Eggink HF, et al. Traumatic lingual ulceration in a newborn: Riga-Fede disease. Ital J Pediatr. 2012;38:20.
27. Carlson DL. Necrotizing sialometaplasia: a practical approach to the diagnosis. Arch Pathol Lab Med. 2009;133(5):692–8.
28. Fava M, Cherubini K, Yurgel L, et al. Necrotizing sialometaplasia of the palate in a cocaine-using patient. A case report. Minerva Stomatol. 2008;57(4):199–202.
29. Imai T, Michizawa M. Necrotizing sialometaplasia in a patient with an eating disorder: palatal ulcer accompanied by dental erosion due to binge-purging. J Oral Maxillofac Surg. 2013;71(5):879–85.
30. Solomon LW, Merzianu M, Sullivan M, et al. Necrotizing sialometaplasia associated with bulimia: case report and literature review. Oral Surg Oral Med Oral Pathol Oral Radiol Endod. 2007;103(2):e39–42.
31. Penner CR, Thompson LD. Necrotizing sialometaplasia. Ear Nose Throat J. 2003;82(7):493–4.
32. Randhawa T, Varghese I, Shameena P, et al. Necrotizing sialometaplasia of tongue. J Oral Maxillofac Pathol. 2009;13(1):35–7.
33. Kaplan I, Alterman M, Kleinman S, et al. The clinical, histologic, and treatment spectrum in necrotizing sialometaplasia. Oral Surg Oral Med Oral Pathol Oral Radiol. 2012;114(5):577–85.
34. Oliveira AMG, Kitakawa D, Carvalho YR, et al. Necrotizing sialometaplasia as a cause of a non-ulcerated nodule in the hard palate: a case report. J Med Case Rep. 2011;5:406.
35. Brannon RB, Fowler CB, Hartman KS. Necrotizing sialometaplasia. A clinicopathologic study of sixty-nine cases and review of the literature. Oral Surg Oral Med Oral Pathol. 1991;72(3):317–25.
36. Dadfarnia T, Mohammed BS, Eltorky MA. Significance of Ki-67 and p 53 immunoexpression in the differential diagnosis of oral necrotizing sialometaplasia and squamous cell carcinoma. Ann Diagn Pathol. 2012;16(3):171–6.
37. Rizkalla H, Toner M. Necrotizing sialometaplasia versus invasive carcinoma of the head and neck: the use of myoepithelial markers and keratin subtypes as an adjunct to diagnosis. Histopathology. 2007;51(2):184–9.
38. Lee DJ, Ahn HK, Koh ES, et al. Necrotizing sialometaplasia accompanied by adenoid cystic carcinoma on the soft palate. Clin Exp Otorhinolaryngol. 2009;2(1):48–51.

Bullous Oral Mucosal Diseases

4

Xin Jin, Xin Zeng, and Wei Li

Keywords
Pemphigus · Pemphigus Vulgaris · Benign Mucous Membrane Pemphigoid · Paraneoplastic Pemphigus · Linear IgA Disease

X. Jin
College of Stomatology, Chongqing Medical University, Chongqing Key Laboratory of Oral Diseases and Biomedical Sciences, Chongqing, China

X. Zeng (✉)
State Key Laboratory of Oral Diseases, National Clinical Research Center for Oral Diseases, Department of Oral Medicine, West China Hospital of Stomatology, Sichuan University, Chengdu, Sichuan, China

W. Li
Department of Dermatology, West China Hospital, Sichuan University, Chengdu, Sichuan, China

Q. Chen, X. Zeng (eds.), *Case Based Oral Mucosal Diseases*,
https://doi.org/10.1007/978-981-13-0286-2_4

4.1 Pemphigus

Case 38 Pemphigus Vulgaris (Involving the Skin and Oral Mucosa)

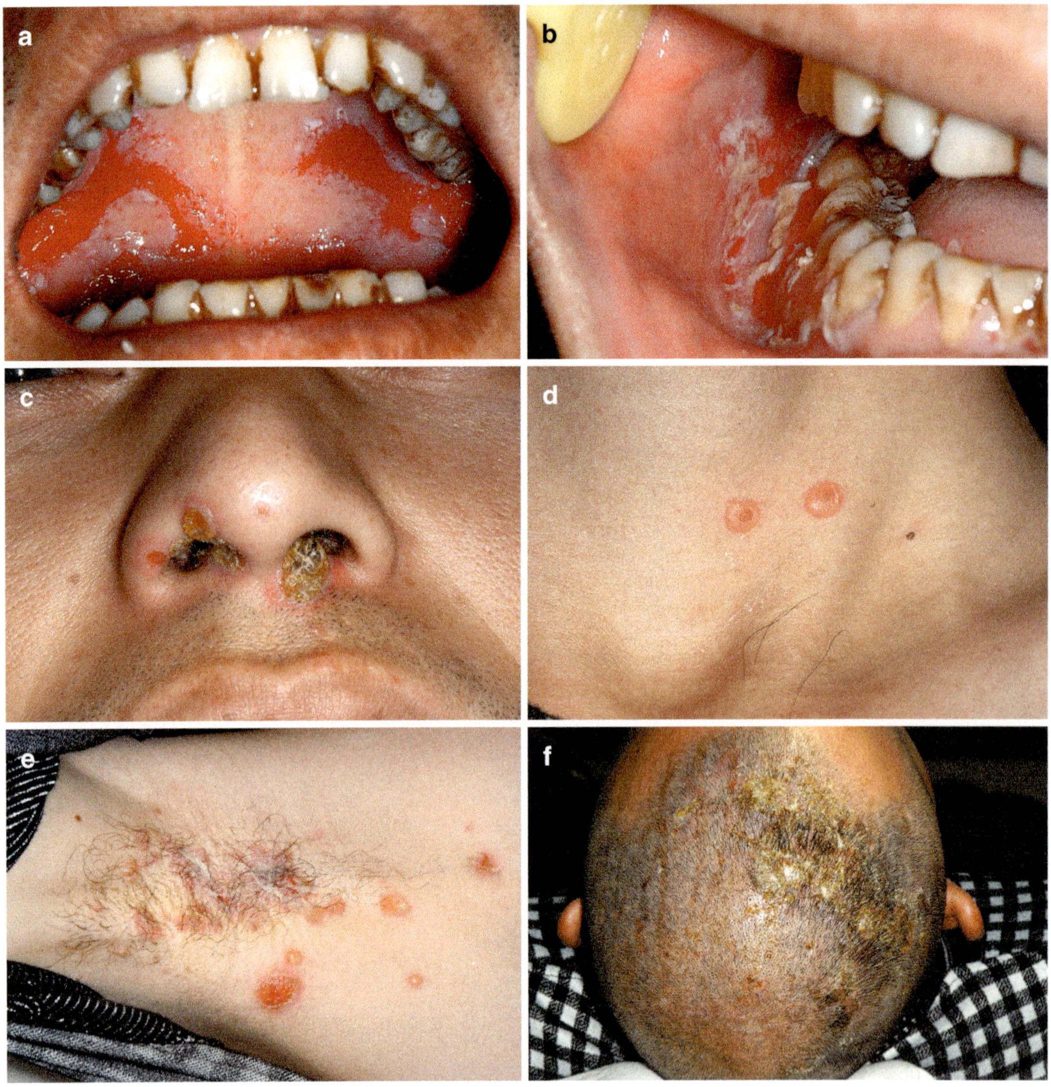

Fig. 4.1 (**a**) Extensive, irregular, and well-defined erosions on the soft palate bilaterally, with a red, clean surface. (**b**) Erosions distributed on the right posterior mandibular buccal gingiva and the nearby buccal mucosa covered by yellowish pseudomembrane. (**c**) Blisters, erosions, and crusts on the nasal skin and mucosa. (**d**) Blisters on the neck. (**e**) Blisters and erosions on the right axilla. (**f**) Erosions and crusts on the scalp

Age: 34 years
Sex: Male
Chief Complaint:
Blisters and bullae on the palate for 3 months
History of Present Illness:
The patient complained that mucosal blisters and bullae appeared on his palate without obvious predisposing causes 3 months ago. Subsequent to the rupture of blister and bullae, painful erosions ensued, which aggravated during eating. He has been diagnosed with fungal stomatitis at a local hospital; however antifungal treatment was ineffective. Ten days ago, blisters appeared on his gingiva, scalp, axillae, and nasal skin. Then the blisters rup-

tured and leave irregularly shaped erosions with a yellowish slough that were refractory.

Past Medical History: None

Allergy: None

Physical Examination:

There were extensive, irregular, and well-defined erosions on the soft palate bilaterally, which had a red, clean surface. No evident inflammatory reaction had been found around the erosions. Multifocal small erosions distributed on the right posterior mandibular buccal gingiva and the nearby buccal mucosa bilaterally, covered by yellowish pseudomembrane which can be removed. Nikolsky's sign was positive. There were blisters, erosions, and crusts on the noses, right axilla, back, neck, and scalp (Fig. 4.1).

Laboratories and Imaging Studies:

1. There was no obvious abnormality in full blood count, blood glucose, and liver and kidney functions.
2. Incisional biopsy of perilesional mucosa which appears normal: Hematoxylin and eosin (HE) staining revealed intraepithelial blister formation which was in accordance with pemphigus vulgaris. Direct immunofluorescence (DIF) microscopy showed the reticular intercellular deposition of IgG and C3.
3. There was no abnormality in chest X-ray and ultrasonography of abdomen.

Diagnosis:

Pemphigus vulgaris

Diagnosis Basis:

1. Chronic onset.
2. Blisters involving skin and mucosa.
3. Characteristics of erosion: (1) clear boundary, (2) irregular shape, (3) clean surface, and (4) no evident inflammatory reaction around the erosions.
4. Positive Nikolsky's sign.
5. The diagnosis was confirmed by HE staining and DIF.

Management:

1. Medication
   Rp.: 2% Sodium bicarbonate solution 250 ml × 1
   Sig.: rinse t.i.d.
   Compound chlorhexidine solution 300 ml × 1
   Sig.: rinse t.i.d.
   Dexamethasone paste 15 g × 1
   Sig.: topical use t.i.d.
2. Aerosol therapy
   Rp.: Dexamethasone sodium phosphate injection 1 ml × 1
   Gentamycin sulfate injection 2 ml × 1
   Vitamin B12 injection 1 ml × 1
   Vitamin C injection 2.5 ml × 1
   Sig.: aerosol therapy b.i.d.
3. The patient was transferred to dermatology department for hospitalization.

Case 39 Pemphigus Vulgaris (Involving the Oral Mucosa Only)

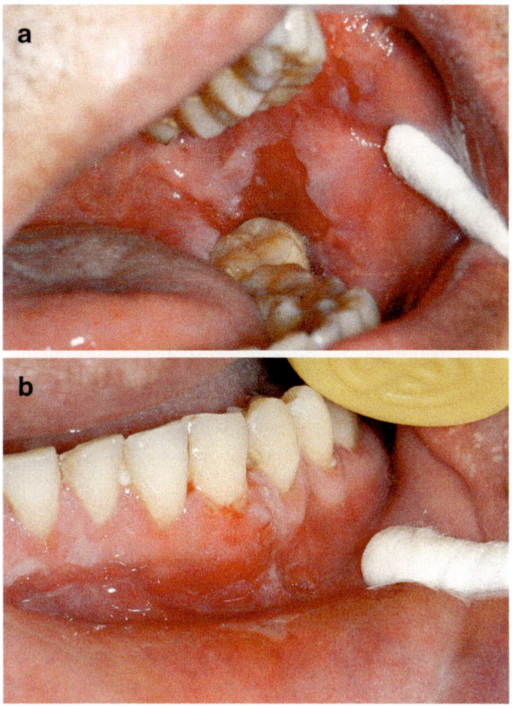

Fig. 4.2 (**a**) Irregular and well-defined erosions involving the left buccal mucosa, with a red, clean surface. (**b**) Irregular erosions covered by pseudomembrane involving the labial mucosa and gingiva

Sex: Male

Age: 41 years

Chief Complaint:

Recurrent oral ulcers for 2 years and ulcers relapsed 1 month ago

History of Present Illness:
He presented to our department with recurrent oral ulcers for 2 years. And he had an episode, every 3–4 months, with one or two ulcers that healed within 10 days. One month ago the condition became worse with multiple ulcers in his mouth which did not heal so far.
Past Medical History: None
Allergy: None
Physical Examination:
Multiple well-defined erosions covered by a few pseudomembranes involved the labial mucosa, left buccal mucosa, ventrum of the tongue, and gingiva, without evident inflammatory reaction around the erosions (Fig. 4.2). Nikolsky's sign was positive. No skin and scalp lesion has been found.
Laboratories and Imaging Studies:

1. There was no obvious abnormality in full blood count, blood glucose, and liver and kidney functions.
2. Incisional biopsy of perilesional mucosa which appears normal: Hematoxylin and eosin (HE) staining revealed intraepithelial blister formation which was in accordance with pemphigus vulgaris. Direct immunofluorescence (DIF) microscopy showed the reticular intercellular deposition of IgG and C3.
3. There was no abnormality in chest X-ray and ultrasonography of abdomen.

Diagnosis:
Pemphigus vulgaris
Diagnosis Basis:

1. Chronic onset.
2. Characteristics of erosion: (1) clear boundary, (2) irregular shape, (3) clean surface, and (4) no evident inflammatory reaction around the erosions.
3. Positive Nikolsky's sign.
4. The diagnosis was confirmed by HE staining and DIF.

Management:

1. Medication
   Rp.: Prednisone acetate 5 mg × 72
   Sig.: 40 mg p.o. q.m. and 20 mg p.o. p.m.
   Calcium carbonate D3 tablets 600 mg × 30
   Sig.: 1tablet p.o. q.d.
   Sucralfate tablets 1 g × 100
   Sig.: 1 g p.o. t.i.d.
   Potassium chloride sustained-release tablets 0.5 g × 24
   Sig.: 0.5 g p.o. b.i.d.
   2% sodium bicarbonate solution 250 ml × 1
   Sig.: rinse t.i.d.
   Compound chlorhexidine solution 300 ml × 1
   Sig.: rinse t.i.d.
   Dexamethasone paste 15 g × 1
   Sig.: topical use t.i.d.
2. Aerosol therapy
   Rp.: Dexamethasone sodium phosphate injection 1 ml × 1
   Gentamycin sulfate injection 2 ml × 1
   Vitamin B12 injection 1 ml × 1
   Vitamin C injection 2.5 ml × 1
   Sig.: aerosol therapy b.i.d.
3. Subsequent visit 1 week later was suggested.

Follow-Up Treatment:
If no new blister is seen 2–4 weeks later after the treatment, the dose of prednisone should be reduced by 10% within 2–4 weeks. If erosions are limited, intralesional injection of mixture of triamcinolone injection and water for injection or 2% lidocaine in the same amount is considered. During the treatment, patients should recheck blood routine, blood glucose, liver and kidney function, and electrolytes one time/1–2 months. If the blister formation and erosions cannot be controlled, the dose of prednisone should be increased, and the patient should be transferred to the department of dermatology.

[Review] Pemphigus
Pemphigus is a group of potentially life-threatening, chronic, and autoimmune disease that is caused by autoantibodies directed against intercellular adhesion substances. The main clinical characteristic is blistering cutaneous and mucosal lesions. Since oral blisters rupture soon after forming, erosive or ulcerated lesions are produced. Oral lesions are most commonly

detected on the buccal mucosa, tongue, and soft palate, while lesions can be seen everywhere of the oral cavity. Pemphigus can be broadly classified into four major types: pemphigus vulgaris, pemphigus vegetans, pemphigus erythematous, and pemphigus foliaceus. The diagnosis of pemphigus requires confirmation by biopsy. The pathologic diagnostic criteria are intraepithelial vesicle formation, acantholysis, and immunological detection of autoantibodies [1].

The etiology of pemphigus vulgaris is unclear. This group of disorders is regarded as autoimmune diseases, due to characteristics of the autoantibodies production against intercellular substances. Desmoglein1 (Dsg1) and desmoglein3 (Dsg3) are desmosomal proteins, which makes the adhesion between epithelial cells. High expression of Dsg3 is presented in the whole epithelial layer of the oral mucosa, while Dsg1 is weakly expressed in all epithelial layers except for the basal cell layer. However, Dsg3 is strongly expressed in the basal and parabasal cell layers within the epidermis, while expression of Dsg1 is observed in all layers of the epidermis. In pemphigus vulgaris, intercellular antibodies are predominantly directed against Dsg3 and less often against Dsg1, leading to the loss of intercellular adhesion of keratinocytes and consequent blister formation. In pemphigus foliaceus, they are predominantly directed against Dsg1 [2]. In some cases, a strong genetic background may be found, such as the Ashkenazi Jews and those of Mediterranean descent [3]. Strong associations with increased expression frequency of some HLA class II alleles have been detected in pemphigus vulgaris. It also may be associated with viral infections. Other stimulating factors reported include garlic foods, infections, and drugs. The thiol group drugs are commonly involved, particularly captopril, penicillamine, and rifampicin [1].

Pemphigus vulgaris is most commonly diagnosed in the forties and fifties, with a male and female prevalence ratio of 1:2. In majority of patients, lesions on the oral mucosa are the initial manifestations, with areas vulnerable to frictional trauma, such as the soft palate, pterygomandibular fold, buccal mucosa, and tongue commonly involved. It is easy to be overlooked and misdiagnosed as herpetic stomatitis or recurrent aphthous ulcer. If the lesions involve the gingiva, doctors may misdiagnose it as exfoliative gingivitis or necrotizing ulcerative gingivitis.

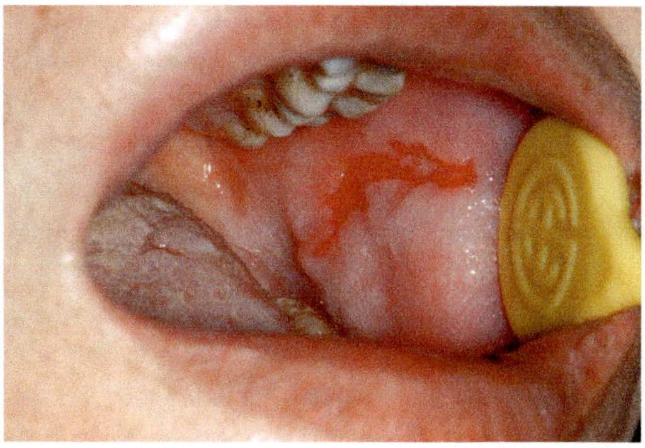

Fig. 4.3 Irregular and well-defined erosions with a red, clean surface involving the left buccal mucosa, without inflamed reaction around the erosions

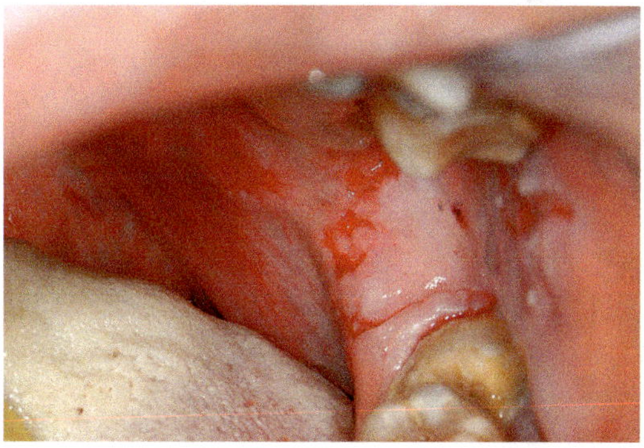

Fig. 4.4 Irregular and well-defined erosions with a red, clean surface involving the left pterygomandibular fold, without inflamed reaction around the erosions

Oral lesions of pemphigus vulgaris appear as small asymptomatic blisters initially. They are thin-walled and easily rupture, then replaced by irregular, sharply outlined, noninfectious erosions with few or without pseudomembrane (Figs. 4.3 and 4.4). Sliding off of the epithelium test is considered to be positive when the epithelium including the blister wall and adjacent mucosa with normal appearance is rubbed off, and then a bright red wound is left. The probe can be inserted painlessly in parallel into the peripheral epithelium of erosions. Nikolsky's sign is elicited by applying tangential pressure with a swab or odontoscope to the normal gingiva.

There is extension of the blister and/or epithelial desquamation in the applied pressure area which is considered positive. Licking of the mucosa can make normal mucosa of normal appearance slough off. All of them are phenomenon of acantholysis which are indicative for primary diagnosis. The final diagnosis is based on examination of HE staining and direct immunofluorescence. Oral lesions have more difficulties in healing than cutaneous lesions. The chronic erosions are usually covered by pseudomembrane. Increased saliva and difficulties in eating and swallowing are the chief complaints. It is worth noting that sometimes the clinical manifestation of pemphigus vulgaris is atypical and easy to be misdiagnosed as recurrent aphthous ulcers. At this point, it is important to examine whether the ulcers are concave or not, which may be indicative of the need for biopsy.

Expect for oral cavity, lesions may affect the sites of conjunctiva, nose, pharynx, larynx, esophagus, and genital. Flaccid bullae are commonly seen in the skin. The flaccid blisters rupture easily and produce red erosions. Slow healing is ordinary state but with no scars [4, 5]. Nikolsky's sign is elicited by tangential pressure with a finger over the normal skin or mucosa. There is extension of the blister and/or removal of epidermis in the applied pressure area which is considered positive. Although the sign is characteristically seen in pemphigus, it can be seen in other diseases, such as pemphigoid in the acute phase and erythema multiform with bullae.

Acantholysis, discontinuous epithelial, and the blisters or cleft formation within the epithelium are the main histological finding. Typical prickle cells, also known as Tzanck cell, can be found by scraping the base of a blister. Both indirect immunofluorescence assays on serum and direct immunofluorescence assays on biopsy tissue show the reticular intercellular deposition of IgG, C3 [6].

Oral cavity is less involved in other types of pemphigus. The oral manifestations of other types of pemphigus were similar to that of pemphigus vulgaris.

Pemphigus vegetans usually affects intertriginous sites such as anogenital and nasolabial mucosa. The papillomatous and verrucous vegetations are commonly formed on the base of blisters. The skin lesions of pemphigus vegetans may resemble exfoliative dermatitis and its prognosis as well. Pemphigus erythematosus resembles cutaneous lupus erythematosus clinically with butterfly lesions on the face.

Glucocorticoids are the first choice for initial treatment. The initial dose of prednisone is identified by the extent and rate of progression of lesions. If lesions are limited to oral mucosa and are not extensive, the single dose of oral prednisone was 40 mg/day at 7:00–8:00 a.m. If oral lesions are extensive, the dose of prednisone was 60–80 mg/day which should be taken twice a day (at 7:00–8:00 a.m. and 2:00–3:00 p.m.). If the condition is controlled, which means that there are no new blisters and existing erosions or ulcers are almost healed, the dose of prednisone should be tapered by 10% reduction of the original dose every 2–4 weeks. And the maintenance dose is 5 mg/day. Patients should not reduce or stop taking glucocorticoids on by themselves.

The long term and high dose of glucocorticoids may induce many adverse effects such as peptic ulcer, diabetes, hypertension, osteoporosis, Cushing's syndrome, a variety of infections, and toxicity of central nervous system. Therefore, regular monitoring of blood pressure, blood glucose, liver and kidney function, fecal occult blood test, electrolyte, etc. are recommended. Adjuvant drugs should be applied properly in order to prevent and mitigate adverse effects. For example, calcium carbonate D3 tablets (one tablet each time, one to two times per day) are used to prevent osteoporosis. To protect gastric mucosa, sucralfate tablets (1 g each time, four times per day) are used. Potassium chloride sustained-release tablets (0.5–1 g each time, one to three times per day) are applied for supplement of potassium according to serum potassium level. Rinsing with 2–4% sodium bicarbonate solution or topical application with nystatin liniment can prevent *Candida albicans* infection.

If the treatment with glucocorticoids is ineffective or the patients have contraindications for glucocorticoids, immunosuppressants can be used as monotherapy or in combination with glucocorticoids, such as azathioprine (1–2 mg/kg/day, to be taken once daily or several times daily) or tripterygium glycosides tablet (1–1.5 mg/kg/day, three times daily).

Topical treatments include antiseptic such as compound chlorhexidine solution; topical glucocorticoids including dexamethasone gargle, dexamethasone paste, triamcinolone acetonide dental paste, and dexamethasone ointment; and antifungal agent such as 2–4% sodium bicarbonate solution and nystatin liniment. Refractory erosions may be treated with intralesional corticosteroid injection (triamcinolone acetonide or compound betamethasone injection mixed with water for injection or 2% lidocaine, multipoint low-dose injection).

For patients with skin lesions and systemic diseases such as diabetes and hypertension, hospitalization in the department of dermatology should be suggested.

4.2 Benign Mucous Membrane Pemphigoid

Case 40 Benign Mucous Membrane Pemphigoid (Bullous Lesion)

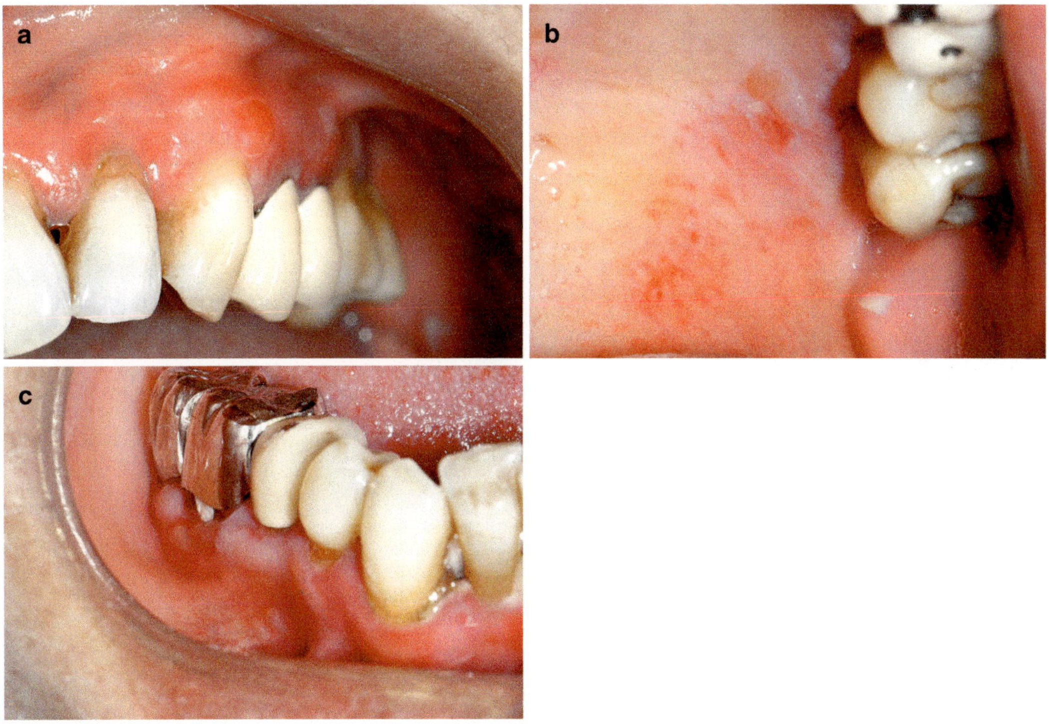

Fig. 4.5 (**a**) Blister and hyperemia on the left maxillary buccal gingiva. (**b**) Blister and erosion on the left maxillary palatal gingiva. (**c**) Erosions on the right mandibular buccal gingiva

Age: 61 years
Sex: Female
Chief Complaints:
Recurrent blisters of the palate and gingiva for 1 month

History of Present Illness:
A 61-year-old female presented to our clinic with recurrent blisters of the palate and gingiva for 1 month. The blisters repeated with an interval of a few days. The erosion was bleeding and painful

after the rupture of blisters, and it could be self-healing. She denied any discomfort of eyes.

Past Medical History: Hepatitis B, cholecystitis, myocardial ischemia, rheumatoid arthritis

Allergy History: Penicillin

Physical Examination:

Multiple small erosions were detected on the marginal gingiva and a blister with the diameter of 4–5 mm on the buccal and palatal side of the maxillary gums, respectively (Fig. 4.5). Nikolsky's sign was negative.

Laboratories and Imaging Studies:

1. There was no obvious abnormality in full blood count, blood glucose, and liver and kidney functions.
2. Hematoxylin and eosin (HE) staining of the gingiva biopsy revealed that stratified squamous epithelium was stripped completely. Direct immunofluorescence (DIF) showed linear deposition of immunoglobulin G and complement C3 along the basement membrane.

Diagnosis:

Benign mucous membrane pemphigoid

Diagnosis Basis:

1. Chronic onset.
2. Vesicles and erosions of gingiva.
3. Nikolsky's sign was negative.
4. The diagnosis was confirmed by HE staining and DIF.

Management:

1. Medication
   Rp.: Tripterygium hypoglaucum tablet 1 g × 100
   Sig.: 2 g p.o. t.i.d.
   Vitamin B6 10 mg × 100 tablets
   Sig.: 5 mg p.o. t.i.d.
   Compound chlorhexidine solution 300 ml × 1
   Sig.: rinse t.i.d.
   Dexamethasone paste 15g × 1
   Sig.: topical use t.i.d.
2. The lesions were dealed with double-diluted triamcinolone acetonide (TA) injection (Sig.: multipoint low-dose intralesional injection st.).
3. Subsequent visit after 2 weeks.

Subsequent Management:

If the lesions have been controlled, the medication for another course of treatment will maintain, and if the control is not reached, prednisone with 20–30 mg/day orally for 7–14 days will be prescribed.

Case 41 Benign Mucous Membrane Pemphigoid (Erosive Lesion)

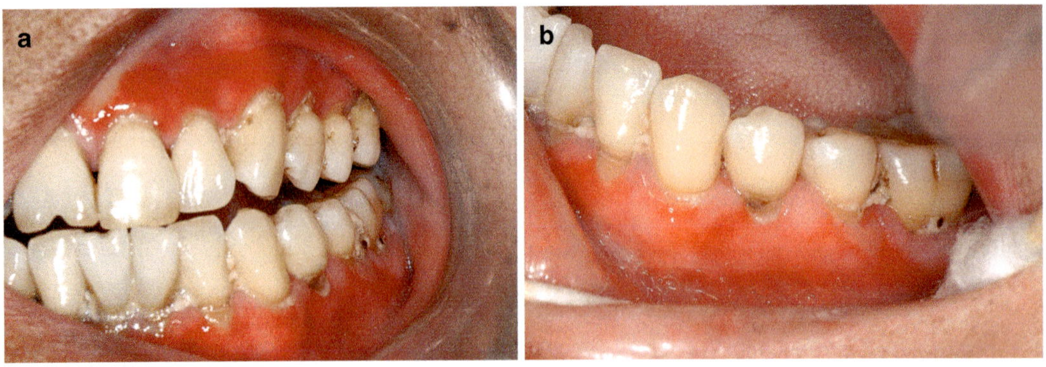

Fig. 4.6 (**a**) Widespread gingival erythema with scattered mung bean size of erosions. (**b**) Erythema with small erosions on the left buccal mandibular gingiva. (**c**) Erythema with small erosions on the right buccal mandibular gingiva. (**d**) Chronic blister and erosion on the posterior soft palate

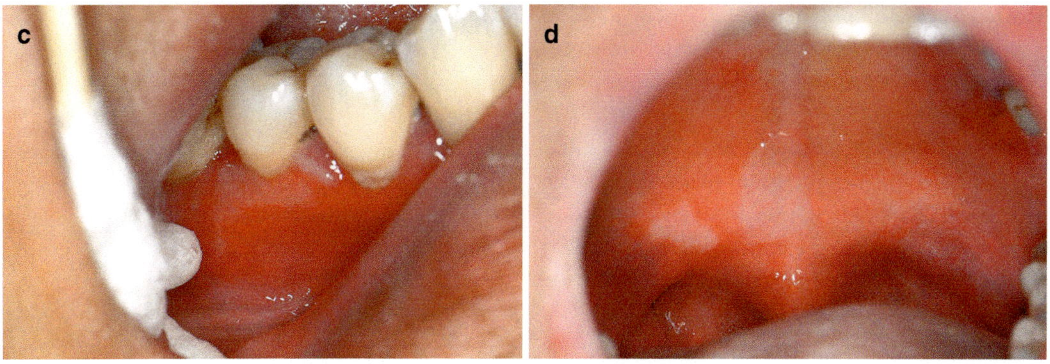

Fig. 4.6 (continued)

Age: 58 years
Sex: Female
Chief Complaints:
Recurrent blood blisters and erosion in the mouth for 1 year
History of Present Illness:
A 58-year-old female presented to our clinic with repeated blood blisters in mouth for 1 year. After the rupture of the blisters, the painful erosions disrupted eating and speaking.
Past Medical History: None
Allergy History: None
Physical Examination:
Widespread gingival erythema was observed with scattered punctiform or mung bean size of erosions. The chronic blister (10 mm × 5 mm) and erosion (5 mm × 3 mm) were found on the posterior soft palate. There was also erosion (10 mm × 5 mm) on the palatal side of the left maxillary gingiva (Fig. 4.6). Nikolsky's sign was negative.
Laboratories and Imaging Studies:

1. There was no obvious abnormality in full blood count, blood glucose, and liver and kidney function.
2. Hematoxylin and eosin (HE) staining of the gingival biopsy revealed that stratified squamous epithelium was stripped completely. Direct immunofluorescence (DIF) showed linear deposition of immunoglobulin G and Complement C3 along the basement membrane.

Diagnosis:
Benign mucous membrane pemphigoid
Diagnosis Basis:

1. Chronic onset.
2. Congestive and erosive gingiva.
3. Nikolsky's sign was negative.
4. The diagnosis was confirmed by HE staining and DIF.

Management:

1. Medication
   Rp.: Prednisone acetate 5 mg × 42 tablets
   Sig.: 30 mg p.o. q.m.
   Calcium carbonate D3 tablets 30 tablets
   Sig.: 1 tablet p.o. q.d.
   Compound chlorhexidine solution 300 ml × 1
   Sig.: rinse t.i.d.
   Dexamethasone paste 15 g × 1
   Sig.: topical use t.i.d.
2. Subsequent visit after 1 week.

Subsequent Management:
If the disease is under control, prednisone acetate could be tapered gradually or replaced with tripterygium hypoglaucum tablet (Sig.: two tablets p.o. t.i.d.). Circumscribed erosions could be dealt with double-diluted triamcinolone acetonide (TA) injection (sig.: multipoint low-dose intralesional injection st.).

[Review] Pemphigoid

Pemphigoid mainly includes benign mucous membrane pemphigoid (MMP) and bullous pemphigoid (BP).

MMP mainly occurs in the elderly. The clinical manifestations are recurrent blisters, skin can also be involved. Due to scar formation left after healing, it is also called cicatricial pemphigoid.

The pathogenesis of MMP is not clear, with complex immune genetic background. The HLA DQB1*0301 may be involved, which plays a role in recognizing the autoantigen (BP180, laminin332, β4-integrin) of basement membrane zone (BMZ). The autoantibody induces complement-mediated release of cytokines and enzyme by acting on the antigen of BMZ or hemidesmosome or induces cytolysis to separate basal cell from the basement membrane [7]. The diagnosis depends on the biopsy and direct immunofluorescence (DIF). The histological pathology reveals the blister or fissure between the epithelium and connective tissue. DIF showed linear deposition of immunoglobulin (Ig) G and complement C3, sometimes accompany with IgA or IgM, along the basement membrane. MMP mainly mediated by IgG, which is different from linear IgA disease [8].

Seventy-five percent of cases of MMP involve the oral mucosa. Gingival lesion is initial and common, and the typical manifestation of it is desquamative gingivitis. Widespread erythema with 2–6 mm vesicles locate on the gingiva, with clear or bloody vesicular fluid. If the lesions occur on the palate or other sites, they often manifest as blisters or erosions after blisters rupture (Figs. 4.7 and 4.8). The fresh erosions are similar to pemphigus vulgaris (PV), covered by the pseudomembrane subsequently. Because of the white stripes around the erosions, it is often misdiagnosed as oral lichen planus (OLP). The pain is less severe than PV. Restriction of mouth opening and microstomia may be induced by the scar at corners of the mouth, due to scar formation left after healing in MMP.

Forty percent of cases of MMP involve the eyes. The initial manifestation is conjunctivitis, which can develop into entropion, trichiasis, synechia, and atrophy of the cornea due to scar formation. Unfortunately, 20% of patients may lose their sight [9]. Therefore, the clinicians should observe closely to the eyes of the patient with MMP. Other common mucosal features include erosions of nose and pharynx, epistaxis, dysphagia, anogenital scar, and adhesion. The skin lesions appear on 20–30% of cases of MMP, which manifest as widespread blisters with thick walls. Blisters are restricted to the scalp and upper limb occasionally, leaving scars after healing [6].

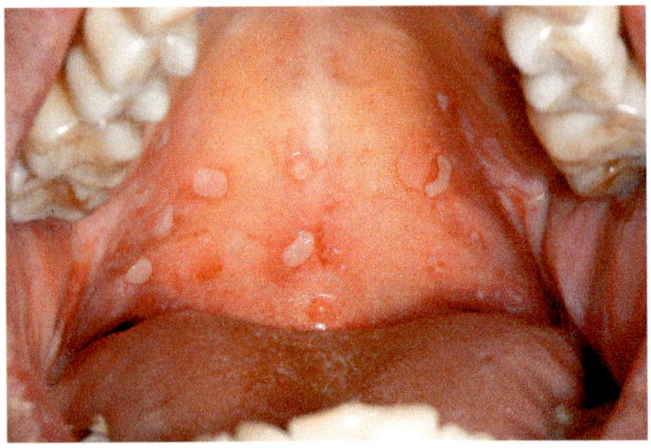

Fig. 4.7 Intact blisters on the posterior palate, with blisters rupture partly

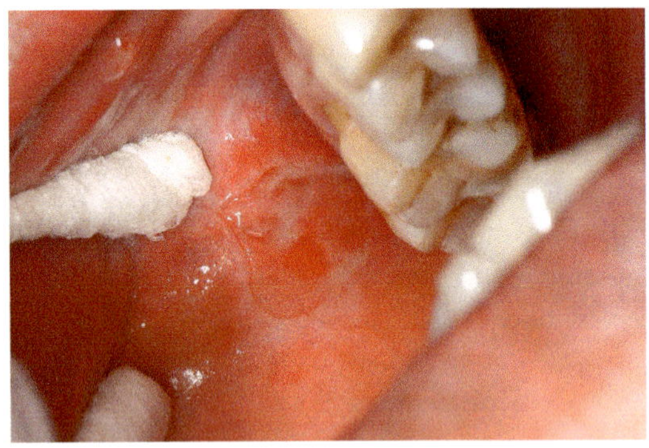

Fig. 4.8 Well-defined erosion on the right buccal mucosa

Bullous pemphigoid (BP) is another type of pemphigoid, which is characterized by tension blisters on the trunk and limbs, without scar occurs after the healing. Involvement of oral cavity is uncommon, with chronic oral ulcers affecting 10–30% of the patients. The precipitating factors include medicine such as sulfasalazine, penicillin, diazepam, furosemide, angiotensin-converting enzyme inhibitors (ACEI), sulfonamides, isoniazid, and ultraviolet (UV), but they are still uncertain. The incidence of BP is also increased as the age increases [6]. It is hard to differentiate between BP and MMP from the histopathology

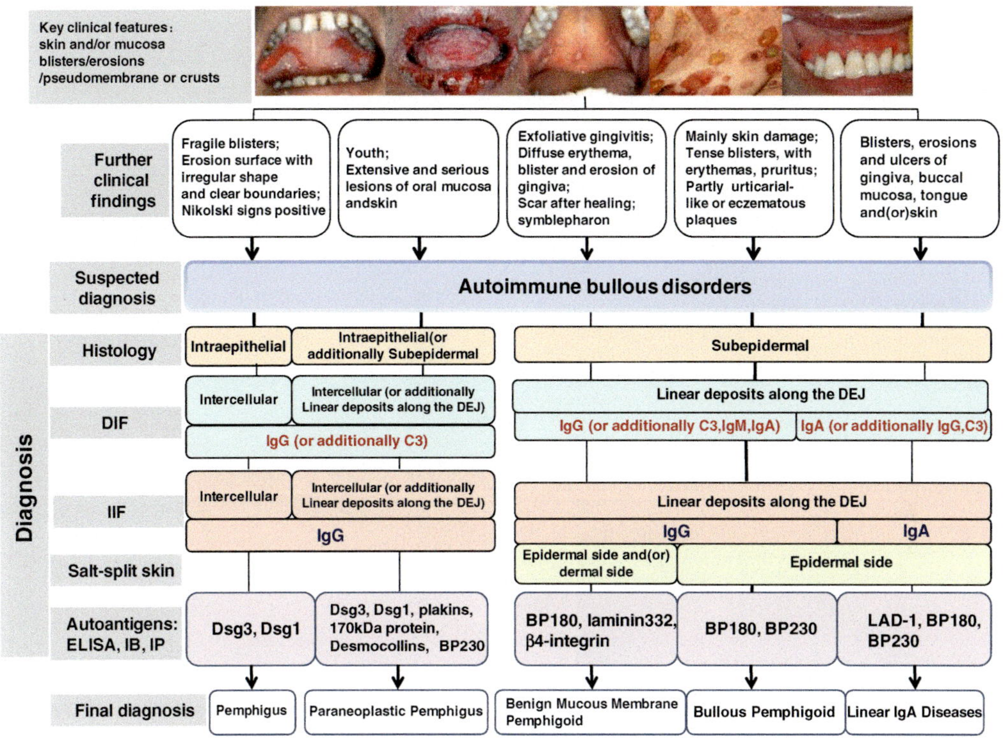

DIF: direct immunofluorescence; IIF: indirect immunofluorescence; DEJ: dermo-epidermal junction; IB: immunoblot; IP: immunoprecipitation

Fig. 4.9 Diagnosis of autoimmune bullous skin diseases

and DIF, but they are slightly different in the clinical manifestations and laboratory tests: (1) the oral lesions are common in MMP, while the cutaneous lesions occur only in BP mostly; (2) scars formation after healing are always in MMP, while not in BP; (3) the autoantigen of MMP are BP180, laminin332, and β4-integrin, while the BP of which are BP180 and BP230; (4) the result of salt split-skin immunofluorescence is different. Therefore, the differential diagnosis depends on the clinical manifestations and laboratory tests (Fig. 4.9).

The systemic therapy of MMP is as follows. If the oral condition is severe, it is necessary to take systemic glucocorticoid into consideration (≤30 mg/day, orally for 7–14 days and then gradually taper). If the oral condition is mild, clinician can choose tripterygium glycoside tablet (1–1.5 mg kg^{-1} day^{-1} t.i.d., orally for 1 month) or tripterygium hypoglaucum tablet (two tablets p.o. t.i.d., orally for 1 month). If the condition is controlled, the tablets can be tapered or given intermittently. In order to relieve the gastrointestinal discomfort, vitamin B6 (5 mg p.o. t.i.d.) can be given simultaneously. If the aforementioned therapy is not effective, minocycline hydrochloride tablets (100 mg p.o. b.i.d.) or combination of tetracycline (250 mg p.o. t.i.d.) and nicotinamide (200 mg p.o. t.i.d. or 500 mg p.o b.i.d.) is another available therapy. Moreover, the dosage should be tapered after 3 months according to the literature.

The topical agents include disinfectants and antiseptics (e.g., compound chlorhexidine solution), glucocorticoid preparation (e.g., dexamethasone solution, dexamethasone paste, triamcinolone acetonide dental paste), and antifungal preparation (e.g., 2–4% sodium bicarbonate solution, nystatin liniment). For the refractory circumscribed erosions, they could be dealed with double-diluted triamcinolone acetonide (TA) injection or compound betamethasone injection (Sig.: multipoint low-dose intralesional injection st.).

During the course of treatment, closely observation of the ocular and cutaneous lesions is required. If the lesions appear, the patients should be advised to visit the ophthalmological and dermatological department.

4.3 Paraneoplastic Pemphigus

Case 42 Paraneoplastic Pemphigus

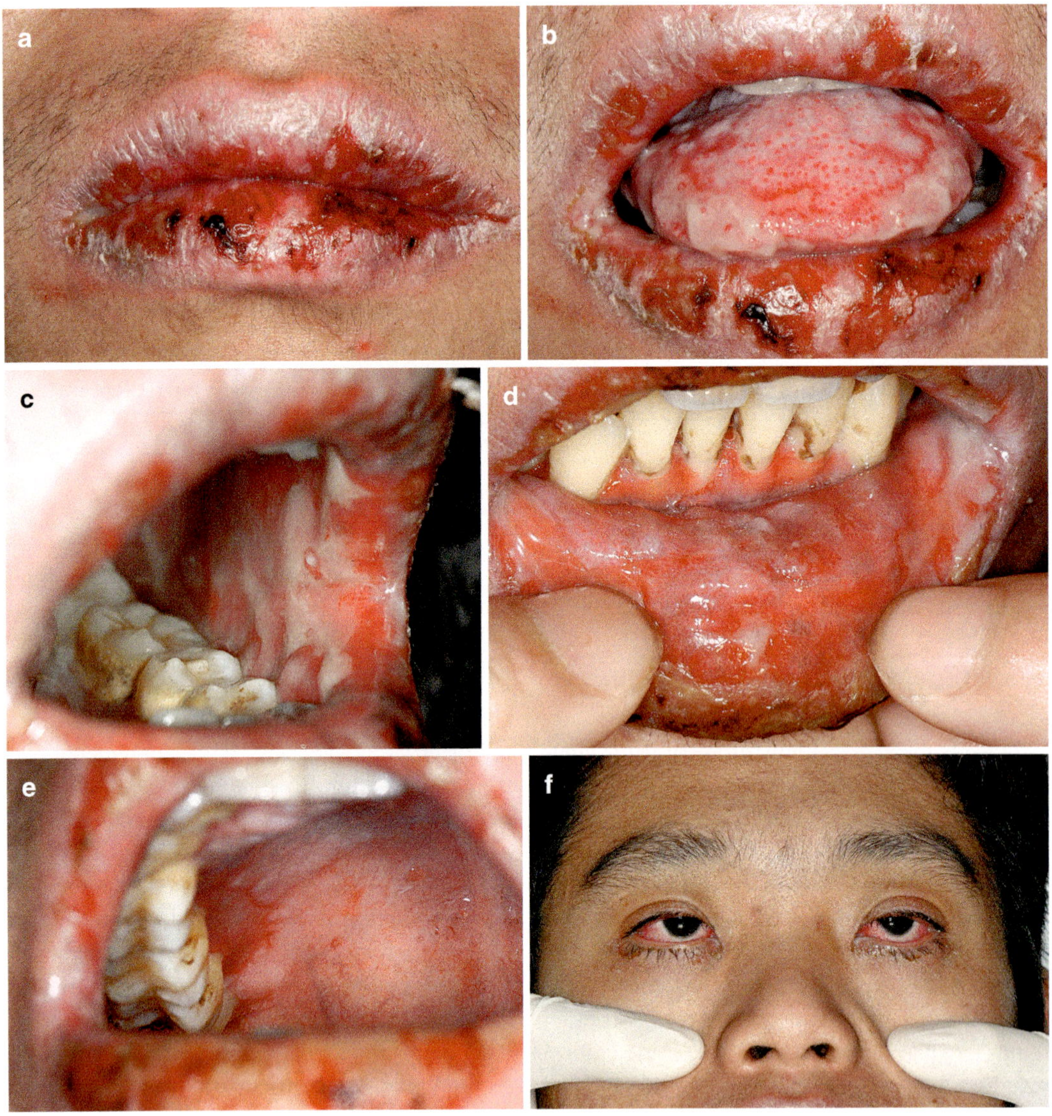

Fig. 4.10 (**a**) Extensive and irregular-shaped erosions on the lips, covered with pseudomembrane. (**b**) Extensive and irregular-shaped erosions on the labial mucosa and tongue, covered with pseudomembrane. (**c**) Extensive and irregular-shaped erosions on the left buccal mucosa, covered with pseudomembrane. (**d**) Extensive and irregular-shaped erosions on the lower labial mucosa, covered with pseudomembrane. (**e**) Extensive and irregular-shaped erosions on the right palate, covered with pseudomembrane. (**f**) Conjunctival congestion. (**g**) Blisters and erosions on the genital mucosa. (**h**) Multiple milia on the chest skin

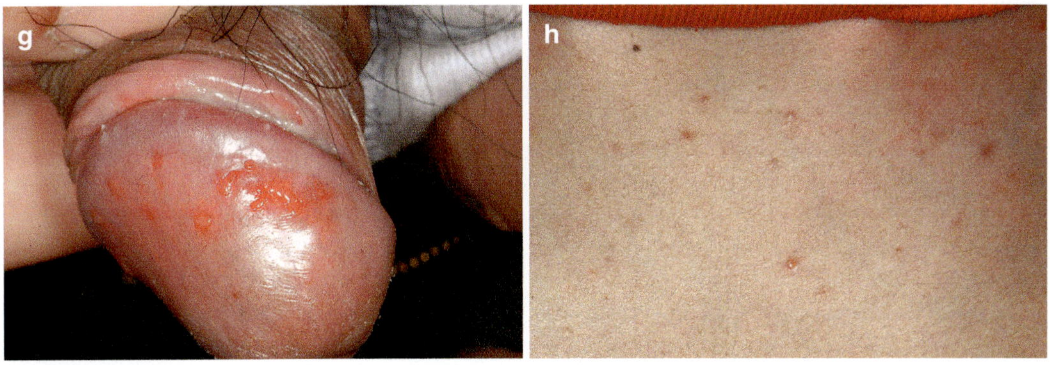

Fig. 10 (continued)

Age: 19 years
Sex: Male
Chief Complaint:
Recurrent oral erosions for 3 months
History of Present Illness:
The patient complained that recurrent oral erosions appeared with serious pain, without obvious predisposing causes for 3 months. His condition improved after each 7-day intravenous infusion. However, erosions always recurred before previous lesions healed completely. He had suffered from blurred vision, photophobia, genital ulcers, and the rash of chest skin for 2 months.
Past Medical History: None
Allergy: None
Physical Examination:
There were extensive and irregular-shaped erosions on the lips, labial mucosa, tongue, buccal mucosa, and palate, which were covered by pseudomembrane (Fig. 4.10a-e). Nikolsky's sign was positive. Conjunctival congestion, multiple milia on the chest skin, and blisters and erosions on the genital mucosa had been found (Fig. 4.10f-h).
Laboratories and Imaging Studies:

1. There was no obvious abnormality in full blood count, blood glucose, and liver and kidney functions.
2. Incisional biopsy of perilesional mucosa which appears normal: Hematoxylin and eosin (HE) staining revealed acantholysis; pemphigus was considered. Direct immunofluorescence (DIF) microscopy showed the reticular intercellular deposition and the linear deposition along the basement membrane of IgG and C3.
3. Cervicothoracic CT showed benign space-occupying lesion in the left neck. Ultrasonography of abdomen revealed no abnormality.
4. Total space-occupying lesion excision was performed and pathologic report was Castleman's disease.

Diagnosis:
Paraneoplastic pemphigus (associated with Castleman's disease)
Diagnosis Basis:

1. The patient was a 19-year-old youth.
2. Extensive and irregular-shaped erosions involved oral mucosa.
3. Nikolsky's sign was positive.
4. The diagnosis was confirmed by HE staining and DIF, especially DIF showed that the deposition of IgG and C3 not only in the intercellular junction but also in the basement membrane zone.
5. A systemic examination revealed Castleman's disease.

Management:

1. Medication
   Rp.: Compound chlorhexidine solution 300 ml × 1
   Sig.: rinse t.i.d.

Dexamethasone paste 15 g × 1
Sig.: topical use t.i.d.

2. Timely treatment of Castleman's disease was suggested and subsequent visit after 2 weeks was required.

[Review] Paraneoplastic Pemphigus

Paraneoplastic pemphigus (PNP) is a life-threatening autoimmune blistering disease, which is associated with neoplassms. It is clinically characterized by serious mucosal erosions (especially oral mucosa) with a polymorphous skin eruption. It was first described in a case series in 1990 by Anhalt et al. PNP has a wide geographic distribution and equal predominance across both genders with the age of onset of 7–76 years old. Fifty-one years is the average age of onset of PNP. Mortality due to the disease has been reported to be as high as 90%. It can affect internal organs, such as the lungs, thyroid, kidney, smooth muscle, and gastrointestinal tract. Such internal organ involvement has led to the proposal that the term, paraneoplastic pemphigus, should be replaced by the term, paraneoplastic autoimmune multiorgan syndrome (PAMS). The heterogeneity in the presentation of the cutaneous manifestations of this disease has led to five different clinical variants: pemphigus-like, bullous pemphigoid-like, erythema multiform-like, graft-versus-host disease-like, and lichen planus-like. If pemphigus-like lesions occurred in the patient with neoplasm, it can be called paraneoplastic pemphigus. It doesn't mean that pemphigus and neoplasm simply coexist in one patient, but means that it is an autoimmune disease with specific serum autoantibodies [10].

There were autoantibodies to multicomponent of plakins family in the serum of patients with PNP. As structural components of desmosomal and hemidesmosomal plaques, plakins play a critical role in the cell adhesion. Periplakins and envoplakins are the most common in PNP/PAMS, followed by desmoplakin I (DP I) and desmoplakin II (DP II). It has been shown in several studies that circulating autoantibodies to the plakin proteins, which has been produced directly by coexisting neoplasms, are responsible for the pathogenesis of PNP/PAMS. The exact mechanisms by which tumor induces PNP/PAMS are unknown. Several hypotheses have been put forward, and they can be classified into five broad categories:

1. Epitope spreading: previously hidden antigens were uncovered by a cell-mediated lichenoid interface dermatitis triggered by tumor.
2. Antigen mimicry: humoral immune response against the tumor cross-reacting with normal epithelial proteins.
3. Cytotoxicity: autoreactive cellular cytotoxicity mediated by $CD8^+$ cytotoxic T lymphocytes, $CD56^+$ natural killer cells, and $CD68^+$ macrophages.
4. Autoantibodies: production of autoantibodies responds to epidermal proteins by the cells from the underlying tumors.
5. Interleukin 6: abundant interleukin 6 secreted due to dysregulation of cytokine production by tumor cells [10].

So far, the most frequently documented neoplasm associated with PNP are B lymphoma, chronic lymphocytic leukemia, thymoma, Castleman's disease, etc. Mucosal lesions are the initial features in most patients. The typical mucosal lesions are similar to the pemphigus-like erosions which is extensive and painful seriously. They often involve the oral cavity, nasopharynx, conjunctiva, anogenital region, and esophagus. The cutaneous lesions usually appear ranging from days to months after the occurrence of mucosal lesions. Mucosal lesions aggravate with the development of the condition. Generally, the response to conventional therapy for pemphigus is poor. Common causes of mortality in PNP include overwhelming sepsis and bronchiolitis obliterans accompanying the Castleman's disease. It is worth noting that the mucocutaneous lesion is usually recognized prior to the neoplasm. A comprehensive search for an underlying neoplasm should be carried out if the diagnosis of paraneoplastic pemphigus is suspected. The examinations include X-ray test, abdominal ultrasound, CT, and serum tumor markers. After the treatment of the underlying neoplasms, the remission of PNP will be obtained [11].

Mucosal lesions of PNP can occur in any part of the oral mucosa such as buccal mucosa, labial mucosa, gingiva and tongue, and nasal mucosa, pharynx, tonsil, vulva mucosa can also be involved. The features of oral lesions include extensive erosions with obvious exudation and severe pain, positive probing test, and positive Nikolsky's sign. In addition, blisters and erosions can occur in the mucosa of digestive tract and respiratory tract, which may lead to the death of respiratory failure. The damage to the eyes may range from mild conjunctivitis to symblepharon accompanied with corneal scarring.

The involvement of skin is extensive, with pain and itching. Multiple manifestations may appear, including scattering or exfoliative erythema, blisters, papules, scales, ulcers, and erosions. Skin lesions occur as erythema initially, such as spotlike, wheal-like, and target-like, followed by blisters and erosions.

Patients with PNP are always suffered from dysphagia, fatigue, muscle pain, which ultimately results in poor general condition.

The histological findings have shown similarities with other known bullous dermatoses, including intraepidermal or subepidermal blistering with no or few mononuclear cells. Direct immunofluorescence (DIF) is considered as one of the main diagnostic criteria for PNP/PAMS, which reveals the deposition of IgG and complement C3 in an intercellular and/or linear pattern. By indirect immunofluorescence (IIF), PNP antibodies stain the simple, columnar, and transitional epithelial tissue substrates (typically rat bladder) in addition to the stratified squamous epithelium. IIF has higher sensitivity and specificity than DIF [10, 12].

PNP should be suspected if the following points occur: a youth suffered from extensive and refractory lesions in the oral mucosa, intercellular and basement membrane deposition of IgG and complement C3 showed in the DIF, and the poor response to the conventional therapy for pemphigus.

The treatments for PNP is mainly target the neoplasms. In patients with a benign tumor, surgical resection would lead to remission or complete resolution of PNP. However, poor prognosis is indicated due to the progressive course of the malignancy. The topical treatment is similar to that of pemphigus.

4.4 Linear IgA Disease

Case 43 Linear IgA Disease

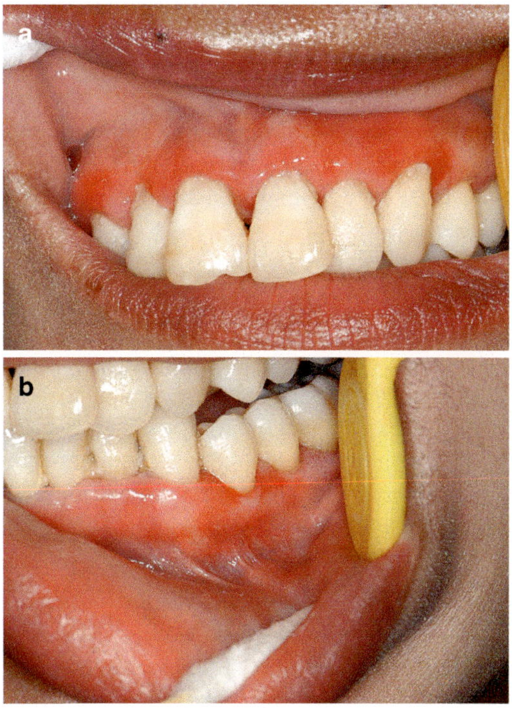

Fig. 4.11 (**a**) Regional erythema and erosions on the anterior maxillary gingiva. (**b**) Localized erythema and erosions on the left mandibular gingiva

Age: 41 years
Sex: Female
Chief Complaints:
Gingival erythema and pain for 2 years
History of Present Illness:
A 41-year-old female presented to our clinic with gingival erythema and pain, as well as difficulty in eating for 2 years. She denied any lesions of skin.
Past Medical History: None
Allergy History: None

Physical Examination:
Obvious erythema and erosions were noticed on the anterior maxillary gingiva. Erosions were located on the buccal mandibular gingiva, with white striae and patches (Fig. 4.11). Nikolsky's sign was negative.
Laboratories and Imaging Studies:

1. There was no obvious abnormality in full blood count, blood glucose, and liver and kidney function.
2. Hematoxylin and eosin (HE) staining of the gingiva biopsy revealed subepidermal blistering, which was accordant with pemphigoid. Direct immunofluorescence (DIF) showed linear deposition of immunoglobulin A (IgA) along the basement membrane. IgG and complement C3 were undetected.

Diagnosis:
Linear IgA disease
Diagnosis Basis:

1. Clinical manifestations were similar to bullous disease (pemphigoid).
2. HE staining of the biopsy was accordant with pemphigoid. DIF showed linear deposition of IgA along the basement membrane.

Management:

1. Medication
   Rp.: Prednisone acetate 5 mg × 35
   Sig.: 25 mg p.o. q.m.
   Zhongtong'an capsules 0.28g × 48
   Sig.: 0.56 g p.o. t.i.d.
   Compound chlorhexidine solution 300 ml × 1
   Sig.: rinse t.i.d.
   Dexamethasone paste 15 g × 1
   Sig.: topical use t.i.d.
2. Intralesional injection was adopted for gingival erythema and erosions: triamcinolone acetonide (TA) injection 40 mg × 1 for multipoint low-dose injection.

Subsequent Management:
If the disease is under control, gradual reduction of prednisone acetate is required for 5 mg per week. Replacement with tripterygium hypoglaucum tablet (two tablets orally, three times a day for 2–4 weeks) could also be applied.

[Review] Linear IgA Disease
Linear IgA disease (LAD), which is also called linear IgA bullous dermatitis (LABD), is an autoimmune bullous disease characterized by linear deposition of IgA along the basement membrane. It is uncommon and can occur at any age. The sex incidence is about equal, or there may be a slight excess of female patients. It can be classified as adult type and children type, with recurrent and chronic clinical features [13].

LAD is an autoimmune disease, which starts spontaneously or drug-induced. The drugs such as vancomycin [14], amlodipine, ampicillin, and sulbactam [15, 16] are the most common triggers. It has been reported that some adult LAD patients accompanied with gluten-sensitive enteropathy [17]. Also it could be induced by the vaccine of HPV [18] according to other studies. But the pathogenesis is still unclear.

The two most characteristic target antigens of LAD are the proteins of 97kD and 120kD, termed the LAD97 and LAD-1, respectively. These proteins present a cleaved portion of the extracellular domain of BP180 [19].

The adult LAD often appears in young and middle-aged people with sudden onset. It is difficult to be distinguished from other bullous diseases due to its nonspecific skin manifestations, with or without mucosal (oral, nasal, genital and ocular) lesions. Nikolsky's sign is negative. The common oral features are blisters and erosions on the buccal mucosa and tongue according to reports [13]. However, two LAD cases we have experienced manifested as erythema and erosions limited to gingiva.

The children LAD often appears in preschool children with sudden onset. It is characterized by recurrent episodes and self-limiting, which could in remission prior to puberty. The cutaneous lesions are extensive and symmetrical, commonly occurring on perioral skin, upper and low limbs, inguinal region, and perineum. Blisters tend to appear on the normal skin or erythema with various degree of pruritus. Nikolsky's sign is negative. The mucosa can also be affected, such as oral erosions and ulcers, nasal obstruction, epistaxis, and conjunctivitis [20].

The histopathology of LAD is subepithelial blister with the destruction of basement membrane zone (BMZ). Direct immunofluorescence (DIF) shows linear deposition of immunoglobulin (Ig) A along the basement membrane with or without the deposition of IgG and complement C3. Indirect immunofluorescence (IIF) shows the negative antibody of BMZ-IgA in most LAD patients' peripheral blood. And even if it is positive, the titer of the antibody is low. However, the antibody is positive in 75% children with LAD.

Because of the nonspecificity of clinical manifestations, the DIF of fresh tissue is the golden standard for the diagnosis of LAD [21].

The lesions of Case 43 in this unit are limited to oral mucosa, which is rare. Two LAD cases we have experienced manifested as erythema and erosions mainly located on gingiva, without cutaneous lesions, which are nonspecific and mild symptoms. It is noteworthy that the LAD limited to oral mucosa may be more common than we imagine. The reason for few reports may be lack of cutaneous lesions and DIF examination, leading to misdiagnosis as other diseases. In order to avoid the misdiagnosis, we should make the DIF as a routine test for the patient with chronic erythematous, erosive, and bullous lesions in the mouth.

Dapsone is effective for LAD, but severe hemolytic anemia should be prevented [22]. The initial dosage is low (0.5 mg kg^{-1} day^{-1}), and the dosage could be increased to 2.5–3.0 mg kg^{-1} day^{-1} for the disease control. The patient who cannot tolerate the dapsone could take sulfadiazine (15–60 mg kg^{-1} day^{-1}) for choice. If sulfadiazine has poor outcome, combined with glucocorticoid could be considered. Topical glucocorticoids should be combined with in patients with mucosal lesions, for the mucosal lesions are often more stubborn than skin. Majority of patients with drug-induced LAD will get remission in 5 weeks after suspected drug withdrawal. LAD often has a good prognosis. Due to the mild symptoms of Case 43, similar therapeutic methods were adopted as we treated pemphigoid.

References

1. Tamgadge S, Tamgadge A, Bhatt DM, Bhalerao S, Pereira T. Pemphigus vulgaris. Contemp Clin Dent. 2011;2(2):134–7.
2. Bystryn JC, Rudolph JL. Pemphigus. Lancet. 2005;366(9479):61–73.
3. Sinha AA. The genetics of pemphigus. Dermatol Clin. 2011;29(3):381–91, vii.
4. Dagistan S, Goregen M, Miloglu O, Cakur B. Oral pemphigus vulgaris: a case report with review of the literature. J Oral Sci. 2008;50(3):359–62.
5. Venugopal SS, Murrell DF. Diagnosis and clinical features of pemphigus vulgaris. Dermatol Clin. 2011;29(3):373–80, vii.
6. Kneisel A, Hertl M. Autoimmune bullous skin diseases. Part 1: Clinical manifestations. J Dtsch Dermatol Ges. 2011;9(10):844–57.
7. Setterfield J, Theron J, Vaughan RW, et al. Mucous membrane pemphigoid: HLA-DQB1*0301 is associated with all clinical sites of involvement and may be linked to antibasement membrane IgG production. Br J Dermatol. 2001;145(3):406–14.
8. Scully C, Lo-Muzio L. Oral mucosal diseases: mucous membrane pemphigoid. Br J Oral Maxillofac Surg. 2008;46(5):358–66.
9. Chan LS, Ahmed AR, Anhalt GJ, et al. The first international consensus on mucous membrane pemphigoid: definition, diagnostic criteria, pathogenic factors, medical treatment, and prognostic indicators. Arch Dermatol. 2002;138(3):370.
10. Frew JW, Murrell DF. Paraneoplastic pemphigus (paraneoplastic autoimmune multiorgan syndrome): clinical presentations and pathogenesis. Dermatol Clin. 2011;29(3):419–25, viii.
11. Sehgal VN, Srivastava G. Paraneoplastic pemphigus/paraneoplastic autoimmune multiorgan syndrome. Int J Dermatol. 2009;48(2):162–9.
12. Nguyen VT, Ndoye A, Bassler KD, et al. Classification, clinical manifestations, and immunopathological mechanisms of the epithelial variant of paraneoplastic autoimmune multiorgan syndrome: a reappraisal of paraneoplastic pemphigus. Arch Dermatol. 2001;137(2):193–206.
13. Venning VA. Linear IgA disease: clinical presentation, diagnosis, and pathogenesis. Dermatol Clin. 2011;32(2):453–8.
14. Selvaraj PK, Khasawneh FA. Linear IgA bullous dermatosis: a rare side effect of vancomycin. Ann Saudi Med. 2012;33(4):1–2.
15. Schafer F, Echeverria X, Gonzalez S. Linear IgA bullous dermatosis induced by ampicillin/sulbactam. Indian J Dermatol Venereol Leprol. 2012;78(2):230.
16. Low L, Zaheri S, Wakelin S. Amlodipine-induced linear IgA disease. Clin Exp Dermatol. 2012;37(6):649.
17. Egan CA, Smith EP, Taylor TB, et al. Linear IgA bullous dermatosis responsive to a gluten-free diet. Am J Gastroenterol. 2001;96(6):1927–9.

18. Ikeya S, Urano S, Tokura Y. Linear IgA bullous dermatosis following human papillomavirus vaccination. Eur J Dermatol. 2012;22(6):787–8.
19. Kasperkiewicz M, Zillikens D, Schmidt E. Pemphigoid diseases: pathogenesis, diagnosis, and treatment. Autoimmunity. 2012;45(1):55–70.
20. Fahad AS, Ammar AR. Unusual clinicopathological and immunological presentation of chronic bullous dermatosis of childhood (linear IgA dermatosis). Indian J Dermatol. 2011;56(56):573–5.
21. Dan H, Lu R, Li W, et al. Linear IgA disease limited to the oral mucosa. J Am Acad Dermatol. 2011;65(3):677–9.
22. Ng SY, Venning VV. Management of linear IgA disease. Dermatol Clin. 2011;29(4):629.

Oral Mucosal Patches Striae Diseases

5

Hongxia Dan, Xin Jin, and Qianming Chen

Keywords
Oral leukoplakia · Oral leukokeratosis · White sponge nevus · Oral lichen planus · Lichenoid reactions · Oral erythroplakia · Oral submucous fibrosis · Discoid lupus erythematosus · Oral Fordyce spots · Morsicatio buccarum et labiorum · Oral potentially malignant disorders

H. Dan
State Key Laboratory of Oral Diseases, National Clinical Research Center for Oral Diseases, Department of Oral Medicine, West China Hospital of Stomatology, Sichuan University, Chengdu, Sichuan, China

X. Jin
College of Stomatology, Chongqing Medical University, Chongqing Key Laboratory of Oral Diseases and Biomedical Sciences, Chongqing, China

Q. Chen (✉)
Changjiang Scholars Program, Ministry of Education, Beijing, China

State Key Laboratory of Oral Diseases, National Clinical Research Center for Oral Diseases, Department of Oral Medicine, West China Hospital of Stomatology, Sichuan University, Chengdu, Sichuan, China
e-mail: qmchen@scu.edu.cn

5.1 Oral Leukoplakia

Case 44 Gingival Leukoplakia (Homogenous Type)

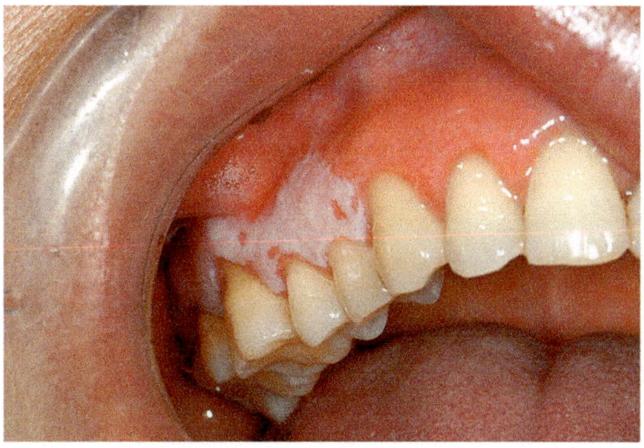

Fig. 5.1 A well-defined homogenous white plaque on the buccal gingiva of the right maxillary premolar and molar teeth

Age: 47 years
Sex: female
Chief Complaints:
A 47-year-old woman complained of color change of the maxillary gingiva for 1 month.
History of Present Illness:
A 47-year-old woman came to our clinic, complaining of a 1-month history of color change of the maxillary gingiva. There was no pain or any obvious discomfort. The patient denied the history of smoking and drinking.
Past Medical History: None.

Q. Chen, X. Zeng (eds.), *Case Based Oral Mucosal Diseases*,
https://doi.org/10.1007/978-981-13-0286-2_5

Allergy: None.

Physical Examination:

A well-defined homogenous white plaque was found on the buccal gingiva of the right maxillary premolar and molar teeth. The size of lesion was approximately 20 mm × 8 mm (Fig. 5.1).

Clinical Impression:

Gingival Leukoplakia (homogenous type)

Laboratory Investigations:

1. Full blood cell count, blood glucose level, and liver and renal function tests revealed no significant abnormalities.
2. An incisional biopsy of the lesion was made. The routine histopathological examination (HE staining) showed the histological changes in accord with oral leukoplakia without epithelial dysplasia.

Diagnosis:

Gingival Leukoplakia (homogenous type)

Diagnosis Basis:

1. Well-defined, raised, white plaque on the mucosa
2. Diagnosis confirmed by histopathological examination (HE staining)

Management:

1. Medication

   Rp.: Thymosin enteric-coated tablets 20 mg × 30 tablets

   Sig.: 20 mg q.d. p.o.

   Beta-carotene 6 mg × 60 tablets

   Sig.: 6 mg b.i.d. p.o.

   Compound danshen dripping pills 360 tablets

   Sig.: 10 tablets t.i.d. p.o.

   Vitamin E 100 mg × 60 tablets

   Sig.: 100 mg q.d. p.o.

   Tretinoin paste 15 g × 1

   Sig.: topical use t.i.d.
2. Follow-up at the frequency of once a month (or more frequent if the condition deteriorates).

Case 45 Proliferative Verrucous Leukoplakia

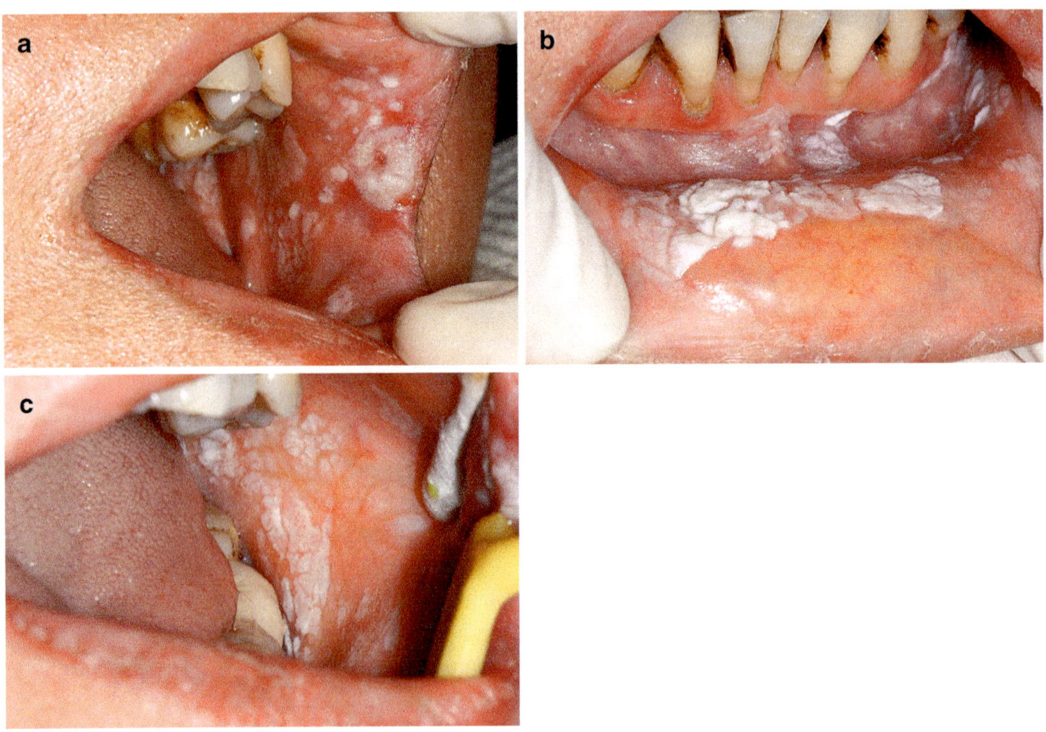

Fig. 5.2 (**a**) A rough, verrucous, highly keratinized whitish lesion was seen on the buccal mucosa close to the left commissure of mouth. (**b**) White plaques, slightly raised and partially verrucous, were observed on the mucosa of the lower lip, gingiva, and vestibular groove of mandibular incisors. (**c**) Whitish plaques, slightly raised and rough, were widely distributed on the left buccal mucosa

Age: 47 years
Sex: female
Chief Complaints:
A 47-year-old woman complained of color change of the left cheek for 5 years.
History of Present Illness:
A 47-year-old woman came to our clinic, complaining of color change of the left cheek for 5 years. The lesion was white, gradually enlarged and extended to the left commissure of the mouth and the lower lip. Pain was mild and occasionally happened while eating.
Physical Examination:
White plaques, slightly raised, rough, some of which verrucous, were widely distributed on the mucosa lining the left cheek, pterygomandibular fold, mandibular vestibular groove, and inner side of the lip (Fig. 5.2a-c). Among these plaques, a lesion inside the lower lip and a lesion inside the left commissure of the mouth were highly keratotic and indurated.
Clinical Impression:
Proliferative Verrucous Leukoplakia
Laboratory Investigations:

1. Routine laboratory tests, including whole blood cell count, blood glucose examination, as well as liver and kidney function panels, were normal.
2. Toluidine blue staining showed negative results except the inner side of the left commissure of the mouth.
3. A lesional biopsy was made inside of the left commissure of the mouth. Findings of routine histopathological examination were in accord with proliferative verrucous leukoplakia with mild-to-moderate epithelial dysplasia.

Diagnosis:
Proliferative Verrucous Leukoplakia
Diagnosis Basis:

1. Multiple proliferative white plaques on the oral mucosa.
2. Findings of histopathological examination.

Management:

1. Surgical resection of the highly keratinized lesions inside the lower lip and the left commissure of the mouth were recommended. Other lesions would be treated by medication.
2. Medication
   Rp.: Thymosin enteric-coated tablets 20 mg × 30 tablets
   Sig.: 20 mg q.d. p.o.
   Beta-carotene 6 mg × 60 tablets
   Sig.: 6 mg b.i.d. p.o.
   Compound danshen dripping pills 360 tablets
   Sig.: 10 tablets t.i.d. p.o.
   Vitamin E 100 mg × 60 tablets
   Sig.: 100 mg q.d. p.o.
   Tretinoin paste 15 g × 1
   Sig.: topical use t.i.d.
3. Follow-up at the frequency of once a month (or more frequent if the condition deteriorates).

Case 46 Malignant Transformation of Oral Leukoplakia

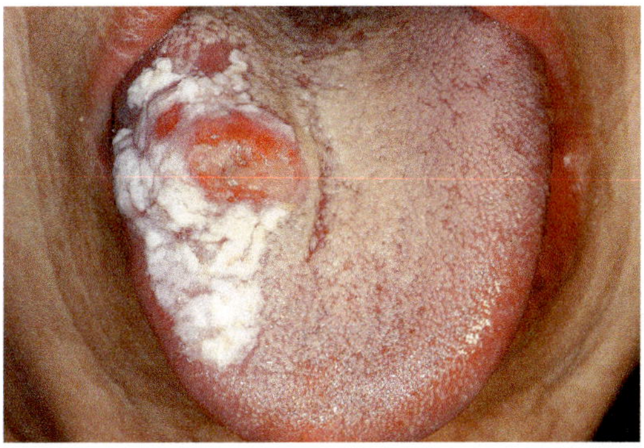

Fig. 5.3 A well-defined whitish plaque with ulceration located on the right dorsal surface of the tongue (Reproduced from Jin et al. 2012)

Age: 63 years
Sex: female
Chief Complaints:
A 63-year-old woman with whitish plaque on the tongue for 7 months
History of Present Illness:
A 63-year-old woman came to our clinic, complaining of whitish plaque on the tongue for 7 months. There wasn't any discomfort other than roughness in the first 6 months. Ulcerative lesions appeared on the inner border of the lesion about 1 month ago. The patient had been suffering from moderate pain since then.

Physical Examination:
A well-defined whitish plaque, 4 cm × 2 cm in size, was observed on the dorsum of the tongue. Two ulcerative lesions with indurated margins, 1.2 cm × 1 cm and 0.4 cm × 0.2 cm in size, were located on the white plaque (Fig. 5.3).
Laboratory Investigations:

1. Routine laboratory tests, including whole blood cell count, blood glucose level, as well as liver and kidney function panels, were normal.
2. A biopsy of the indurated margin of the ulcer was made. Findings of routine histopathological examination were in accord with oral squamous cell carcinoma.

Diagnosis:
Malignant Transformation of Oral Leukoplakia
Diagnosis Basis:

1. Well-defined, whitish plaque on the oral mucosa.
2. Ulcerative lesions with indurated margins on the white plaque.
3. Findings of histopathological examination.

Management:

1. The patient was referred to the Department of Oral and Maxillofacial Surgery of our hospital for further examinations and treatment.
2. Frequent follow-up after the surgery was recommended.

[Review] Oral Leukoplakia
Oral leukoplakia (OLK) is defined as a whitish patch or plaque that cannot be clinically or histologically diagnosed as any other disease. It is the most common type of oral potentially malignant lesion. The prevalence of oral leukoplakia ranges from 0.4% to 0.7%. There is no gender preference or a preference for men [1]. The onset of the disease usually happens between the ages of 40 and 60. Some studies suggest that OLK is mostly commonly seen on the inner surface of the commissure of the mouth, while other studies show that the gingiva and lingual mucosa are more commonly affected. Epidemiological data indicates that the development of leukoplakia may be affected by factors such as region of residence, ethnic groups, and smoking habits [2].

OLK can be classified into two major types: homogeneous type and nonhomogeneous type. Homogeneous OLK appears as a well-defined, flat, or wrinkled white plaque (Fig. 5.4). According to the appearance of the lesion, nonhomogeneous OLK can be further divided into three subtypes: speckled (Fig. 5.5), ulcerated (Fig. 5.6), and verrucous (Fig. 5.7). Speckled OLK has an appearance of whitish patches with a nodular surface or whitish patches interspersed with erythematous mucosa; ulcerative OLK has ulcers or erosions on the white plaques; verrucous OLK has exophytic thorns or papillae. Nonhomogeneous OLK was more closely associated with epithelial dysplasia and cancer [3].

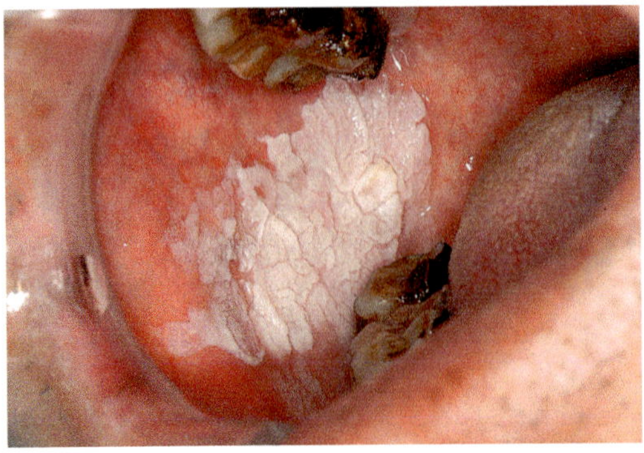

Fig. 5.4 Well-defined wrinkled leukoplakia on the left buccal mucosa. Histological findings were in accord with leukoplakia without epithelial dysplasia

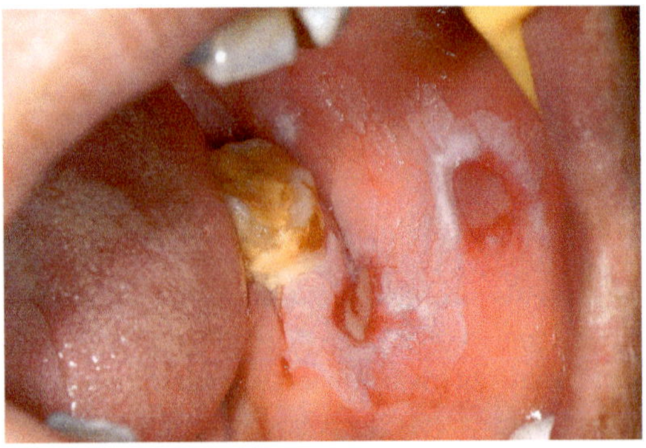

Fig. 5.6 Ulcerated leukoplakia on the left buccal mucosa. Histological findings were in accord with leukoplakia with moderate to severe epithelial dysplasia

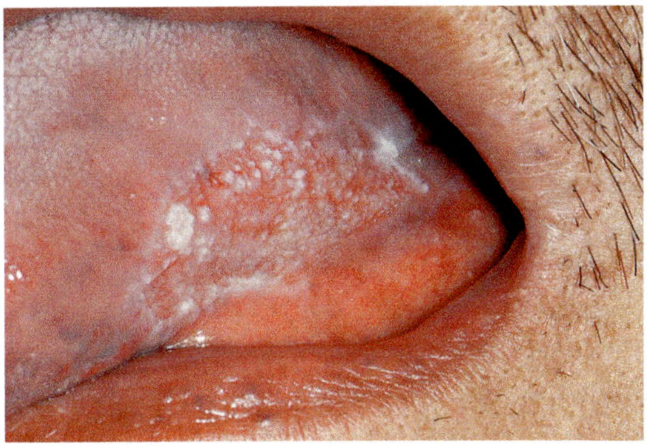

Fig. 5.5 Speckled OLK on the left side of the tongue. Histological findings were in accord with leukoplakia with mild epithelial dysplasia

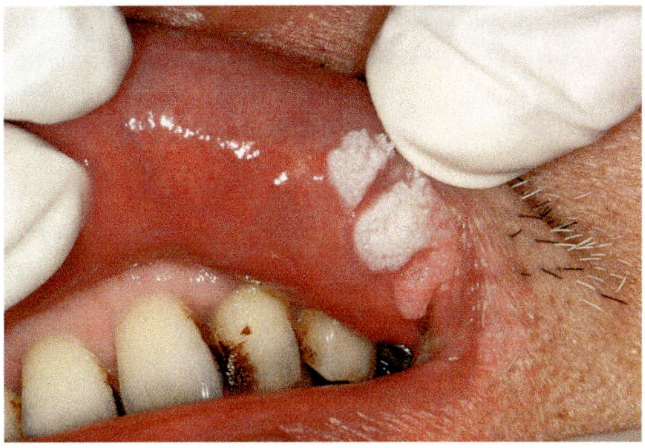

Fig. 5.7 Verrucous leukoplakia on the left upper lip. Histological findings were in accord with leukoplakia with moderate epithelial dysplasia

Proliferative verrucous leukoplakia (PVL), a special type of OLK, usually has multiple lesions which are characterized by chronic proliferation and intractability. The reported malignant transformation rate of PVL is up to 100%. PVL is most common in middle-aged women. The typical lesion is a well-defined verrucous white plaque, which usually starts on the gingiva and then spreads to other regions of the mouth [3]. It is very difficult to be differentiated from verrucous carcinoma. The pathological process of PVL may start as simple keratosis and then develop to leukoplakia or even invasive squamous cell carcinoma. The histological morphology of PVL usually overlaps with other types of OLK, but the abnormal keratinization is more severe. PVL usually has no or only mild epithelial dysplasia at early stages of the disease. If the lesion is verrucous leukoplakia with severe dysplasia, it is more appropriate to be diagnosed as carcinoma in situ rather than PVL [4].

The reported malignant transformation rate of OLK varies from 0.13% to 17.5% in a follow-up time that ranges from 1 to 30 years [2]. This variation could be a result of different research methods, such as the choice of the control group, length of the follow-up period, and different smoking habits. There are many factors that may be related to the risk of malignant transformation. Some researchers in India suggested that the malignant transformation rate of OLK was higher in men than in women, which may be associated with tobacco chewing and smoking [5]. There were other studies indicating that non-smoking female patients had a higher risk of malignant transformation compared with other patients. Elder people had a higher risk of malignant transformation than people in a younger age group [6]. Leukoplakia on the ventral surface of the tongue and the floor of the mouth is associated with a risk of malignant transformation up to 43%, probably due to higher permeability of these areas that leads to increased exposure to carcinogens in saliva and the oral cavity. Compared with homogeneous OLK, nonhomogeneous OLK has higher risk of malignant transformation. Cancer development can happen in 80% of patients with PVL [3].In addition, lesions larger than 200 square mm or lesions dispersedly distributed are also considered to be at high risk.

Epithelial dysplasia reflects the abnormal differentiation of the epithelium. It is present in 1–30% of OLK cases. It was reported that up to 36% of OLK with dysplasia would develop to squamous cell carcinoma [7]. The grade of epithelial dysplasia is important in the treatment and prognosis prediction of OLK. However, the judgment of the severity of epithelial dysplasia can be very subjective. Lesions with moderate to severe dysplasia do not necessarily develop into squamous cell carcinoma, some of them may be resected at the time of biopsy and some of them may get better as time goes by. On the other hand, malignant transformation can also occur in OLK without dysplasia [8]. Therefore, it is difficult to predict the risk of malignant transformation of an individual patient.

The development of OLK is related to local irritation factors and some infections. Tobacco chewing, smoking, and betel nut chewing are common local irritation factors, all of which are associated with the development of leukoplakia. There is much debate about whether *Candida* infection is the etiological factor of OLK or just a type of secondary infection. Different types of *Candida* species have been isolated from nonhomogeneous OLK with epithelial dysplasia. Eradication of *Candida* does not lead to vanishing of the lesion but may facilitate the transformation of high-risk nonhomogeneous OLK to low-risk homogenous OLK [9]. HPV is probably associated with the occurrence and malignant transformation of OLK. PVL is closely related with HPV infection. Infection of HPV-16 is an independent risk factor of malignant transformation of OLK [10]. EBV has been related with various cancers. Some studies suggested that it might play a part in oral carcinogenesis. However, no solid evidence has been found regarding the relationship between OLK and EBV [11].

Elucidation of the mechanisms of cancer development can help us with the prediction of the malignant transformation of OLK, with or without epithelial dysplasia. The development of OLK is associated with various molecular abnormalities, such as aneuploidy, aberrant telomerase activity, and loss of heterozygosity (LOH).

LOH in the chromosome of tumor suppressor gene has some predictive value for malignant transformation risk of OLK. LOH at 3p, 4q, 8p, 9p, 11q, 13q, and 17p loci have been reported to be associated with increased risk of malignant transformation. LOH does not appear in OLK with low risk of malignant transformation [12].

The DNA ploidy provides information on the degree of genetic instability and aberrations. In OLK with dysplasia, diploid cells are considered to be at low risk, tetraploid cells are considered to be at mediate risk, while aneuploid cells is considered to be at high risk of malignant transformation [13].

Genes associated with dysplasia include p53, cyclooxygenase 2, prostaglandin E synthase, and so on. *p53* is a tumor suppressor gene. Wild-type *p53* can induce apoptosis, but the mutant type inhibits apoptosis [14].

Protein markers associated with malignant transformation of OLK include integrins, the CD44 family, cell cycle regulators, matrix metalloproteinase 11, vascular endothelial growth factor, etc. [3]. However, all of these markers are still being studied. Until now, no recognized markers can be widely applied clinically.

Diagnosis of OLK is established after ruling out other well-defined entities that may appear as whitish plaques on the oral mucosa, such as linea alba, leukoedema, white sponge nevus, morsicatio buccarum, contact stomatitis, verrucous carcinoma, oral hairy leukoplakia, oral lichen planus, oral lesions of discoid erythematosus, and secondary syphilis. A biopsy should be conducted if no remission is achieved in 2–4 weeks after removing the local irritation factors. Biopsy not only rules out other well-defined diseases histologically but also gives us information about the existence and grade of epithelial dysplasia. This is the basis of the diagnosis and treatment of OLK. The site of biopsy is usually determined based on the findings of the physical examination, but the results of supplementary techniques, such as toluidine blue staining and auto-immunofluorescence, may help the doctor with the judgment.

Various factors should be considered when the treatment plan of OLK is formulated. Common factors include type of lesion, site, size, severity of dysplasia, and reaction to drugs. The initial treatment is to eliminate local irritation factors such as smoking, residual roots, or sharp edges of teeth. If the lesion is homogeneous, small, and located in non-hazardous sites, with no or mild epithelial dysplasia, it can be treated using topical agents only. Retinoids, such as tretinoin paste and 0.1–0.3% retinoic acid ointment, can be applied to the white plaques once or twice per day. Application of the agent to erosive or erythematous lesions should be avoided. Vitamin A and D drops or vitamin E can also be applied, three to four times per day.

If the lesion is large, with multiple sites involved or moderate epithelial dysplasia, systemic medication regimen could be adopted, such as thymosin enteric-coated tablets (20 mg, q.d. or b.i.d.), antioxidants beta-carotene (6 mg, q.d. or b.i.d.), vitamin E (0.1 g, q.d.), and compound danshen dropping pill (ten pills, t.i.d.). The above treatment can be used for 1 month or longer if needed. Regular follow-up visits should be scheduled every 1–2 months.

If the lesion is located in high-risk sites, or nonhomogeneous, or with severe dysplasia, surgical resection should be considered. However, tissue surrounding the white plaques, even with a normal appearance, could be altered molecularly. Thus, complete resection of the lesion does not necessarily mean that it could not recur. Regular follow-up visits should be scheduled.

5.2 Oral Leukokeratosis

Case 47 Oral Leukokeratosis

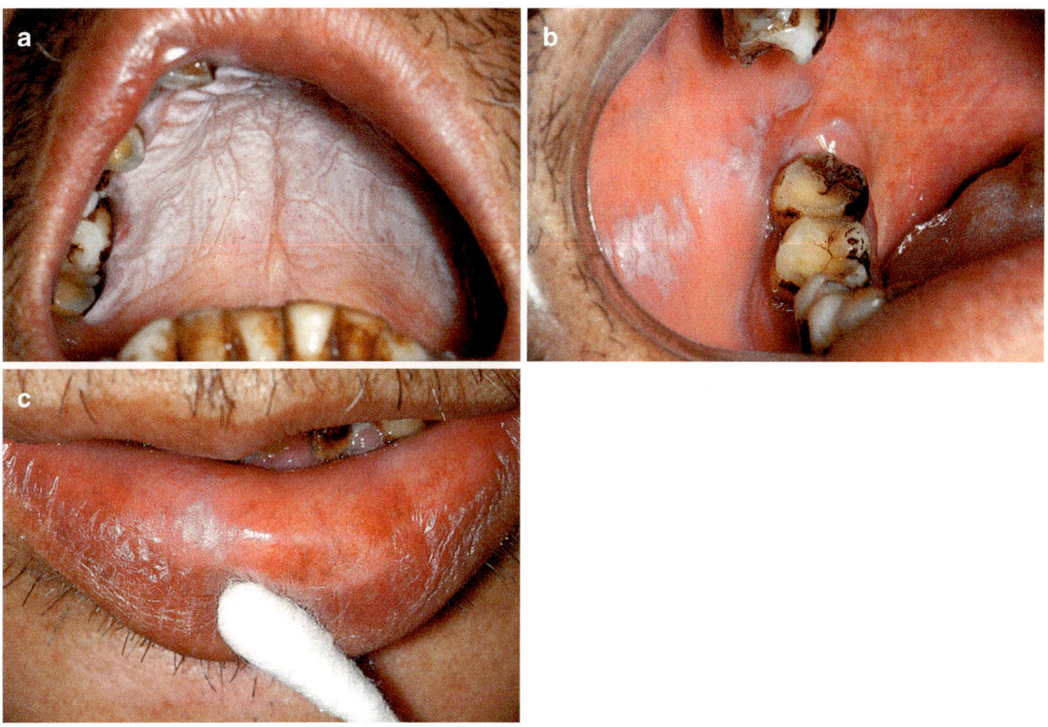

Fig. 5.8 (**a**) Homogeneous white patches widely distributed on the hard palate. Openings of the palatine glands were very clear on the whitish background. (**b**) White patches, flat and ill-demarcated, distributed along the linea alba of the right buccal mucosa. (**c**) Soybean-sized white patch, rough and ill-demarcated, was observed on the mucosa of the right lower lip, almost the location where cigarettes were hold

Age: 59 years
Sex: Male
Chief Complaints:
A 59-year-old man with whitish patches on the palate and cheeks for 4 days
History of Present Illness:
A 59-year-old man complained that he found some white patches on his palate and cheeks 4 days ago. There wasn't any discomfort other than roughness. The patient had been smoking 20–40 cigarettes per day for 40 years.
Past Medical History: Myocardial ischemia.
Allergy: None.
Physical Examination:
Homogeneous white patches widely distributed on the hard palate could be observed. Openings of the palatine glands were very clear on the whitish background (Fig. 5.8a). White patches, flat and ill-demarcated, were distributed along the linea alba of the right buccal mucosa (Fig. 5.8b). Soybean-sized white patch, rough and ill-demarcated, was observed on the mucosa of the right lower lip, almost the location where cigarettes were hold (Fig. 5.8c).
Diagnosis:
Oral leukokeratosis.
Diagnosis Basis:

1. Flat, ill-defined whitish patches on the oral mucosa.
2. The lesions were located on various parts of the oral mucosa.
3. Smoking habits.

Management:

1. The patient was suggested to quit smoking.
2. Medication
   Rp.: Vitamin E 100 mg × 60 tablets
   Sig.: 100 mg q.d. p.o.
   Vitamin A and D drops 15 ml × 1 tube
   Sig.: topical application t.i.d.
3. Regular follow-up was recommended.

[Review] Oral Leukokeratosis, Leukoedema, and Linea Alba

Leukokeratosis is a type of white plaques or patches on the oral mucosa caused by long-term frictional, thermal, chemical stimulation. The stimulations often come from ill-fitting denture, malocclusion, residual root and crown, poor brushing techniques, long-term smoking, and sharp edges of teeth. Labial, buccal, and lingual mucosae are most commonly affected (Fig. 5.9). Partial or complete remission of the lesion can be achieved if the causative factor is eliminated.

Widely distributed keratosis caused by long-term smoking is also called nicotine stomatitis. It's commonly seen on the palatal and buccal mucosa, probably due to chemical and thermal stimulations.

Leukokeratosis often presents as ill-demarcated milky white plaques or patches, with a soft and smooth surface. Epithelial hyperkeratosis is the principal histological change.

The primary treatment is to eliminate the irritation factors, such as quit smoking; remove the residual crown, root and elongated tooth; and eliminate the ill-fitting denture. No risk of malignant transformation of leukokeratosis has been reported [15, 16].

Leukoedema is a type of mucosal change commonly seen on oral mucosa, the cause of which is unknown. There is a high predilection for African-Americans but no gender preference [17]. Tobacco smoking and betel nut chewing are reported factors that can increase the range of the lesion. Similar changes can also be observed on other mucosal surfaces such as the larynx and vagina. Clinically, the lesion looks like the surface of the mucosa is covered by a diffuse, grayish white, or milky veil. Sometimes the mucosal surface can be wrinkled, which will disappear if the mucosa is stretched (Fig. 5.10). The histopathological feature is intracellular edema of spinous cells and thickening of epithelium. Patients with leukoedema seldom have any discomfort. No malignant transformation of this condition has been reported. There's no need for treatment [16].

Linea alba refers to an asymptomatic linear elevation on the buccal mucosa, level with the occlusal plane. It usually extends from the angle of the mouth to the molar teeth (Fig. 5.11). It is commonly seen in adults and is probably caused by irritation from the teeth. Similar white line could also appear along the border of the tongue due to long-term stimulation from the lingual edge of mandibular teeth. The pathological feature is hyperkeratosis. No treatment is needed, and spontaneous remission can be achieved in some cases [16].

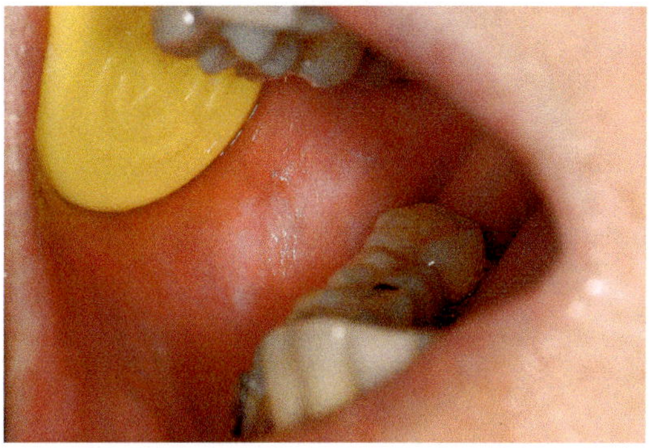

Fig. 5.9 White patches, flat, dispersed, and ill-demarcated, were found on the right buccal mucosa

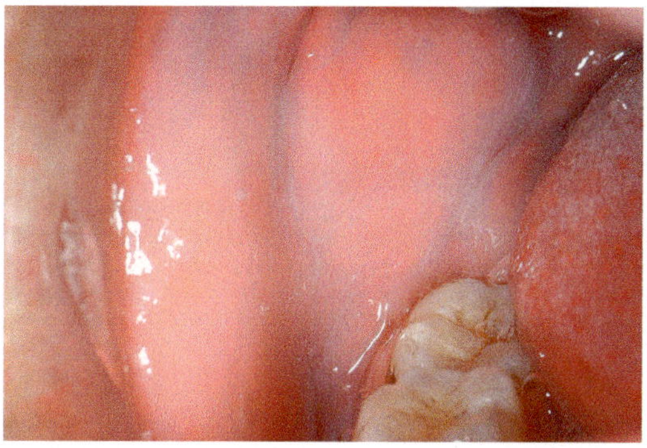

Fig. 5.10 Right buccal mucosa with a diffuse, grayish white, milky, and wrinkled surface

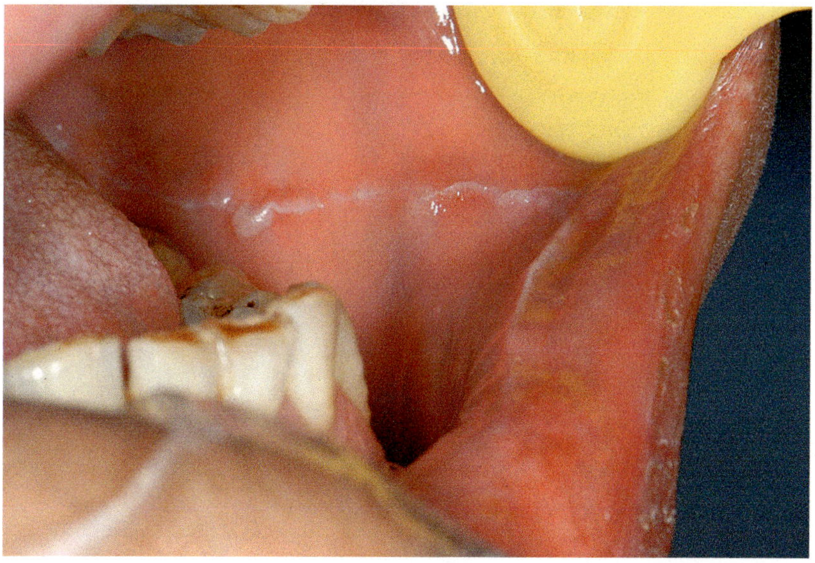

Fig. 5.11 Linear elevation at the level of occlusal line on the inner surface of the left buccal mucosa

5.3 White Sponge Nevus

Case 48 White Sponge Nevus

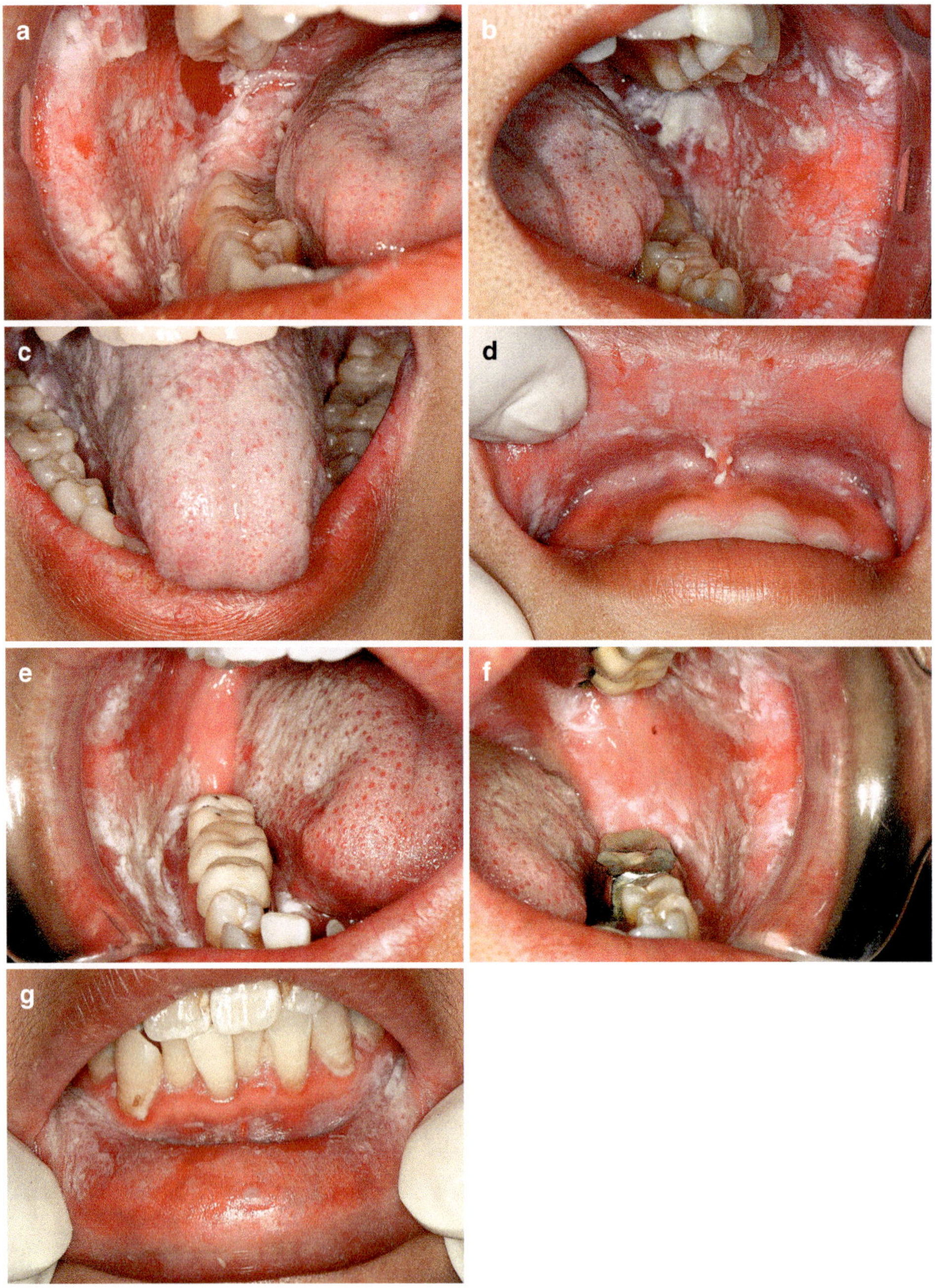

Fig. 5.12 (**a**) White spongy patches widely distributed on the right buccal mucosa. (**b**) White spongy patches widely distributed on the left buccal mucosa. (**c**) White spongy patches widely distributed on the dorsum of the tongue. (**d**) White spongy patches widely distributed on the upper lip. (**e**) The mother of the patient also had white spongy lesions on the right buccal mucosa. (**f**) The mother of the patient also had white spongy lesions on the left buccal mucosa. (**g**) The mother of the patient also had white spongy lesions on the lower lip and mucosa lining on the vestibular groove of the mandibular incisors

Age: 17 years
Sex: Female
Chief Complaints:
A 17-year-old girl with white plaques in the mouth for 10 years
History of Present Illness:
A 17-year-old girl came to our clinic, complaining that she had white plaques in the mouth for 10 years. There wasn't any discomfort. The white patches got thicker when she had a cold. Her mother also had similar symptoms for more than 1 year. Both the patient and her mother denied any history of recurrent fever and rapid weight loss.
Past Medical History: None.
Allergy: None.
Physical Examination:
White spongy patches were widely distributed on the oral mucosa. Part of them can be erased, leaving a normal or erythematous surface (Fig. 5.12a–d). Her mother also had similar lesions on the oral mucosa (Fig. 5.12e–g).
Clinical Impression:
White sponge nevus

Laboratory Investigations:

1. Whole blood cell count didn't reveal any abnormality. Anti-HIV antibody was negative.
2. A lesional biopsy was made on the left buccal mucosa. Findings of routine histological examination (HE staining) was in accord with white sponge nevus.

Diagnosis:
White sponge nevus
Diagnosis Basis:

1. Lesions presented early in life.
2. Family history.
3. Widely distributed white spongy patches on the oral mucosa
4. Findings of histological examination.

Management:
The cause and prognosis of the disease was explained. No treatment was recommended.

Case 49 White Sponge Nevus

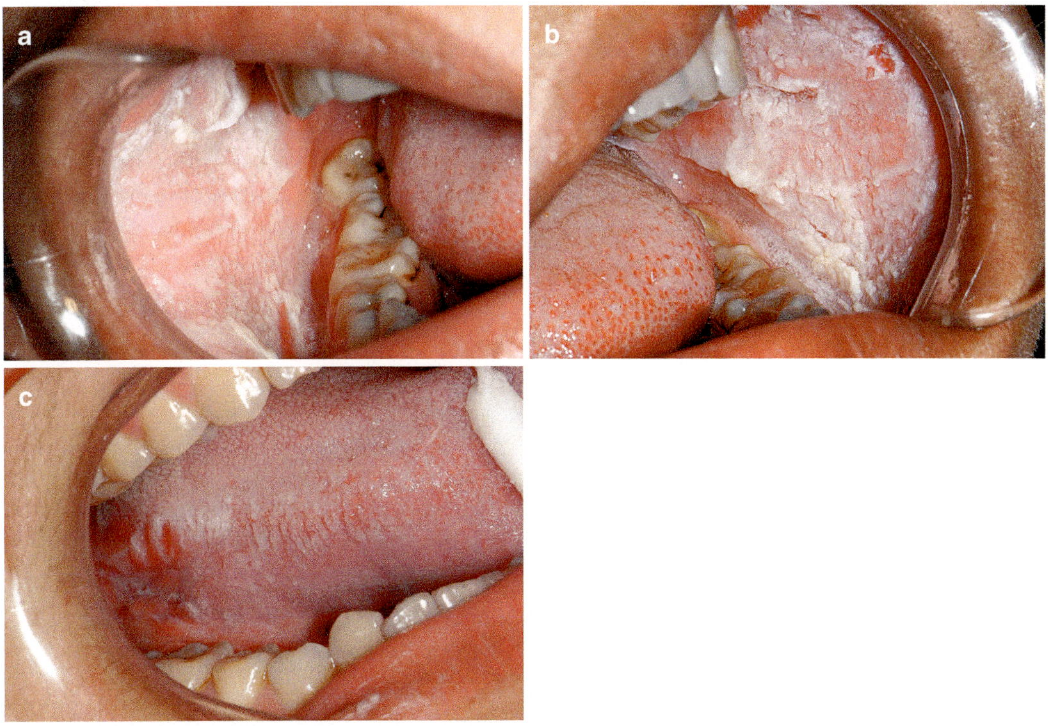

Fig. 5.13 (**a**) White spongy patches widely distributed on the right buccal mucosa. (**b**) White spongy patches widely distributed on the left buccal mucosa. (**c**) White spongy patches widely distributed along the border of the tongue

Age: 20 years
Sex: Female
Chief Complaints:
A 20-year-old woman with white plaques on the oral mucosa for 9 years
History of Present Illness:
A 20-year-old woman complained that she had white plaques on the oral mucosa for 9 years. There wasn't any discomfort other than dryness. Her sister also had similar lesions on the oral mucosa.
Past Medical History: Hepatitis B.
Allergy: None.
Physical Examination:
White spongy patches were widely distributed on the lateral border of the tongue, buccal mucosa, soft palate, and floor of the mouth. Part of them can be erased, leaving an erythematous surface (Fig. 5.13).
Clinical Impression:
White sponge nevus
Laboratory Investigations:

1. Whole blood cell count didn't reveal any abnormality. Anti-HIV antibody was negative.
2. A lesional biopsy was made on the right buccal mucosa. Findings of routine histological examination (HE staining) was in accord with white sponge nevus.

Diagnosis:
White sponge nevus
Diagnosis Basis:

1. Lesions presented early in life.
2. Family history.
3. Widely distributed white spongy patches on the oral mucosa
4. Findings of histological examination.

Management:
The cause and prognosis of the disease was explained. No treatment was recommended.

[Review] White Sponge Nevus
White sponge nevus is considered as an autosomal dominant disease resulting from point mutation of either keratin 4 or keratin 13 genes [18–20]. A family history may be noticed.

Lesions usually appear before puberty, presenting as bilaterally distributed soft white spongy patches on the mucosa. The patches may be partially erased, without causing any erosion. Buccal mucosa is most commonly affected. Lesions may also be found on the lip, tongue, and the floor of the mouth. The mucosa of the esophagus, larynx, nasal cavity, and anogenital area may also be involved [16, 21].

The characteristic pathological findings include parakeratosis, thickening of the epithelium, and intracellular edema with perinuclear condensation of keratin [21].

The diagnosis is based on clinical manifestations and family history. Histological examination is adopted when it is difficult to be differentiated from other white lesions. This disorder hasn't been associated with any risk of malignant transformation. No treatment is needed if the patient doesn't report any discomfort.

5.4 Oral Lichen Planus

Case 50 Oral Lichen Planus (Non-erosive Type)

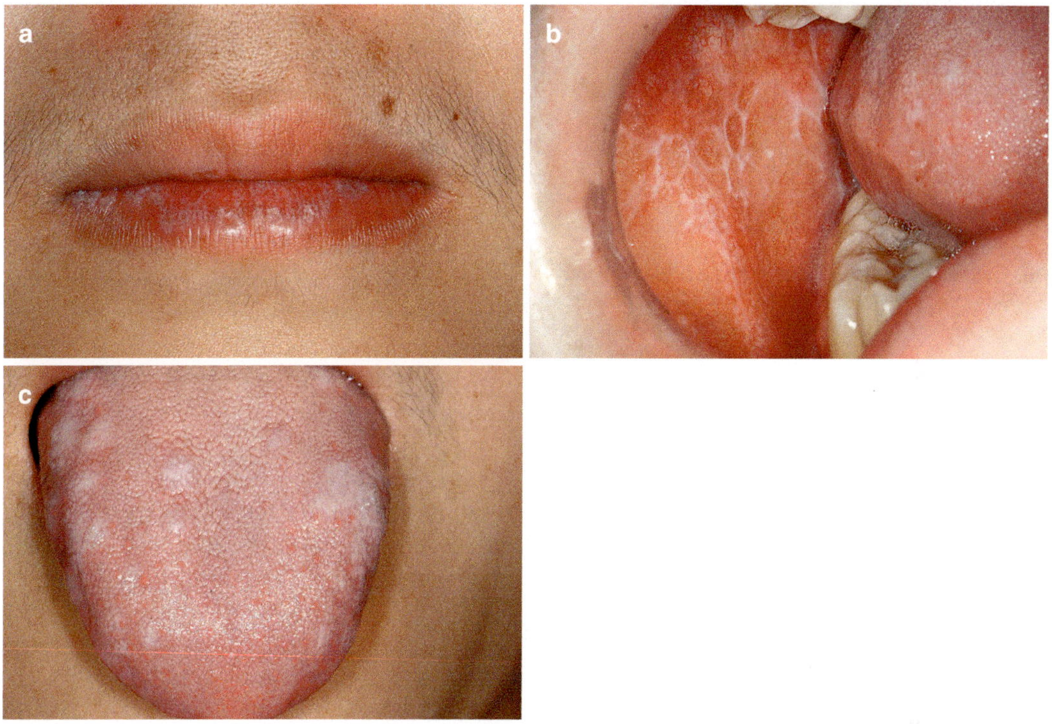

Fig. 5.14 (**a**) Pearl white streaks on the lower lip. (**b**) Pearl white streaks on the right buccal mucosa. (**c**) Pearl white patches on the dorsum of the tongue

Age: 23 years
Sex: Female
Chief Complaints:
A 23-year-old woman with pain while eating spicy food for more than 1 year
History of Present Illness:
A 23-year-old woman came with a complaint of pain on the tongue when she was eating hot or spicy food for more than 1 year. There was no spontaneous pain.
Past Medical History: None.
Allergy: None.
Physical Examination:
Pearl white lacy streaks and patches were seen on the lower lip, left and right buccal mucosa, and dorsum of the tongue (Fig. 5.14). There was no erythematous or erosive lesion. No abnormality was found on the fingernails and skin.

Diagnosis:
Oral lichen planus (non-erosive type)
Diagnosis Basis:

1. Pearl white lacy streaks and patches.
2. No obvious inducing factors.

Management:

1. Medication
   Rp.: Thymosin enteric-coated tablets 20 mg × 30 tablets
   Sig.: 20 mg q.d. p.o.
   Beta-carotene 6 mg × 60 tablets
   Sig.: 6 mg q.d. p.o.
   Dexamethasone paste 15 g × 1
   Sig.: topical use t.i.d.
2. Regular follow-up visits were suggested.

Case 51 Oral Lichen Planus (Erosive Type)

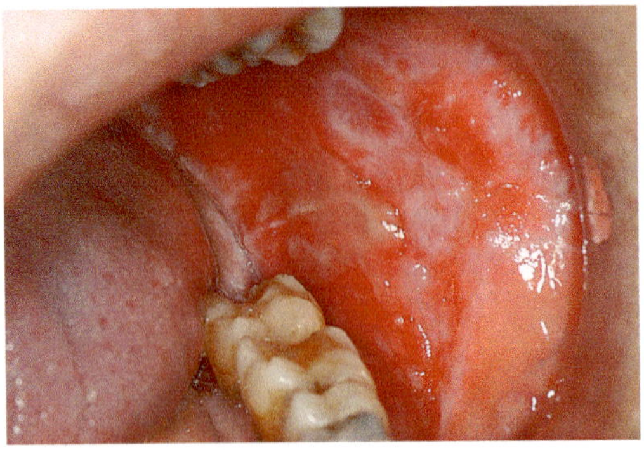

Fig. 5.15 Pearl white lacy streaks and patches with interspersed erythematous and erosive lesions on the buccal mucosa

Age: 58 years
Sex: Female
Chief Complaints:
A 58-year-old woman with erosion and pain on the buccal mucosa for 2 months
History of Present Illness:
A 58-year-old woman complained of erosion and pain on the buccal mucosa for 2 months. The pain got worse when she was eating hot or spicy food.
Past Medical History: None.
Allergy: None.
Physical Examination:
Pearl white lacy streaks and patches with interspersed erythematous and erosive lesions were seen on the buccal mucosa. No abnormality was found on the fingernails and skin (Fig. 5.15).
Diagnosis:
Oral lichen planus (erosive type).
Diagnosis Basis:

1. Pearl white lacy streaks and patches with erythematous and erosive lesions.
2. No obvious inducing factors.

Management:

1. Medication
   Rp.: Prednisone acetate tablets 5 mg × 35 tablets
   Sig.: 25 mg q.m. p.o.
   Compound chlorhexidine solution 300 ml × 1
   Sig.: rinse t.i.d.
   Dexamethasone paste 15 g × 1
   Sig.: topical use t.i.d.
2. Aerosol therapy
   Rp.: Dexamethasone sodium phosphate injection 1 ml × 1
   Gentamycin sulfate injection 2 ml × 1
   Vitamin B12 injection 1 ml × 1
   Vitamin C injection 2.5 ml × 1
   Sig.: aerosol therapy b.i.d.
3. A follow-up visit after 1 week was scheduled.

Follow-Up Treatment:
In the follow-up visit, the erosions got localized, intra-lesional injection of triamcinolone acetonide was given, and the oral medication was switched to tripterygium hypoglaucum tablets (two tablets t.i.d. p.o.).

[Review] Oral Lichen Planus

Oral lichen planus (OLP) is a chronic inflammatory disorder of the oral mucosa. It affects about 0.5–3% of the population, especially women aged from 30 to 60 years. Compared with the normal oral mucosa, OLP has a higher risk of cancer development and is thus classified by the World Health Organization as one of the oral potentially malignant disorders [22].

Although the etiology of OLP is still unclear, the association of immune dysregulation with the pathogenesis of this disease is widely accepted. The primary event of this process is the interaction between endogenous and exogenous factors (antigens, drugs, viruses, psychological stress [23], and so on) with keratinocytes (KCs), which then leads to degranulation of mast cells, activation of macrophages, and release of proinflammatory cytokines such as tumor necrosis factor-α (TNF-α). TNF-α not only affects T-lymphocyte homing but also induces the expression of adhesion molecules by endothelial cells and KCs. The expression of adhesion molecules promotes the infiltration of lymphocytes, which further promote degranulation of mast cells and produce interferon-γ (IFN-γ), leading to extension of the lesion. IFN-γ not only upregulates expression of major histocompatibility complex (MHC) class I but also induces expression of

MHC class II by KCs. Modified surface antigens of KCs can be recognized by Langerhans cells (LC) and presented to T lymphocytes. KCs then become the target of cytotoxic T cells. Damaged keratinocytes release cytokines which could further stimulate the differentiation and chemotaxis of Langerhans cells, as well as the growth of T lymphocytes.

Although the relationship between genetic factors and OLP is still controversial, studies have shown that gene polymorphisms of several cytokines, such as TNF-α and interleukin (IL)-10, may be associated with individual's susceptibility to OLP [24–27].

Studies on the association between OLP and infective factors mainly focus on hepatitis C virus (HCV) infection. Researches carried out in different regions provide us with different results, some of them are contradictory [28–31]. The association of OLP and HCV infection HCV is still controversial [32].Some researchers suggested that patients with or without HCV had different hereditary basis, which might be related with the allele of HLA-DR6 gene [32].

There are six types of OLP lesions: papular, reticular, plaque-like, atrophic, erosive/ulcerative, and bullous. Reticular OLP usually presents as asymptomatic pearl white lacy streaks distributed in a reticular or circular pattern (Fig. 5.16). This type of lesion is most commonly seen on the buccal mucosa but can also be observed on the lips, gingiva, and tongue. Papular OLP is clinically characterized by small white dots on the mucosa (Fig. 5.17), which usually intermingles with other forms of OLP. Plaque-like OLP often locates on the buccal mucosa and dorsal surface of the tongue. This type of lesion is usually smooth, flat, or slightly elevated, similar to homogeneous oral leukoplakia (Figs. 5.18 and 5.19). Atrophic OLP is most frequently observed

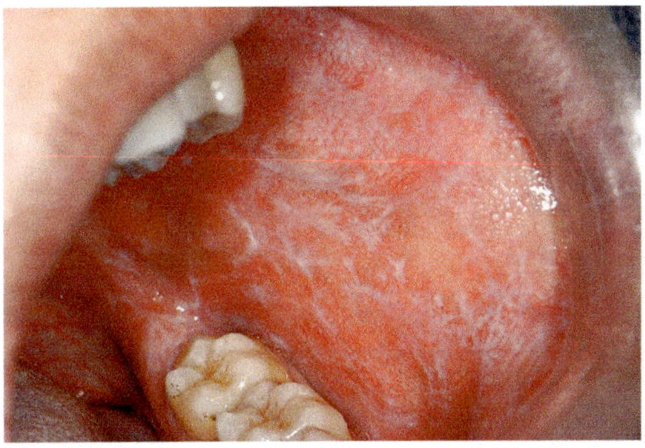

Fig. 5.16 Reticular form: pearl white lacy streaks on left buccal mucosa

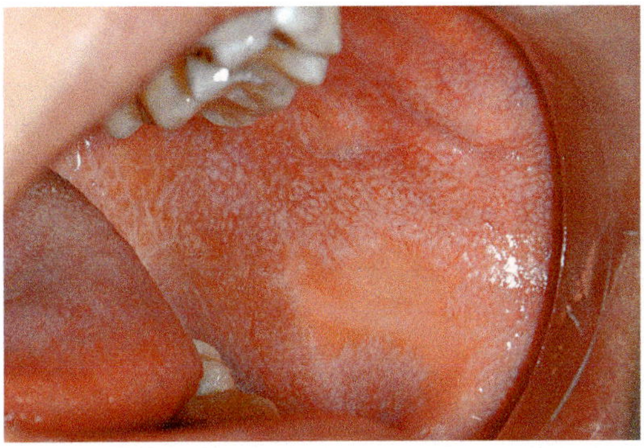

Fig. 5.17 Papular form: lots of white dots densely distributed on the left buccal mucosa

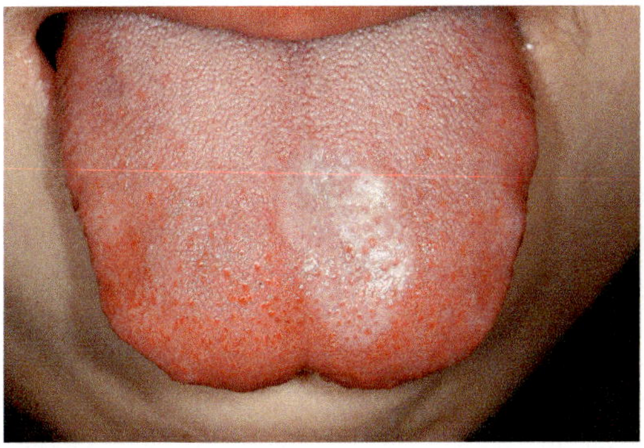

Fig. 5.18 Plaque-like form: single pearl white patch on dorsum of the tongue

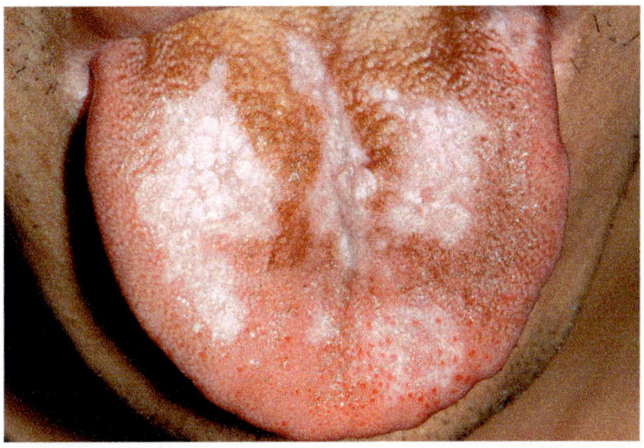

Fig. 5.19 Plaque-like form: multiple pearl white patches on dorsum of the tongue, flat or slightly elevated

on dorsum of the tongue, presenting as atrophy of lingual papilla surrounded by white streaks (Fig. 5.20). Patients with atrophic OLP may have burning sensation and pain while eating. Erosive/ulcerative OLP are characterized by erosive/ulcerative lesions surrounded by white streaks [33].The bullous lesions in OLP are usually quite small, with a diameter of about 2 mm; sometimes larger bulla can also be seen (Fig. 5.21). The forms mentioned above can be divided into two major types: erosive type and non-erosive type.

Some OLP patients have skin lesions, with predilection for the flexor aspects of the extremities. Cutaneous lesions are mostly symmetrical, presenting as flat violaceous papules. The papules can get confluent and form patches or plaques that are slightly elevated, well-demarcated, with a waxy luster and white streaks (Wickham's striae) (Figs. 5.22 and 5.23). Skin lesions can be itchy. If the scalp is involved, hair follicles can be destroyed, leading to alopecia. Affected nails/toenails are usually thin, wrinkled, and reluster, with tiny scales, longitudinal grooves, pits, and ridges (Fig. 5.22). Skin of the scrotum is occasionally involved [33].

OLP is considered as an oral potentially malignant disorder (Fig. 5.24); however, due to the heterogenicity of different studies, the reported frequency of malignant transformation varies a lot. A recent study carried out by a Chinese group showed that the malignant transformation rate of OLP was less than 1% [34]. Since malignant transformation was frequently found at locations distant to OLP lesions, some researchers thought

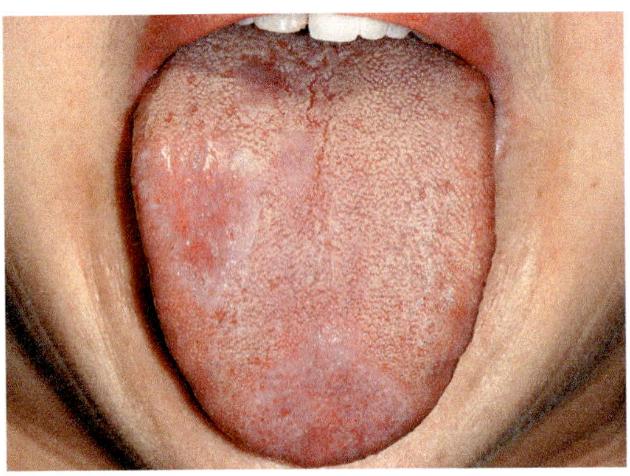

Fig. 5.20 Atrophic form: atrophy of lingual papilla surrounded by pearl white streaks

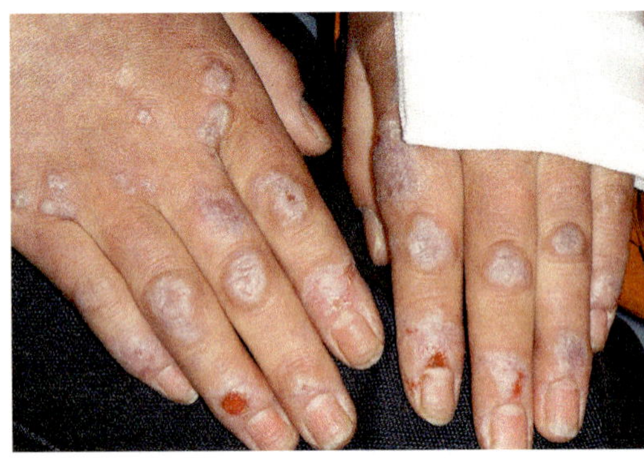

Fig. 5.22 Skin and nail/toenail lesions: violaceous papules forming patches or flat-topped plaques with a waxy luster and white streaks; atrophic nails with longitudinal grooves

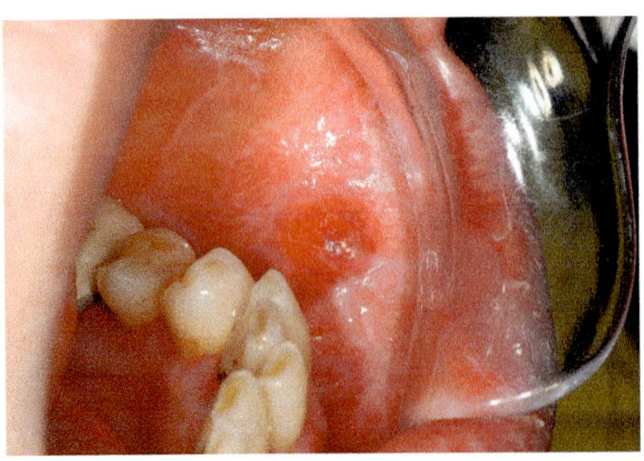

Fig. 5.21 Bullous form: bullous lesions of various sizes surrounded by pearl white streaks on the inner surface of the left lower lip

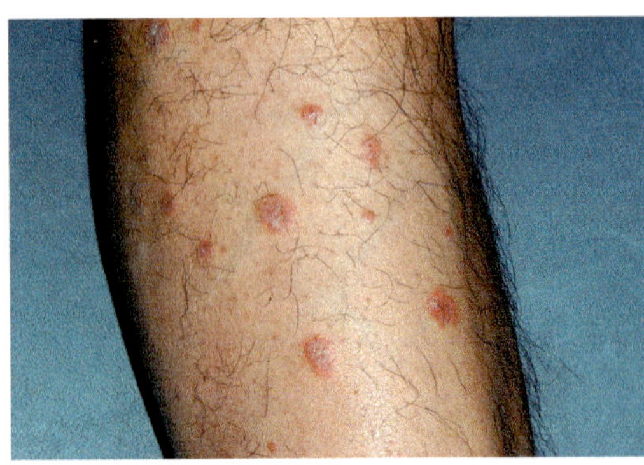

Fig. 5.23 Skin lesions: violaceous flat papules on the skin of the leg

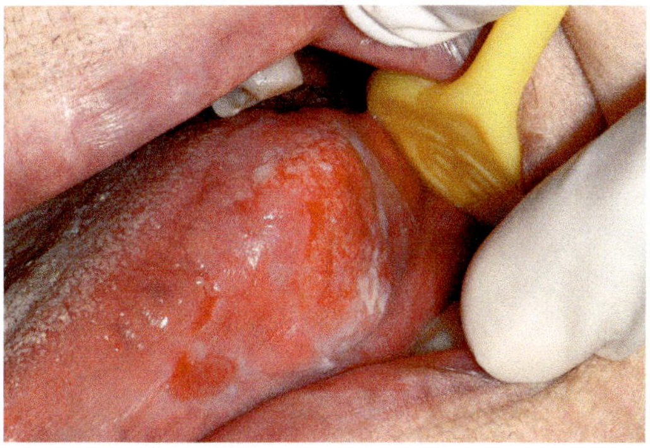

Fig. 5.24 Malignant transformation of OLP on the lateral and ventral surface of the tongue

that malignant transformation might be a result of external factors rather than the natural terminate of OLP. They also believed that those cases with malignant transformation might not be OLP but lichenoid reactions [35]. In short, the risk of malignant transformation is low in OLP. Besides elimination of irritation factors, regular follow-up visits at the frequency of at least twice a year are recommended.

The treatment goal of OLP is to facilitate healing of erosion and ulceration, alleviate pain and discomfort, and reduce the risk of malignant transformation.

For patients with asymptomatic non-erosive OLP, no treatment but regular follow-up visits are recommended.

For patients with non-erosive OLP and no discomfort other than roughness, the following medication regimens may be used: compound danshen dripping pill (10 pills t.i.d. p.o.), β-carotene capsules (6 mg q.d./b.i.d. p.o.), or vitamin E capsules (100 mg q.d. p.o.), used continuously for 1 month. Cod liver oil, vitamin A and D drops, and vitamin E can be applied topically 3–4 times a day. If the lesions are extremely keratotic and thick, 0.1–0.3% acitretin oral paste or 1% viaminate oral paste can be applied topically once or twice a day.

For patients with non-erosive OLP and pain while eating, if immunodeficiency is indicated, medications containing immunopotentiators may be used: transfer factor capsules (6 mg t.i.d. p.o.), thymosin enteric-coated tablets (20 mg q.d./b.i.d./t.i.d. p.o.), pidotimod (400 mg q.d./b.i.d. p.o.), or bacillus Calmette-Guerin polysaccharide nucleic acid injection (1 ml q.o.d. i.m.), used for a month. Topical treatment agents such as 0.01% chlorhexidine mouth wash and compound borax solution (diluted fivefold with water before use) can be used three times a day. Glucocorticoids like dexamethasone paste, prednisolone acetate solution, triamcinolone acetonide (diluted fivefold with water before use), triamcinolone acetonide dental paste, and dexamethasone ointment can be applied topically three times a day.

For patients with a limited number of small erosive lesions, triamcinolone acetonide injection or compound betamethasone injection combined with sterile water or 2% lidocaine (at a ratio of 1:1) can be used for intra-lesional injection. Oral medications and topical agents are similar to those used for patients with non-erosive OLP and pain while eating.

For patients with larger or multiple small erosive lesions, triamcinolone acetonide injection or compound betamethasone injection combined with sterile water or 2% lidocaine (at a ratio of 1:1) can be used for intra-lesional injection. Tripterygium hypoglaucum tablets (two tablets t.i.d. for 2 weeks or longer) can be used. Topical agents are similar to those used for patients with non-erosive OLP and pain while eating.

For patients with widespread erosive lesions, systemic prednisone acetate (15–30 mg daily, in a single morning dose, for 1–2 weeks) can be used in combination with aerosol therapy (dexamethasone sodium phosphate injection, gentamycin sulfate injection, vitamin C injection, and vitamin B12 injection, once or twice a day for 3–5 days). Once the erosive lesions are controlled, the medication regimen can be switched to tripterygium hypoglaucum tablets (two tablets t.i.d. for 2 weeks or longer) or tripterygium glycosides tablets (1–1.5 mg/kg/day, divided to three doses, for 2 weeks or longer). Topical agents are similar to those used for patients with non-erosive OLP and pain while eating. Moreover, 2–4% sodium bicarbonate mouthwash and nystatin liniment can also be used topically.

5.5 Lichenoid Reactions

Case 52 Lichenoid Reaction Caused by Dental Amalgam

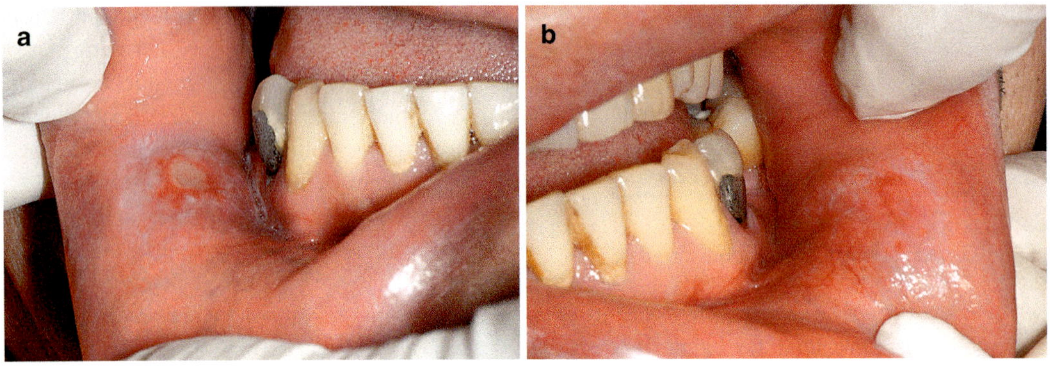

Fig. 5.25 (**a**) White striae and ulcerative lesion on the mucosa next to the amalgam restoration. (**b**) White striae on the mucosa next to the amalgam restoration

Age: 41 years
Sex: Male
Chief Complaints:
A 41-year-old man with white striae on the oral mucosa for more than 3 months
History of Present Illness:
A 41-year-old man complained of white striae on the oral mucosa for more than 3 months. There was no discomfort until 1 week ago, when an ulcer appeared in the center of the lesion.
Past Medical History:
The patient had his teeth filled 6 months ago. He denied any history of systemic diseases.
Allergy: None.
Physical Examination:
White striae were observed on the mucosa close to the amalgam restorations on the buccal side of mandibular first premolar teeth (Fig. 5.25a-b); an ulcer with a diameter of 4 mm was seen in the center of the white lesion on the right side.

Diagnosis:
Lichenoid reaction.
Diagnosis Basis:

1. White striae and ulcer in the center.
2. Amalgam restorations right next to the lesion.
3. Lesions disappeared after the amalgam restorations were replaced with resin.

Management:

1. Medication
   Rp.: Dexamethasone paste 15 g × 1
   Sig.: topical use t.i.d.
2. Amalgam restorations were replaced with resin.

Follow-Up Treatment:
One month after amalgam restorations were replaced with resin, the lesion regression was observed.

Case 53 Lichenoid Reaction (Chronic Graft-Versus-Host Disease)

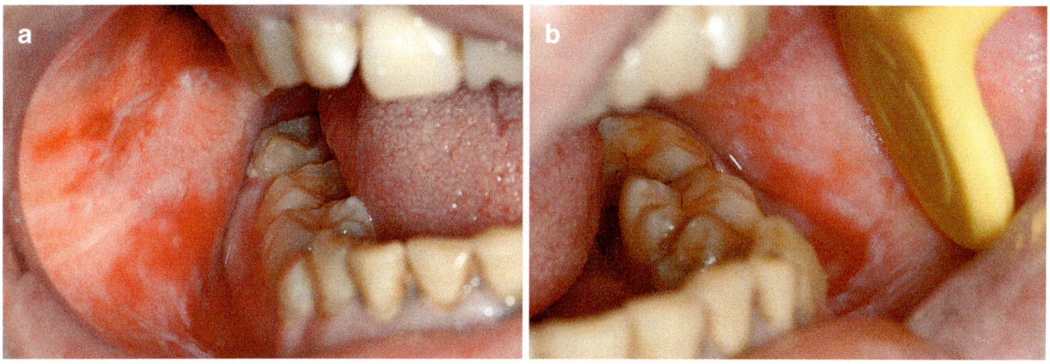

Fig. 5.26 (**a**) White striae with interspersed erythema on the right buccal mucosa. (**b**) White striae on the left buccal mucosa, with erythematous and erosive lesions on the mucosa lining the vestibular groove of the left mandibular molars

Age: 43 years
Sex: Male
Chief Complaints:
A 43-year-old man with recurrent erosions and pain of the oral mucosa for 6 months
History of Present Illness:
A 43-year-old man complained that he had been suffering from recurrent erosions and pain of the oral mucosa since he had bone marrow transplantation 6 months ago. The symptoms could be partially relieved when he used mouth rinses prescribed by local doctors.
Past Medical History:
Bone marrow transplantation 6 months ago due to leukemia.
Allergy: None.
Physical Examination:
White striae with interspersed erythematous lesions were observed on the buccal mucosa; erosion with a size of 12 mm × 4 mm was seen on the mucosa lining the vestibular groove of the left mandibular molars (Fig. 5.26a-b).
Diagnosis:
Lichenoid reaction (chronic graft-versus-host disease)
Diagnosis Basis:

1. White striae with interspersed erythematous lesions and erosion on the buccal mucosa.
2. Lesions appeared after bone marrow transplantation.

Management:

1. Medication
   Rp.: Compound chlorhexidine solution 300 ml × 1
   Sig.: rinse t.i.d.
   Dexamethasone paste 15 g × 1
   Sig.: topical use t.i.d.
   Triamcinolone acetonide (TA) injection 40 mg × 1
   Sig.: Intra-lesional injection at the dose of 8 mg/site s.t.

[Review] Lichenoid Reactions
Lichenoid reactions may involve the skin and oral mucosa. Oral lichenoid reactions (OLR) present as lesions similar to OLP, such as white streaks, white patches, and erythematous/ulcerative lesions. According to the etiological factors, OLR can be classified into three types: oral lichenoid contact lesions, oral lichenoid drug reactions, and oral lichenoid reactions of graft-versus-host disease (GVHD) [36].

Oral lichenoid contact lesion is a special type of allergic contact stomatitis. It belongs to the group of delayed hypersensitivity reactions. The lesions are usually right next to dental restoration materials, such as dental amalgam. Partial or total remission can be achieved shortly after elimination of the irritation [37].

Oral lichenoid drug reactions are often induced by medications such as β-blockers, angiotensin-converting enzyme inhibitors, non-steroidal anti-inflammatory agents, and methyldopa and hypoglycemic agents [38].

GVHD is quite common in patients receiving either peripheral blood stem cell or bone marrow stem cell transplantation [39]. Patients receiving organ transplantation can also develop GVHD. The risk of GVHD is higher when the host is unrelated with the donor or when the donor or host is old. Acute GVHD typically presents as erythematous eruptions, diarrhea, and/or hepatitis, which most commonly occur within the first 3–4 months. Chronic GVHD (cGVHD) can affect almost all the major organ systems. The skin, conjunctiva, oral and vaginal mucosa, liver, and salivary and lacrimal glands are most commonly involved [40].The number of patients receiving allogenic hematopoietic cell transplantation each year is around 15,000 worldwide. The estimated incidence of cGVHD is about 40–70% in patients who survived the initial transplantation [40].

Oral lesions occur in 45–83% of cGVHD cases. Lichenoid lesions and dryness of the oral mucosa are two of the most common oral manifestations. The former can last for a long time and can be difficult to be differentiated from OLP clinically and histologically [22, 41].

The primary treatment of oral lichenoid contact lesions and oral lichenoid drug reactions is to eliminate the irritation factors, such as replacing the dental restoration material and changing the medication regimen. The treatment goal of oral GVHD is to relieve pain and eating difficulty and to improve the life quality of patients. To control the existing lichenoid reactions, topical therapy similar to that used for erosive OLP is recommended.

5.6 Oral Erythroplakia

Case 54 Oral Erythroplakia

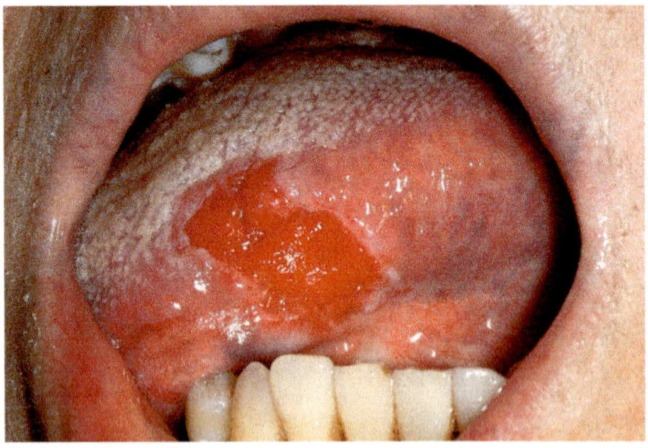

Fig. 5.27 A soft, well-defined erythematous lesion with a slightly rough surface on the lingual mucosa

Age: 63 years
Sex: Female
Chief Complaints:
A 63-year-old woman with pain on the tongue for 1 year
History of Present Illness:
A 63-year-old woman complained of pain on the tongue for 1 year. The patient was diagnosed with oral lichen planus at a local hospital and had been taking traditional Chinese medicine since then. However, no improvement had been achieved and the pain was getting worse.
Past Medical History: None.
Allergy: None.
Physical Examination:
A soft, well-defined erythematous lesion with a slightly rough surface was observed on the left ventral and lateral surface of the tongue (Fig. 5.27).

Laboratory Investigations:
A lesional biopsy was made on left margin of the tongue, and histopathological findings were in accord with erythroplakia with mild-to-moderate epithelial dysplasia.
Diagnosis:
Oral erythroplakia
Diagnosis Basis:

1. Well-defined erythematous lesion on the oral mucosa.
2. Findings of histopathological examination.

Management:
The patient was referred to the Department of Oral and Maxillofacial Surgery for further examinations and treatment.

Case 55 Malignant Transformation of Oral Erythroleukoplakia

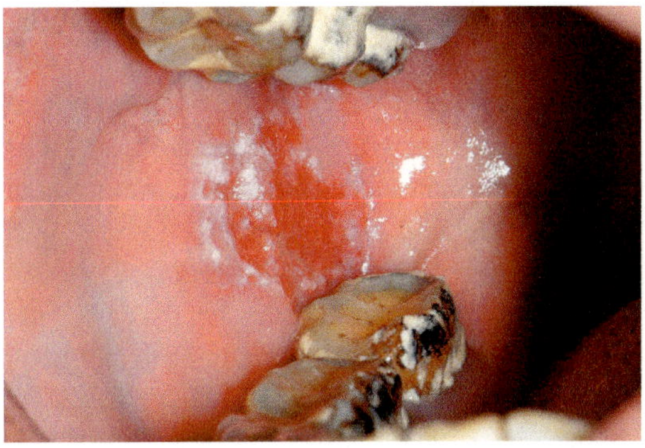

Fig. 5.28 A well-defined erythematous lesion with interspersed white dots and erosions was observed on the right buccal mucosa

Age: 45 years
Sex: Male
Chief Complaints:
A 45-year-old man with pain on the right cheek for 6 months
History of Present Illness:
A 45-year-old man complained of pain on the right cheek for 6 months. The patient also had pain when he was eating. He had been using some over-the-counter oral paste, but no improvement had been achieved.
Past Medical History: None.
Allergy: None.
Physical Examination:
A well-defined erythematous lesion with interspersed erosions was observed on the right cheek. The anterior part of the lesion was accompanied with some irregular white dots (Fig. 5.28).
Laboratory Investigations:
A lesional biopsy was made on the right buccal mucosa, and histopathological findings suggested carcinoma in situ with focal infiltration into the lamina propria.
Diagnosis:
Carcinoma in situ (malignant transformation of oral erythroleukoplakia)
Diagnosis Basis:

1. Well-defined erythematous lesion with irregular white dots.
2. Findings of histopathological examination.

Management:
The patient was referred to the Department of Oral and Maxillofacial Surgery for further examinations and treatments.

[Review] Oral Erythroplakia
According to Kramer et al., the definition of oral erythroplakia is "any lesion of the oral mucosa that presents as bright red velvety plaques which cannot be characterized clinically or pathologically as any other recognizable condition" [42]. In an article by Villa et al., several studies on the prevalence of oral erythroplakia carried out between 1971 and 2007 were analyzed; the reported prevalence ranges from 0.02% to 0.2% (mean prevalence, 0.11%), and the estimated malignant transformation rate was 44.9% [43, 44]. Oral erythroplakia usually affects middle-aged and senior citizens. No gender preference has been observed.

The etiology and pathogenesis of oral erythroplakia is still unclear. Most patients have history of smoking and excessive drinking. Besides, aberrant DNA content (DNA aneuploidy), mutation of p53 gene, human papillomavirus, and candida infection may also contribute to the development of this disorder. There is no consensus whether oral erythroplakia is a primary disease or a disease that evolves from oral leukoplakia [45].

Oral erythroplakia most commonly locates on the ventral surface of the tongue, the floor of the mouth, the palate, and the tonsillar fossa. The patients usually complain of pain or a burning sensation on the mucosa. A typical lesion of oral erythroplakia is a bright red velvety plaque with a smooth, speckled, or nodular surface. The lesion is usually well-defined, and the red color doesn't fade under pressure. The lesions won't disappear after anti-infective therapy. Sometimes, the red lesion is interspersed with yellow-white spots. The lesion is usually single and soft. However, it may become indurated during the process of malignant transformation [46]. Oral erythroplakia is divided into three subtypes according to the clinical manifestation:

1. Homogeneous erythroplakia: well-defined red lesion with a smooth surface, either flat or slightly raised, with a diameter of less than 2 cm; usually locates on the buccal or palatal mucosa; normal mucosa may be seen in the lesion (Fig. 5.29).
2. Interspersed erythroplakia: white spots interspersed among an erythematous lesion, similar to lichen planus.
3. Granular or speckled erythroplakia: granules can be observed on the erythematous lesion. This is the most common type of oral erythroplakia which can affect almost any part of the oral mucosa. The histological examination often shows carcinoma in situ or invasive cancer.

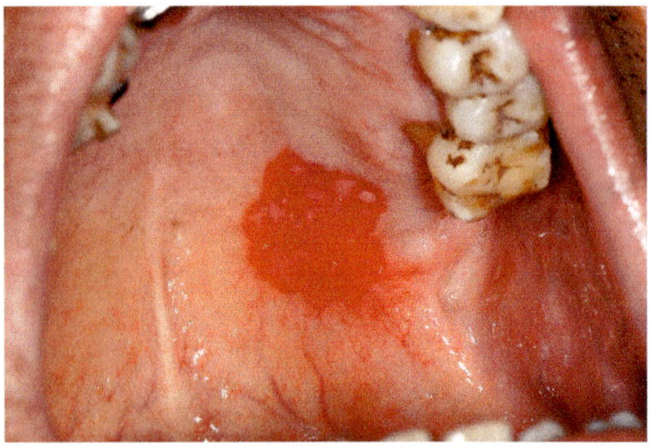

Fig. 5.29 Homogeneous erythroplakia: well-defined red lesion with a smooth surface and with normal mucosa scattered in the lesion

Under histological examination, oral erythroplakia often present as epithelial atrophy, lack of cuticle, and epithelium dysplasia. Cancer in situ or squamous cell carcinoma can be observed in some advanced cases [43]. Some researchers proposed that atrophy of the epithelium and the exposed microvasculature might account for the red appearance of the lesion. However, this hypothesis could not explain the thickening of the epithelium in some parts of the lesion [47].

Oral erythroplakia is a diagnosis of exclusion. It should be differentiated from several oral mucosal diseases, such as stomatitis associated with local irritation, erythematous candidiasis, oral lichen planus, chronic discoid lupus erythematosus, medicamentous reaction, and syphilitic mucous patches. The first thing is to remove the irritating factor. Anti-infective therapy may be followed. Two percent sodium bicarbonate solution and nystatin suspension can be used if fungal infection is suspected. If non-fungal infection or traumatic stomatitis is considered, mouthwash such as compound chlorhexidine solution, compound borax solution (using 1:5 dilution), or 1% povidone iodine solution can be used; topical corticosteroids such as dexamethasone ointment, prednisolone suspension, and triamcinolone acetonide oral paste can also be applied. Moreover, intra-lesional injection of triamcinolone acetonide can be performed. If the lesion doesn't heal or improve in 10–14 days, a lesional biopsy is strongly recommended [48].

Once the diagnosis of oral erythroplakia is confirmed, the recommended treatment is surgical excision. Nevertheless, there is no widely accepted guideline regarding the range of excision. Few data on the recurrence of this disease are available [49]. Comprehensive evaluation of the related symptoms and clinical signs, early detection of the disease, long-term follow-up, and reasonable biopsy should be applied to prevent malignant transformation [50].

5.7 Oral Submucous Fibrosis

Case 56 Oral Submucous Fibrosis

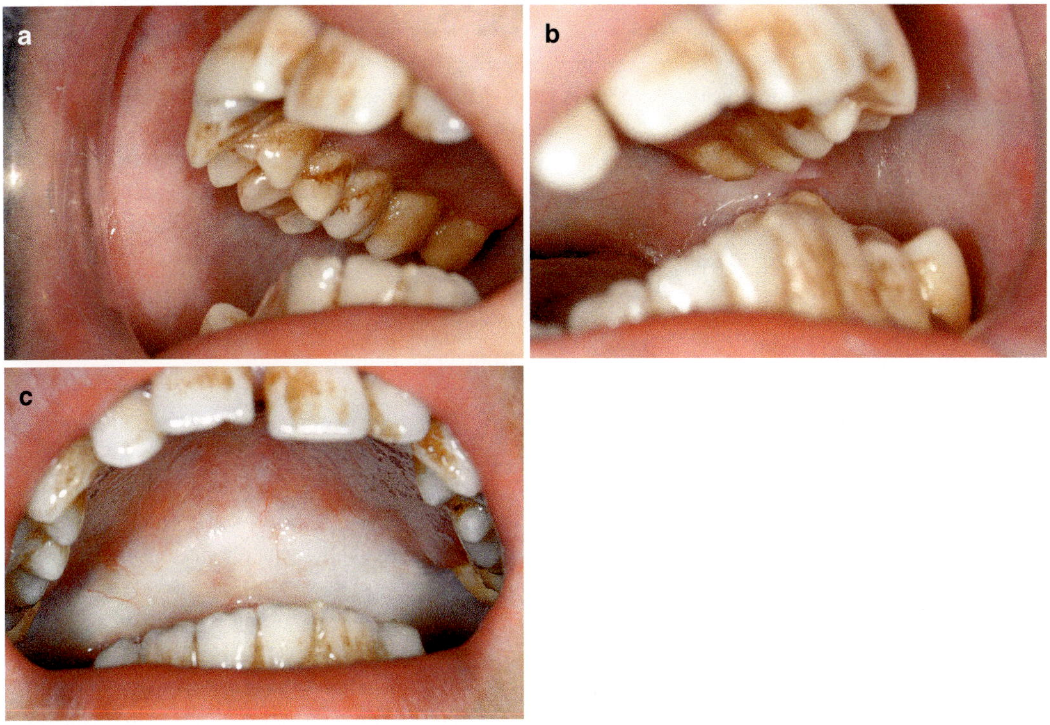

Fig. 5.30 (**a**) Blanching of right buccal mucosa. (**b**) Blanching of left buccal mucosa. (**c**) Blanching of the palatal mucosa

Age: 25 years
Sex: Male
Chief Complaints:
A 25-year-old man with pain eating hot or spicy food for 2 years and restriction of mouth opening for 2 months
History of Present Illness:
A 25-year-old man complained of a burning sensation on the oral mucosa when he was eating hot or spicy food and brushing his teeth over the past 2 years. He also had progressive restriction of mouth opening for 2 months. He had been smoking for 7 years and had a long-standing habit of chewing betel quid for around 6 years.
Past Medical History: Superficial gastritis.
Allergy: None.
Physical Examination:
Buccal mucosa and the posterior portion of the soft palate were extensively blanched and rigid with palpable fibrous bands underneath (Fig. 5.30a-c). Mouth opening was restricted to about the width of two fingers.
Laboratories and Imaging Studies:
A lesional biopsy was made on the right buccal mucosa. Histological findings indicated the diagnosis oral submucous fibrosis.
Diagnosis:
Oral submucous fibrosis (OSF)
Diagnosis Basis:

1. History of betel quid chewing.
2. Restriction of mouth opening.
3. Blanched fibrotic oral mucosa with palpable fibrotic bands.
4. Findings of histopathological examination.

Management:

1. Medication
   Rp.: Triamcinolone acetonide (TA) injection 40 mg × 1
      Sig.: Intra-lesional injection at the dose of 6 mg/site s.t.

Tripterygium hypoglaucum tablet 1 g × 200 tablets
Sig.: 2 g t.i.d. p.o.
Compound danshen dripping pill 600 tablets
Sig.: 10 tablets t.i.d. p.o.
Compound chlorhexidine solution 300 ml × 1
Sig.: rinse t.i.d.
Dexamethasone paste15g × 1
Sig.: topical use t.i.d.

2. The patient was instructed to discontinue the habit of chewing betel quid, and a follow-up visit was scheduled.

Follow-Up Treatment:
Once the remission of the burning sensation and restriction of mouth opening was achieved, regular follow-up visits were suggested.

[Review] Oral Submucous Fibrosis
Oral submucous fibrosis (OSF) is a chronic, progressive disease characterized by collagen accumulation in lamina propria and submucosal tissue. Oral cavity, oropharynx, and the upper section of the esophagus can be involved. Blanching of the oral mucosa and stiffness of the submucosal connective tissue is commonly detected. Formation of thick bands of collagen can be seen in advanced stage of this disease, leading to restriction of mouth opening. OSF predominantly affects the Asian population, especially people from India, Sri Lanka, Taiwan, and Hunan Province of China. No gender preference is observed. In 1996, it was reported that about 2.5 million people were suffering from this disease worldwide; the prevalence was still increasing, probably due to growing consumption of areca nut [51].

Evidences from epidemiologic studies confirmed betel quid chewing as the major risk of OSF. The development of OSF is related to the frequency and duration of betel quid chewing. Case-control studies suggested that the incidence rate of OSF in the subjects below the age of 21 was almost twice as that in the subjects between 21 and 40. In the younger group, it took around 3.5 years to develop the disease from the start of the habit, while in the older group, it took about 6.5 years [52]. Since OSF is mainly characterized by submucous fibrosis and hyalinization, most studies on the pathogenesis of this disease are focused on metabolism and pathological change of the extracellular matrix. In essence, the disease is a collagen metabolic disorder due to interruption of the collagen synthesis and degradation equilibrium.

Areca nut contains various chemical components. Among all these components, arecoline makes the most important contribution to the development of OSF, while flavonoid components like tannins have a synergistic role. Extracts of areca nut or chemically purified arecoline could stimulate the proliferation and collagen production of fibroblasts in vitro. When stimulated by arecoline, fibroblasts from OSF patients produce more collagen fibers compared with normal fibroblasts, which is probably associated with mutation of the fibroblast in OSF [53, 54].

Apart from increase of collagen formation, reduction of collagen degradation also contributes to the development OSF. Tannin and crude extract of areca nut hampers the collagenase activity. Another study revealed that type III collagen was almost entirely replaced by type I collagen as the disease progressed. Due to alteration of molecular structures, collagen fibers from OSF could be more difficult to degrade than normal ones [55, 56].

Collagen degradation by fibroblast phagocytosis is important in physiological renewal of extracellular matrix. In OSF, this process was disturbed. The capability of collagen phagocytosis by fibroblasts is hampered by arecoline and nicotine in a dose-dependent manner [57]. Interruption of the balance between matrix metalloproteinases (MMPs) and tissue inhibitors of matrix metalloproteinases (TIMPs) may also lead to cumulative deposition of extracellular matrix [58, 59].

Altered cytokine secretions have also been noticed in OSF. Decrease or absence of IFN-γ production and increase of interleukin-1 and interleukin-6 production might be related with the development of OSF. Increased expression of platelet-derived growth factor, transforming growth factor-β, and basic fibroblast growth factor could also be observed in OSF tissue [60].

Circulating immunocomplex, immunoglobulin, and various autoantibodies could be detected in the sera of OSF patients. It was revealed that the serum levels of antinuclear antibody, anti-smooth muscle antibody, and anti-gastric parietal cell antibody were significantly higher in OSF patients than in healthy controls. Increased levels of immunocomplex and serum immunoglobins have also been reported. These all support the role of immunological factor in the development of OSF [61].

The studies of the role of genetic factors in OSF have been focused on gene polymorphisms and their association with the susceptibility of OSF. Gene polymorphisms of TNF-α has been associated with risk of OSF. Major histocompatibility complex class I chain-related gene A (MICA) has also been related with this disease [62].

Areca nut contains a large amount of copper. Compared with healthy subjects, patients with OSF have higher concentration of soluble copper in the saliva and the oral mucosa. The effect of copper on collagen formation is dependent on lysyl oxidase, which is upregulated in OSF tissue. In vitro studies have shown that the increase of copper concentration could promote the proliferation of fibroblasts. However, since no fibrosis of the visceral organs has been found using ultrasonic examination and copper level in the excrement of OSF patients is within the normal range, the effect of copper on fibroblasts is probably localized to the oral mucosa [63, 64].

OSF is considered as one of the oral potentially malignant disorders. The reported malignant transformation rate ranges from 7% to 13%. In a follow-up duration of 17 years, the malignant transformation rate of OSF was about 7.6%.

Areca nut has been considered as a chemical carcinogen. The genotoxic and mutagenic effects of areca nut are closely related with polyphenols, alkaloids, and areca nut-specific nitrosamines. Moreover, slaked lime in the quid could enhance the level of reactive oxygen species and then lead to oxidative DNA damage. The risk of malignant transformation could be further enhanced by factors such as older age, nutritional deficiency, trauma, tobacco smoking, and genetic susceptibility. Furthermore, due to epithelial atrophy and reduced vascularity underneath the epithelium, the permeability of the carcinogen will be facilitated, while the absorption will be hindered. These combined effects will result in extended exposure of the oral mucosa to carcinogens [65].

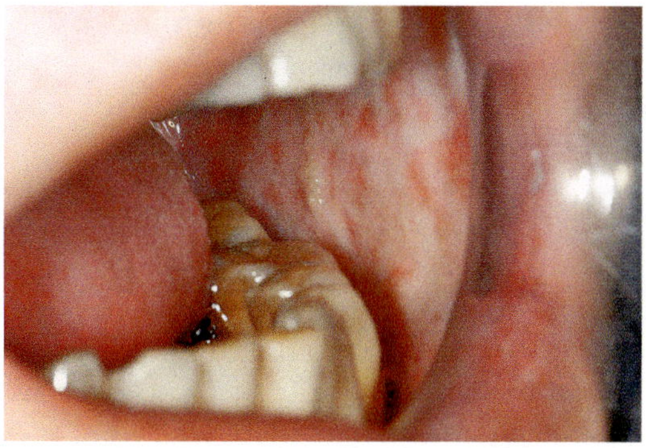

Fig. 5.31 Marble-like appearance of the buccal mucosa

The clinical manifestations of OSF depend on the development of the disease. Burning sensation and intolerance to irritative food and beverages are commonly reported at the early stage. Vesicles and erosion may be present, followed by induration of the oral mucosa involving the lip, tongue, buccal mucosa, and palate. Restriction of mouth opening to various degrees can be observed. The characteristic clinical manifestations include blanching and opacity of the oral mucosa with a marble-like appearance (Fig. 5.31). Fibrous bands could be found by palpation. Epithelial dysplasia can be found in OSF lesions, which may later result in malignant transformation. Due to restriction of mouth opening caused by the disease, early diagnosis of cancer can be difficult [65].

The diagnosis of OSF is based on history of betel quid chewing and typical clinical manifestations, which can further be confirmed by histopathological findings.

Quitting betel quid chewing is necessary for the treatment of OSF. An optional treatment regimen commonly used by the authors is as follows: tripterygium hypoglaucum tablet (2 g t.i.d. p.o.) and compound danshen dripping pill (10 pills t.i.d. p.o.) consecutively for 1 month, local corticosteroids such as dexamethasone paste or triamcinolone acetonide oral paste, and intra-lesional injection of triamcinolone acetonide at the dose of 6 mg/site if necessary.

5.8 Discoid Lupus Erythematosus

Case 57 Discoid Lupus Erythematosus

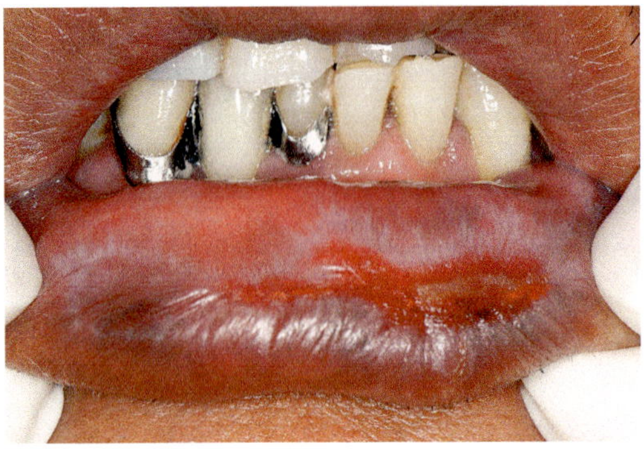

Fig. 5.32 Erythematous lesion on the lower lip, with radiating keratotic striae along the mucosal side and pigmentation along the cutaneous side of the lesion

Age: 58 years
Sex: Male
Chief Complaints:
A 58-year-old man with recurrent ulceration, bleeding, and pain in the lower lip for 6 months
History of Present Illness:
A 58-year-old man complained of recurrent ulceration, bleeding, and pain in the lower lip for 6 months. The lesion took about 14 days to heal but usually recurred after 1 month.
Past Medical History: None.
Allergy: None.
Physical Examination:
An 8 mm × 3 mm erosive and erythematous lesion coved with blood crust was found on the lower lip. The erythematous lesion is surrounded with short white streaks in a radial pattern. Pigmentation could be observed on the skin side of the lesion (Fig. 5.32).
Laboratory Investigations:
Routine laboratory tests, including whole blood cell count, blood glucose examination, as well as liver and kidney function panels, were normal.
Diagnosis:
Chronic discoid lupus erythematosus (CDLE).
Diagnosis Basis:

1. Erosive and erythematous lesion on the lower lip.
2. White striae radiating from the border of the lesion.
3. Pigmentation.

Management:

1. Medication
   Rp.: Triamcinolone acetonide (TA) injection 40 mg × 1
      Sig.: Intra-lesional injection at the dose of 6 mg/site s.t.
      Hydroxychloroquine 0.1 g × 28 tablets
      Sig.: 0.1 g b.i.d. p.o.
      Vitamin B6 10 mg × 100 tablets
      Sig.: 5 mg b.i.d. p.o.
      Compound chlorhexidine solution 300 ml × 1
      Sig.: labial hydropathic compress t.i.d.
      Dexamethasone paste 15 g × 1
      Sig.: topical use t.i.d.
2. A follow-up visit after 2 weeks was scheduled. The patient was advised to avoid exposure to sunlight or eating spicy food.

Follow-Up Treatment:
If complete or partial remission was achieved in the follow-up visit, the treatment plan can be switched to the following regimen: total glucosides of paeony capsules (0.6 g b.i.d./t.i.d. p.o. for about 3–4 weeks). If no improvement was achieved, the treatment plan can be switched to a regimen with tripterygium hypoglaucum tablet (2 g t.i.d. p.o.) or thalidomide (75 mg q.d. p.o.) for about 2 weeks.

[Review] Discoid Lupus Erythematosus (DLE)

Discoid lupus erythematosus (DLE) is a chronic cutaneous lupus erythematosus featured by discoid erythematous-to-violaceous plaques involving the skin and mucosa. It usually affects the sun-exposed skin, primarily the facial region [66]. DLE is more likely to affect women than men. There is a slight racial predilection for people of African descents. The common age of disease onset is around 20–40 years.

The etiology of DLE remains obscure, although a number of factors have been suggested. Among them, sunlight has been confirmed to be associated with the development and exacerbation of DLE. Photosensitivity to ultraviolet is quite common in patients with DLE, which may be associated with the interactions between T cells and heat shock proteins (HSPs).

One hypothesis is that HSPs are unveiled by UV radiation; this process is followed by interaction of HSPs with accumulated T cells, leading to liquefactive degeneration of basal epithelial cells [67].

Genetic background also played an important part in the pathogenesis of DLE. Several haplotypes, such as human histocompatibility (HLA) -B7, B8, and Cw7, have been related with individual's susceptibility to DLE. HLA-DQA-0102 and HLA-DRB-1601 alleles have also been considered as potential genetic marker for DLE [68, 69]. Recently, genome-wide association studies (GWAS) have shed a new light on the genetic background of systemic lupus erythematosus (SLE). Nevertheless, it is still uncertain whether those genes recognized by GWAS have exactly the same role in the development of DLE.

Several observations suggest that DLE may be affected by hormones. For instance, the incidence of DLE is higher in women and the severity of DLE in women's menstrual cycle, pregnancy, and menopause [70].

Even though defined autoantibodies of SLE are not often detected in DLE, tissue binding of immunoglobulins and complements are usually found at the dermo-epidermal junction. Therefore, DLE is considered as a chronic autoimmune mucocutaneous disorder. However, it is still debatable whether these deposits directly participate in the pathogenesis of DLE or are just secondary to the development of DLE lesions. It is noticeable that increased immunoglobulin production has been reported in DLE, most of which are induced by activation of B cells, indicating that humoral and cellular immune responses are both involved in DLE [67] .

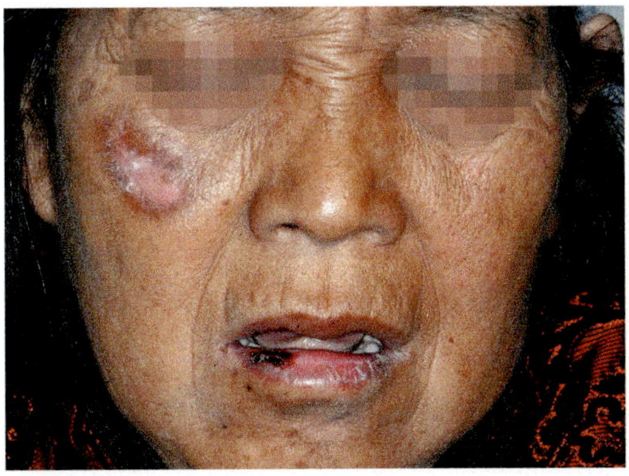

Fig. 5.33 DLE lesions involving the lower lip and the skin of the right cheek. Erosive lesion with radiating white striae and blood crust was observed on the lower lip, while atrophic lesion with central hypopigmentation and peripheral hyperpigmentation was observed on the skin of the right cheek

The skin lesion of DLE usually emerged in the form of an erythematous papule and then followed by hyperkeratosis with follicular plugging. Pigmentary changes may happen. The center of the lesion is usually atrophic and hypopigmented, while the periphery is often hyperpigmented. The face, scalp, ears, and chest are frequently affected. The lesions are persistent and may produce scarring [71] (Fig. 5.33).

Approximately 20% of the patients with DLE have oral lesions, with or without skin involvement [67, 72]. The vermilion, buccal mucosa, and tongue are commonly affected. Although the lesions most often locate on the lower lip, both the upper and lower lip can be involved at the same time (Figs. 5.34, 5.35, and 5.36). The typical lesion is a well-demarcated plaque with central erythema surrounded with short white streaks in a radial pattern. The cutaneous side of the lesion could be pigmented, with or without white striae. The borderline of mucosa and skin can be blurry, and the lesion has a tendency to invade into the skin.

The diagnosis of DLE may be made according to the clinical appearance and be further confirmed by histopathological findings.

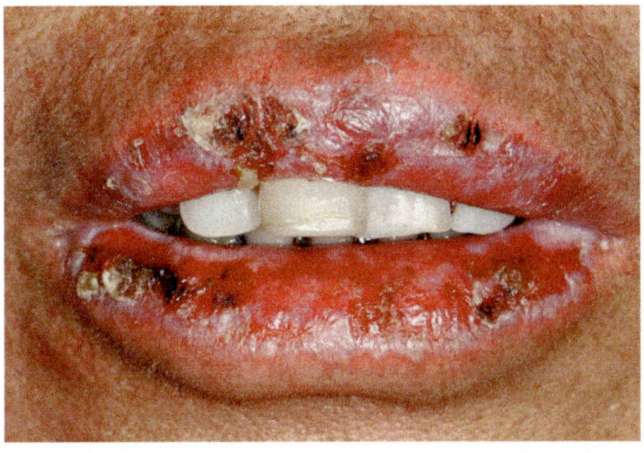

Fig. 5.34 DLE lesions involving the upper and lower lips

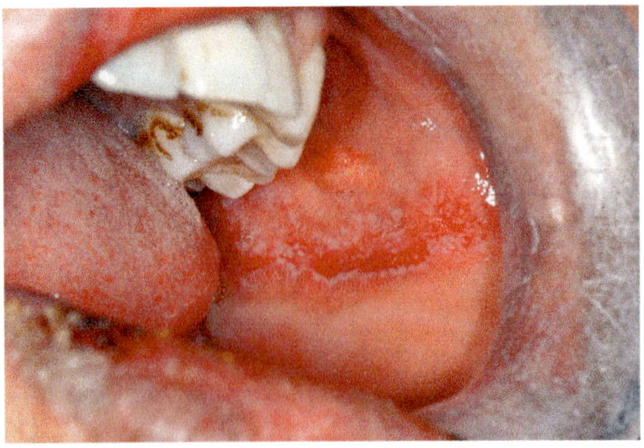

Fig. 5.35 DLE lesion on the left buccal mucosa

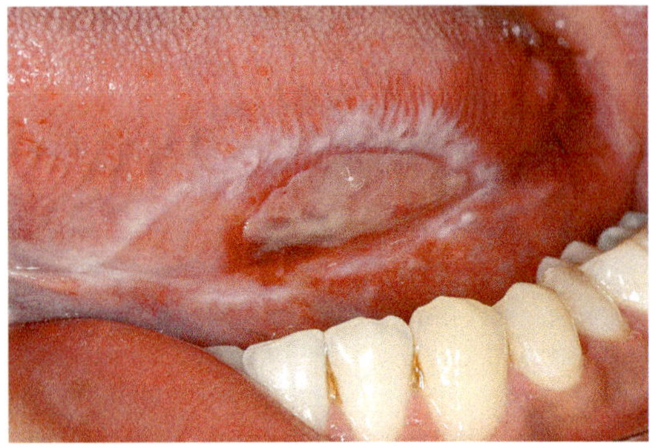

Fig. 5.36 DLE lesion on the ventrum of the tongue

Typical histopathological changes include vacuolar degeneration of basal cells, lymphocyte infiltration surrounding the blood vessels, and appendages in the dermis. Epidermal atrophy, hyperkeratosis with follicular plugging, and vascular dilation with colloid bodies may be observed [67].

Direct immunofluorescence (DIF) can be used for the differential diagnosis of DLE and other diseases. Linear or granular deposits of immunoglobulins and complement components along the dermo-epidermal junction may be detected.

DLE is classified as one of the oral potentially malignant disorders by World Health Organization. Although the incidence of DLE is higher in women and people of African descents, the malignant transformation is more likely to happen in European males. It has been reported that in a follow-up period of 26–41 years, 3.3% of the patients developed squamous cell carcinoma [73]. In another retrospective study, 6 out of 87 patients with diagnosis of oral DLE developed oral cancer [74].

Around 5% of DLE cases may develop to SLE, especially patients with HLA-B8 [75]. Identified clinical risk factors include widespread DLE lesions, telangiectasias, arthritis, arthralgias, and Raynaud's phenomenon. Laboratory risk factors include anemia, leucopenia, thrombocytopenia, high erythrocyte sedimentation rates (ESRs), high levels of anticardiolipin antibodies, high titres of antinuclear antibodies (ANAs), and positive DIF findings in skin with normal appearance. More aggressive treatments and frequent follow-up may be necessary for the management of patients at high risk. The patient may also be referred to rheumatologists or nephrologists when necessary. It has been reported that treatment with hydroxychloroquine or chloroquine at an early stage could delay the occurrence of SLE in DLE patients and may prevent or alleviate damage to peripheral organs [76] .

The recommended first-line systemic therapy for DLE is hydroxychloroquine (0.1 g b.i.d. for 2 weeks or longer). Vitamin B6 (5 mg b.i.d.) is supposed to be taken at the same time to ameliorate gastrointestinal reaction. Besides, thalidomide (50–100 mg q.d.) or tripterygium hypoglaucum tablets (2 g t.i.d. for 2 weeks or longer) can also be used. Systemic prednisone acetate (15–25 mg daily, in a single morning dose, for 5–7 days) is often given in short courses to patients with widespread lesions or acute exacerbation, before switching the treatment plan to the reagents mentioned above. Total glucosides of paeony capsules (0.6 g b.i.d./t.i.d. for 3 weeks or longer) can be used by patients with mild symptoms. Topical agents that had been reported effective for DLE include mouth rinse and liniments. Mouth rinses, including compound chlorhexidine solution, compound borax solution (diluted fivefold with water before use), and 1% povidone iodine solution, can be used for hydropathic compress, three times a day. Liniments are mainly topical corticosteroids, such as dexamethasone paste, prednisolone acetate suspension, triamcinolone acetonide, triamcinolone acetonide oral paste, and dexamethasone ointment. Additionally, triamcinolone acetonide injection or compound betamethasone injection combined with sterile water or 2% lidocaine (at a ratio of 1:1) can be used for intra-lesional injection. Aerosol therapy with dexamethasone sodium phosphate injection, gentamycin sulfate injection, vitamin C injection, and Vitamin B12 injection, once or twice a day for 3–5 days, is an optional topical therapy. Moreover, sun exposure must be minimized by avoiding the peak hours for sun exposure and by wearing protective clothing and high efficiency sunscreens. Diet containing large amount of spicy food and seafood should be avoided. A regular follow-up is necessary to prevent potentially malignant transformation.

5.9 Oral Fordyce Spots

Case 58 Oral Fordyce Spots

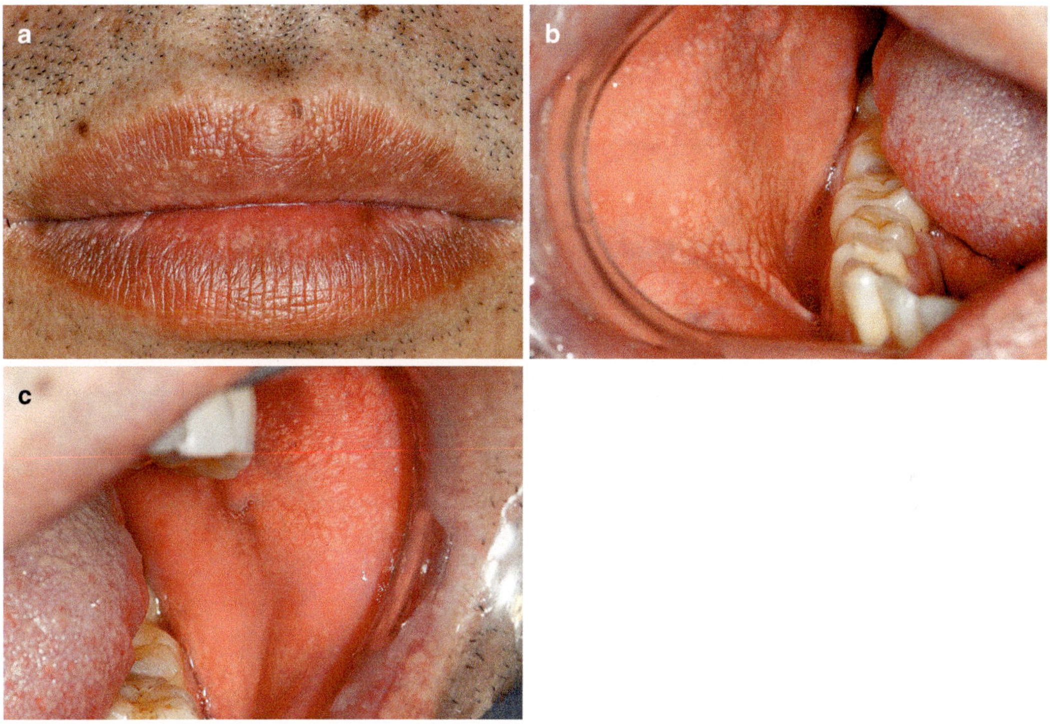

Fig. 5.37 (**a**) Yellowish-white spots were observed on the vermillion. (**b**) Yellowish-white spots on the right buccal mucosa. (**c**) Yellowish-white spots on the left buccal mucosa

Age: 50 years
Sex: Male
Chief Complaints:
A 50-year-old man with "white spots" on the lip and buccal mucosa for 2 days
History of Present Illness:
A 50-year-old man came to the clinic after he found painless "white spots" on the lip and buccal mucosa 2 days ago.
Past Medical History: None.
Allergy: None.
Physical Examination:
Multiple yellowish-white granules were found on the vermillion and the buccal mucosa (Fig. 5.37a-c). No erythematous or ulcerative lesions were observed.
Diagnosis:
Oral Fordyce spots.
Diagnosis Basis:

1. Involvement of buccal mucosa and the lips.
2. Asymptomatic yellowish-white granules on the oral mucosa.

Management:
Explain the cause and prognosis of the disease to the patient.

[Review] Oral Fordyce Spots
Oral Fordyce spots (FSs) are ectopic sebaceous glands. They appear as yellow or yellowish-white painless granules with a smooth and soft surface, about 1–3 mm in dimension. They can be scattered on the mucosa or distributed in aggregates and are most commonly seen on the vermilion of upper lip, buccal mucosa, and the retromolar area, often bilaterally [77].

Oral FSs are usually not biopsied as they can be readily diagnosed based on the clinical features. When examined under a microscope, they have appearance similar to normal sebaceous glands, but usually don't have hair follicles or ducts that connect to the surface of the oral mucosa.

Oral FSs usually appear after puberty, probably due to the changes of hormone levels. However, some investigations have indicated that the formation of ectopic sebaceous glands might be related with the nervous system. Factors like insulin-like growth factor and corticotrophin-releasing hormone may induce the formation of ectopic sebaceous glands by facilitating the growth of nervous fibers. Valid research data on the etiology of this disorder is still lacking [77–80].

It is not necessary to treat oral FSs. If the granules must be removed due to cosmetic reasons, carbon dioxide super-pulsed laser can be a safe and effective treatment option [81].

5.10 Morsicatio Buccarum et Labiorum

Case 59 Morsicatio Buccarum et Labiorum

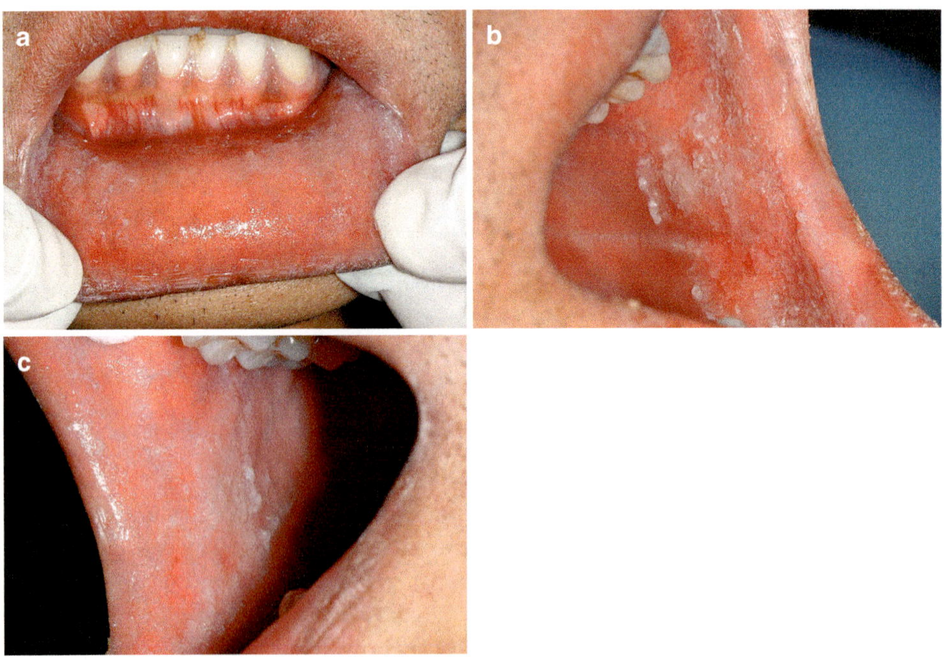

Fig. 5.38 (**a**) The inner surface of the lower lip was covered by squama that was partially attached to the epithelium. In the area where the squama was peeled off, the underneath mucosa was intact and didn't have any significant color change or ulceration. (**b**) The left buccal mucosa was covered by squama that was partially attached to the epithelium. In the area where the squama was peeled off, the underneath mucosa was intact and didn't have any significant color change or ulceration. (**c**) The right buccal mucosa was covered by squama that was partially attached to the epithelium. In the area where the squama was peeled off, the underneath mucosa was intact and didn't have any significant color change or ulceration

Age: 24 years
Sex: Male
Chief Complaints:
A 24-year-old man with rough feeling on the inner surface of lips and the buccal mucosa for 1 year
History of Present Illness:
A 24-year-old man came to our clinic, complaining of 1-year history of chronic desquamation and rough feeling on the inner surface of lips and the buccal mucosa. History of habitual cheek and lip biting was reported. Treatment with vitamin B_2, folic acid, acetylspiramycin tablets, cydiodine buccal tablets, and bezoar antidotal pills did not show any significant effect.
Past Medical History: None.
Allergy: None.
Physical Examination:
The inner surface of the lips and the buccal mucosa were covered with squama that was partially attached to the epithelium (Fig. 5.38a-c). The squama could be wiped off without any pain using a cotton stick and didn't cause any significant color change, bleeding, or ulceration on the underneath mucosa.
Diagnosis:
Morsicatio buccarum et labiorum.
Diagnosis Basis:

1. Buccal mucosa and inner surface of lips covered with squama that could be wiped off without any pain or subsequent bleeding or ulceration.
2. History of habitual cheek and lip biting.

Management:

1. Medication
   Rp.: Vitamin E 0.1 g × 60
   Sig.: topical use t.i.d.
2. Stop habitual cheek and lip biting.

[Review] Morsicatio Buccarum et Labiorum
Morsicatio buccarum et labiorum is caused by self-injury, and the target of injury is oral mucosa. It appears as whitish squama on the oral mucosa and can be difficult to be distinguished from other mucosal disorders, such as oral lichen planus, oral candidiasis, and white sponge nevus. Some studies suggest that it is most common in adolescents aged 15–19 years. The lesions are more often bilateral [82].

Morsicatio buccarum et labiorum often affects parts of the oral mucosa that are in direct contact with the teeth, such as the lower lip and the buccal mucosa. The mucosa is covered with loose squama that can be peeled off without causing any significant color change, bleeding, or ulceration of the underneath mucosa. The patients usually don't have any discomfort other than a rough feeling on the mucosa involved [83].

Morsicatio buccarum et labiorum is a form of self-induced injury. It is closely related with psychological factors. Some researchers think that the compulsion represents aggressive feelings or a form of self-punishment. The habit is often combined with teeth grinding. Some investigators think that some form of surface irregularity, such as oral white sponge nevus or linea alba, precedes the onset of the cheek biting.. The patients may feel compelled to remove these lesions, which is how the habit begins. Some patients with this disorder are unaware of the habits. Questioning the patient's family members or close friends who have witnessed the habits can help the clinicians to obtain necessary information [84].

The diagnosis of morsicatio buccarum et labiorum is often based on clinical manifestations and the history of habitual cheek and/or lip biting. Pathological characteristics of this disorder are acanthosis of the epithelium with superficial erosion lined by an irregular, frayed layer of parakeratosis. The surface is basophilic because of accumulated cellular debris and bacteria on the intact epithelium and among torn fragments. Beneath the erosion there is a necrotic layer of cells with characteristic eosinophilic staining [85].

The lesions of morsicatio buccarum et labiorum can heal spontaneously without any sequela if the patient can quit the habit. Topical agents, such as vitamin E, can be used to reduce the roughness of the mucosa affected. The patient should be referred to a psychologist or psychiatrist if needed.

References

1. Banoczy J, Gintner Z, Dombi C. Tobacco use and oral leukoplakia. J Dent Educ. 2001;65(4):322–7.
2. Amagasa T, Yamashiro M, Uzawa N. Oral premalignant lesions: from a clinical perspective. Int J Clin Oncol. 2011;16(1):5–14.
3. Martorell-Calatayud A, Botella-Estrada R, Bagan-Sebastian JV, Sanmartin-Jimenez O, Guillen-Barona C. Oral leukoplakia: clinical, histopathologic, and molecular features and therapeutic approach. Actas Dermosifiliogr. 2009;100(8):669–84.
4. Ge L, Zhou HM, Zeng X, Wu LY, Lin M. A case report on canceration of proliferative verrucous leukoplakia. Hua Xi Kou Qiang Yi Xue Za Zhi. 2007;25(3):310–2.
5. Gupta PC, Mehta FS, Daftary DK, et al. Incidence rates of oral cancer and natural history of oral precancerous lesions in a 10-year follow-up study of Indian villagers. Community Dent Oral Epidemiol. 1980;8(6):283–333.
6. Banoczy J. Follow-up studies in oral leukoplakia. J Maxillofac Surg. 1977;5(1):69–75.
7. Larsson A, Warfvinge G. Malignant transformation of oral lichen planus. Oral Oncol. 2003;39(6):630–1.
8. Cowan CG, Gregg TA, Napier SS, McKenna SM, Kee F. Potentially malignant oral lesions in northern Ireland: a 20-year population-based perspective of malignant transformation. Oral Dis. 2001;7(1):18–24.
9. Reibel J. Prognosis of oral pre-malignant lesions: significance of clinical, histopathological, and molecular biological characteristics. Crit Rev Oral Biol Med. 2003;14(1):47–62.
10. D'Souza G, Kreimer AR, Viscidi R, et al. Case-control study of human papillomavirus and oropharyngeal cancer. N Engl J Med. 2007;356(19):1944–56.
11. Bagan JV, Jimenez Y, Murillo J, et al. Epstein-Barr virus in oral proliferative verrucous leukoplakia and squamous cell carcinoma: a preliminary study. Med Oral Patol Oral Cir Bucal. 2008;13(2):E110–3.
12. Zhang L, Rosin MP. Loss of heterozygosity: a potential tool in management of oral premalignant lesions. J Oral Pathol Med. 2001;30(9):513–20.
13. Sudbo J, Lippman SM, Lee JJ, et al. The influence of resection and aneuploidy on mortality in oral leukoplakia. N Engl J Med. 2004;350(14):1405–13.
14. Poeta ML, Manola J, Goldwasser MA, et al. TP53 mutations and survival in squamous-cell carcinoma of the head and neck. N Engl J Med. 2007;357(25):2552–61.
15. Bouquot JE, Gorlin RJ. Leukoplakia, lichen planus, and other oral keratoses in 23,616 white Americans over the age of 35 years. Oral Surg Oral Med Oral Pathol. 1986;61(4):373–81.
16. Bhattacharyya I, Chehal HK. White lesions. Otolaryngol Clin N Am. 2011;44(1):109–31, vi.
17. Martin JL. Leukoedema: an epidemiological study in white and African Americans. J Tenn Dent Assoc. 1997;77(1):18–21.
18. Damm DD. Bilateral white cheeks. White sponge nevus. Gen Dent. 2010;58(6):539–40.
19. Zhang JM, Yang ZW, Chen RY, Gao P, Zhang YR, Zhang LF. Two new mutations in the keratin 4 gene causing oral white sponge nevus in Chinese family. Oral Dis. 2009;15(1):100–5.
20. Shibuya Y, Zhang J, Yokoo S, Umeda M, Komori T. Constitutional mutation of keratin 13 gene in familial white sponge nevus. Oral Surg Oral Med Oral Pathol Oral Radiol Endod. 2003;96(5):561–5.
21. Cutlan JE, Saunders N, Olsen SH, Fullen DR. White sponge nevus presenting as genital lesions in a 28-year-old female. J Cutan Pathol. 2010;37(3):386–9.
22. Farhi D, Dupin N. Pathophysiology, etiologic factors, and clinical management of oral lichen planus, part I: facts and controversies. Clin Dermatol. 2010;28(1):100–8.
23. Li ZW, Zhou Y, Zhao M. Progresses in studies on association between psychological factors and oral lichen plans. Zhonghua Kou Qiang Yi Xue Za Zhi. 2009;44(4):250–2.
24. Krasowska D, Chodorowska G, Koziol-Monrewka M, et al. The -308 promoter polymorphism in the tumour necrosis factor gene in patients with lichen planus. Acta Derm Venereol. 2005;85(5):400–3.
25. Bai J, Jiang L, Lin M, et al. Association of polymorphisms in the tumor necrosis factor-alpha and interleukin-10 genes with oral lichen planus: a study in Chinese cohort with Han ethnicity. J Interf Cytokine Res. 2009;29(7):381–8.
26. Xavier GM, de Sa AR, Guimaraes AL, et al. Investigation of functional gene polymorphisms interleukin-1 beta, interleukin-6, inerleukin-10 and tumor necrosis factor in individuals with oral lichen planus. J Oral Pathol Med. 2007;36(8):467–81.
27. Kimkong I, Hirankarn N, Nakkuntod J, et al. Tumor necrosis factor-alpha gene polymorphisms and susceptibility to oral lichen planus. Oral Dis. 2011;17(2):206–9.
28. Stojanovice L, Lunder T, Poljak M, et al. Lack of evidence for hepatitis C virus infection in association with lichen planus. Int J Dermatol. 2008;47(12):1250–6.
29. Zhou Y, Jiang L, Liu J, et al. The prevalence of hepatitis C virus infection in oral lichen planus in an ethnic Chinese cohort of 232 patients. Int J Oral Sci. 2010;2(2):90–7.
30. Gimenez-Garcia R, Perez-Castrillon JL. Lichen planus and hepatitis C virus infection. J Eur Acad Dermatol Venereol. 2003;17(3):291–5.
31. Beaird LM, Kahloon N, Franco J, et al. Incidence of hepatitis C in lichen planus. J Am Acad Dermatol. 2001;44(2):311–2.
32. Lodi G, Scully C, Carrozzo M, Griffiths M, Sugerman PB, Thongprasom K. Current controversies in oral lichen planus: report of an international consensus meeting. Part 1. Viral infections and etiopathogenesis. Oral Surg Oral Med Oral Pathol Oral Radiol Endod. 2005;100(1):40–51.
33. Sousa FA, Rosa LE. Oral lichen planus: clinical and histopathological considerations. Braz J Otorhinolaryngol. 2008;74(2):284–92.
34. Shen ZY, Liu W, Feng JQ, Zhou HW, Zhou ZT. Squamous cell carcinoma development in pre-

viously diagnosed oral lichen planus: de novo or transformation. Oral Surg Oral Med Oral Pathol Oral Radiol Endod. 2011;112(5):592–6.
35. Krutchkoff DJ, Cutler L, Laskowski S. Oral lichen planus: the evidence regarding potential malignant transformation. J Oral Pathol. 1978;7(1):1–7.
36. Ismail SB, Kumar SK, Zain RB. Oral lichen planus and lichenoid reactions: etiopathogenesis, diagnosis, management and malignant transformation. J Oral Sci. 2007;49(2):89–106.
37. Schlosser BJ. Lichen planus and lichenoid reactions of the oral mucosa. Dermatol Ther. 2010;23(3):251–67.
38. Crincoli V, Di BMB, Scivetti M, Lucchese A, Tecco S, Festa F. Oral lichen planus: update on etiopathogenesis, diagnosis and treatment. Immunopharmacol Immunotoxicol. 2011;33(1):11–20.
39. Mohty M, Kuentz M, Michallet M, et al. Chronic graft-versus-host disease after allogeneic blood stem cell transplantation: long-term results of a randomized study. Blood. 2002;100(9):3128–34.
40. Imanguli MM, Alevizos I, Brown R, Pavletic SZ, Atkinson JC. Oral graft-versus-host disease. Oral Dis. 2008;14(5):396–412.
41. Flowers ME, Parker PM, Johnston LJ, et al. Comparison of chronic graft-versus-host disease after transplantation of peripheral blood stem cells versus bone marrow in allogeneic recipients: long-term follow-up of a randomized trial. Blood. 2002;100(2):415–9.
42. Kramer IR, Lucas RB, Pindborg JJ, Sobin LH. Definition of leukoplakia and related lesions: an aid to studies on oral precancer. Oral Surg Oral Med Oral Pathol. 1978;46(4):518–39.
43. Villa A, Villa C, Abati S. Oral cancer and oral erythroplakia: an update and implication for clinicians. Aust Dent J. 2011;56(3):253–6.
44. Hashibe M, Mathew B, Kuruvilla B, et al. Chewing tobacco, alcohol, and the risk of erythroplakia. Cancer Epidemiol Biomark Prev. 2000;9(7):639–45.
45. Reichart PA, Philipsen HP. Oral erythroplakia—a review. Oral Oncol. 2005;41(6):551–61.
46. Hosni ES, Salum FG, Cherubini K, Yurgel LS, Figueiredo MA. Oral erythroplakia and speckled leukoplakia: retrospective analysis of 13 cases. Braz J Otorhinolaryngol. 2009;75(2):295–9.
47. Shear M. Erythroplakia of the mouth. Int Dent J. 1972;22(4):460–73.
48. Duvvi SK, Thomas L, Vijayanand S, Reddy KT. Two-week rule for suspected head and neck cancer. A study of compliance and effectiveness. J Eval Clin Pract. 2006;12(6):591–4.
49. van der Waal I. Potentially malignant disorders of the oral and oropharyngeal mucosa; terminology, classification and present concepts of management. Oral Oncol. 2009;45(4–5):317–23.
50. Mignogna MD, Fedele S. Oral cancer screening: 5 minutes to save a life. Lancet. 2005;365(9475):1905–6.
51. Auluck A, Rosin MP, Zhang L, Sumanth KN. Oral submucous fibrosis, a clinically benign but potentially malignant disease: report of 3 cases and review of the literature. J Can Dent Assoc. 2008;74(8):735–40.
52. Ranganathan K, Devi MU, Joshua E, Kirankumar K, Saraswathi TR. Oral submucous fibrosis: a case-control study in Chennai, South India. J Oral Pathol Med. 2004;33(5):274–7.
53. Harvey W, Scutt A, Meghji S, Canniff JP. Stimulation of human buccal mucosa fibroblasts in vitro by betel-nut alkaloids. Arch Oral Biol. 1986;31(1):45–9.
54. Meghji S, Scutt A, Harvey W, Canniff JP. An in-vitro comparison of human fibroblasts from normal and oral submucous fibrosis tissue. Arch Oral Biol. 1987;32(3):213–5.
55. Utsunomiya H, Tilakaratne WM, Oshiro K, et al. Extracellular matrix remodeling in oral submucous fibrosis: its stage-specific modes revealed by immunohistochemistry and in situ hybridization. J Oral Pathol Med. 2005;34(8):498–507.
56. Kuo MY, Chen HM, Hahn LJ, Hsieh CC, Chiang CP. Collagen biosynthesis in human oral submucous fibrosis fibroblast cultures. J Dent Res. 1995;74(11):1783–8.
57. Shieh DH, Chiang LC, Lee CH, Yang YH, Shieh TY. Effects of arecoline, safrole, and nicotine on collagen phagocytosis by human buccal mucosal fibroblasts as a possible mechanism for oral submucous fibrosis in Taiwan. J Oral Pathol Med. 2004;33(9):581–7.
58. Shieh DH, Chiang LC, Shieh TY. Augmented mRNA expression of tissue inhibitor of metalloproteinase-1 in buccal mucosal fibroblasts by arecoline and safrole as a possible pathogenesis for oral submucous fibrosis. Oral Oncol. 2003;39(7):728–35.
59. Chang YC, Yang SF, Tai KW, Chou MY, Hsieh YS. Increased tissue inhibitor of metalloproteinase-1 expression and inhibition of gelatinase A activity in buccal mucosal fibroblasts by arecoline as possible mechanisms for oral submucous fibrosis. Oral Oncol. 2002;38(2):195–200.
60. Haque MF, Harris M, Meghji S, Barrett AW. Immunolocalization of cytokines and growth factors in oral submucous fibrosis. Cytokine. 1998;10(9):713–9.
61. Chiang CP, Hsieh RP, Chen TH, et al. High incidence of autoantibodies in Taiwanese patients with oral submucous fibrosis. J Oral Pathol Med. 2002;31(7):402–9.
62. Tilakaratne WM, Klinikowski MF, Saku T, Peters TJ, Warnakulasuriya S. Oral submucous fibrosis: review on aetiology and pathogenesis. Oral Oncol. 2006;42(6):561–8.
63. Ma RH, Tsai CC, Shieh TY. Increased lysyl oxidase activity in fibroblasts cultured from oral submucous fibrosis associated with areca nut chewing in Taiwan. J Oral Pathol Med. 1995;24(9):407–12.
64. Rajendran R, Kumari KR, Kumar AS. Liver ultrasound and faecal copper estimation in oral submucous fibrosis. Indian J Dent Res. 2003;14(1):13–21.
65. Angadi PV, Rao SS. Areca nut in pathogenesis of oral submucous fibrosis: revisited. Oral Maxillofac Surg. 2011;15(1):1–9.
66. Tebbe B. Clinical course and prognosis of cutaneous lupus erythematosus. Clin Dermatol. 2004;22(2):121–4.

67. Donnelly AM, Halbert AR, Rohr JB. Discoid lupus erythematosus. Australas J Dermatol. 1995;36(1):3–10; quiz 11–2.
68. Knop J, Bonsmann G, Kind P, et al. Antigens of the major histocompatibility complex in patients with chronic discoid lupus erythematosus. Br J Dermatol. 1990;122(6):723–8.
69. Volc-Platzer B, Anegg B, Milota S, Pickl W, Fischer G. Accumulation of gamma delta T cells in chronic cutaneous lupus erythematosus. J Invest Dermatol. 1993;100(1):84S–91S.
70. Yell JA, Burge SM. The effect of hormonal changes on cutaneous disease in lupus erythematosus. Br J Dermatol. 1993;129(1):18–22.
71. Hordinsky M. Cicatricial alopecia: discoid lupus erythematosus. Dermatol Ther. 2008;21(4):245–8.
72. Burge SM, Frith PA, Juniper RP, Wojnarowska F. Mucosal involvement in systemic and chronic cutaneous lupus erythematosus. Br J Dermatol. 1989;121(6): 727–41.
73. Dhingra M, Bhalla M, Thami GP, Mittal P. Metastasizing squamous cell carcinoma arising from chronic discoid lupus erythematosus plaque of recent onset. Indian J Dermatol Venereol Leprol. 2011;77(5):626.
74. Liu W, Shen ZY, Wang LJ, et al. Malignant potential of oral and labial chronic discoid lupus erythematosus: a clinicopathological study of 87 cases. Histopathology. 2011;59(2):292–8.
75. Harper JG, Pilcher MF, Szlam S, Lind DS. Squamous cell carcinoma in an African American with discoid lupus erythematosus: a case report and review of the literature. South Med J. 2010;103(3):256–9.
76. Chong BF, Song J, Olsen NJ. Determining risk factors for developing systemic lupus erythematosus in discoid lupus erythematosus patients. Br J Dermatol. 2012;166(1):29–35.
77. Mansur AT, Aydingoz IE. Unilateral buccal Fordyce spots with ipsilateral facial paralysis: a sign of neuro-sebaceous connection? Acta Derm Venereol. 2012;92(2):177–8.
78. Yuan H, et al. Corticotrophin-releasing hormone (CRH) facilitates axon outgrowth. Spinal Cord. 2010;48(12):850–6.
79. Toyoda M, Nakamura M, Morohashi M. Neuropeptides and sebaceous glands. Eur J Dermatol. 2002;12(5): 422–7.
80. Deplewski D, Rosenfield RL. Growth hormone and insulin-like growth factors have different effects on sebaceous cell growth and differentiation. Endocrinology. 1999;140(9):4089–94.
81. Ocampo-Candiani J, et al. Treatment of Fordyce spots with CO2 laser. Dermatol Surg. 2003;29(8):869–71.
82. Glass LF, Maize JC. Morsicatio buccarum et labiorum (excessive cheek and lip biting). Am J Dermatopathol. 1991;13(3):271–4.
83. Wang JY, Liu WZ, Li XY, Li ZW, Zeng X. Morsicatio buccarum et labiorum: two cases report. Hua Xi Kou Qiang Yi Xue Za Zhi. 2009;27(6):681–2. 685
84. Damm DD, Fantasia JE. Bilateral white lesions of buccal mucosa. Morsicatio buccarum. Gen Dent. 2006;54(6):442. 444
85. Sewerin I. A clinical and epidemiologic study morsicatio buccarum-labiorum. Scand J Dent Res. 1971;79(2):73–80.

Labiolingual Diseases

6

Lu Jiang, Xin Jin, and Qianming Chen

Keywords
Cheilitis · Eczematous Cheilitis · Exfoliative Cheilitis · Cheilitis Glandularis · Cheilitis Granulomatosa · Angular Cheilitis · Geographic Glossitis · Fissured Tongue · Atrophic Glossitis · Median Rhomboid Glossitis · Lingual Papillitis · Coated Tongue · Burning Mouth Syndrome

L. Jiang
State Key Laboratory of Oral Diseases, National Clinical Research Center for Oral Diseases, Department of Oral Medicine, West China Hospital of Stomatology, Sichuan University, Chengdu, Sichuan, China

X. Jin
College of Stomatology, Chongqing Medical University, Chongqing Key Laboratory of Oral Diseases and Biomedical Sciences, Chongqing, China

Q. Chen (✉)
Changjiang Scholars Program, Ministry of Education, Beijing, China

State Key Laboratory of Oral Diseases, National Clinical Research Center for Oral Diseases, Department of Oral Medicine, West China Hospital of Stomatology, Sichuan University, Chengdu, Sichuan, China
e-mail: qmchen@scu.edu.cn

6.1 Cheilitis

Case 60 Eczematous Cheilitis

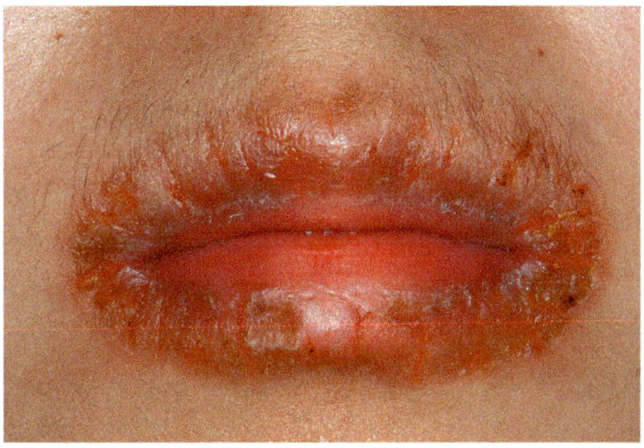

Fig. 6.1 Many scattered vertical fissures distributed on mucosa of upper and lower lips, with exudate and yellow crust

Age: 17 years
Sex: Male
Chief Complaints:
A 17-year-old boy complained of cracked lips associated with pain for 2 months
History of Present Illness:
A 17-year-old boy presented to our clinic complaining of dry and scaly lips, which were followed by painful, cracked, and bleeding lesions for the past 2 months. He habitually licked his lips.
Past Medical History: None
Allergy: None

Q. Chen, X. Zeng (eds.), *Case Based Oral Mucosal Diseases*,
https://doi.org/10.1007/978-981-13-0286-2_6

Physical Examination:
Multiple vertical rhagades, redness, effusions, and yellow crusts were observed on the upper and lower lips (Fig. 6.1). There was no cutaneous involvement.
Diagnosis:
Eczematous cheilitis
Diagnosis Basis:
This patient had eczema, erosions, redness, edema, and rhagades on the lips, giving adequate clues to the diagnosis.
Management:

1. Aerosol therapy
   Rp.: Dexamethasone sodium phosphate injection 1 ml × 1
   Gentamycin sulfate injection 2 ml × 1
   Vitamin B12 injection 1 ml × 1
   Vitamin C injection 2.5 ml × 1
   Sig.: aerosol therapy b.i.d.
2. Medication
   Rp.: Prednisone acetate 5 mg × 15 tablets
   Sig.: 15 mg p.o. q.m.
   Multivitamin formula with minerals 60 tablets
   Sig.: 1 tablet q.d. p.o.
   Compound chlorhexidine solution 300 ml × 1
   Sig.: local hydropathic compresses t.i.d.
   Dexamethasone paste 15 g × 1
   Sig.: topical use t.i.d.
3. We advised the patient not to lick his lips to prevent avulsion of his lip lesions. He was also advised to pay attention to his diet to avoid worsening of symptoms.

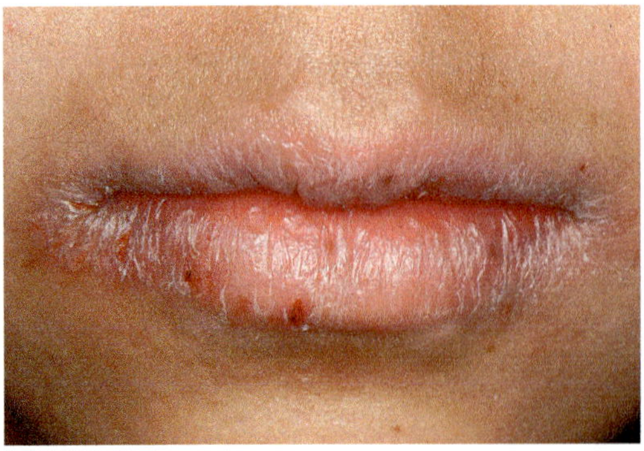

Fig. 6.2 Dryness of upper and lower lips, more scales visible, with some shallow chapping

Case 61 Exfoliative Cheilitis
Age: 22 years
Sex: Female
Chief Complaints:
A 22-year-old woman complained of dry and scaly lips for 3 years
History of Present Illness:
A 22-year-old woman presented to our clinic complaining of dry and scaly lips with slight itching for the past 3 years.
Past Medical History: None
Allergy: None
Physical Examination:
Dryness, scaling, and small rhagades were present on the upper and lower lips (Fig. 6.2). There was no cutaneous involvement.
Diagnosis:
Exfoliative cheilitis
Diagnosis Basis:
The patient complained of dryness and scales on the lips, providing clues pointing to the diagnosis.
Management:

1. Medication
   Rp.: Multivitamin formula with minerals 60 tablets
   Sig.: 1 tablet q.d. p.o.
   Compound chlorhexidine solution 300 ml × 1
   Sig.: local hydropathic compresses t.i.d.
   Compound triamcinolone acetonide cream 5 g × 1
   Sig.: topical use t.i.d.
2. We advised the patient not to lick her lips to prevent avulsion of the lesions on her lips. She was also advised to pay attention to her diet to prevent exacerbation of symptoms.

Case 62 Cheilitis Glandularis

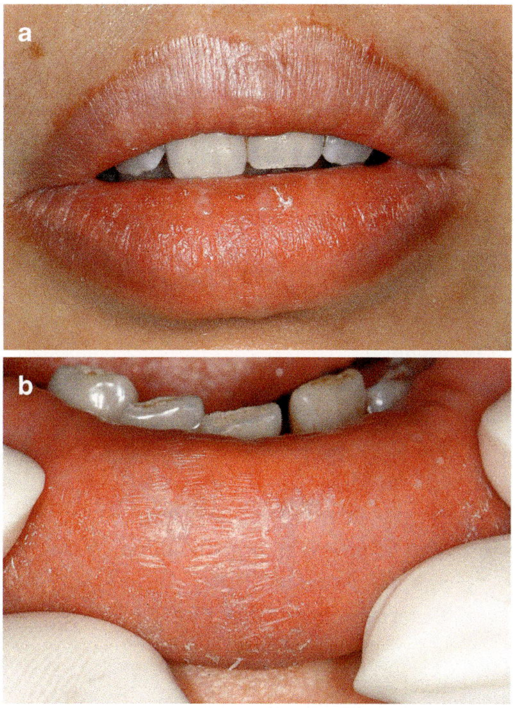

Fig. 6.3 (**a**) Dryness and slight swelling of lower lip, small granules visible in vermilion labial mucosa, and clear, transparent mucous exudate visible upon manual compression. (**b**) Clear, transparent mucous exudate visible upon manual compression of inner mucosa of lower lip

Age: 41 years
Sex: Female
Chief Complaints:
A 41-year-old woman complained of peeling of her lips for over 30 years
History of Present Illness:
A 41-year-old woman presented to our clinic with recurrent peeling of her lips with exudation of viscous fluid and a feeling of adhesion between the lips for over 30 years. She had no other symptoms, such as dryness, pain, or itching.
Past Medical History: None
Allergy: None.
Physical Examination:
Mild dryness and small scales were present on the upper and lower lips. Oral cavity examination revealed multiple nodules on the vermilion border of the upper lip and the inner aspect of the lower labial mucous membrane (Fig. 6.3a). Enlarged ostia that secreted clear tenacious mucus were visible (Fig. 6.3b).
Diagnosis:
Cheilitis glandularis
Diagnosis Basis:

1. The patient had some typical symptoms, such as a feeling of adhesion between the lips, peeling, and clear fluid secretion.
2. Oral cavity examination revealed multiple nodules on the labial mucous membrane. Enlarged ostia that secreted clear tenacious mucus were visible.

Management:

1. Medication
   Rp.: Multivitamin formula with minerals 60 tablets
   Sig.: 1 tablet q.d. p.o.
   Compound chlorhexidine solution 300 ml × 1
   Sig.: local hydropathic compresses t.i.d.
   Dexamethasone paste 15 g × 1
   Sig.: topical use t.i.d.
2. We advised the patient not to lick her lips to prevent avulsion of the lip lesions. She was also advised to pay attention to her diet to avoid worsening of symptoms.

Case 63 Cheilitis Granulomatosa (Melkersson-Rosenthal Syndrome)

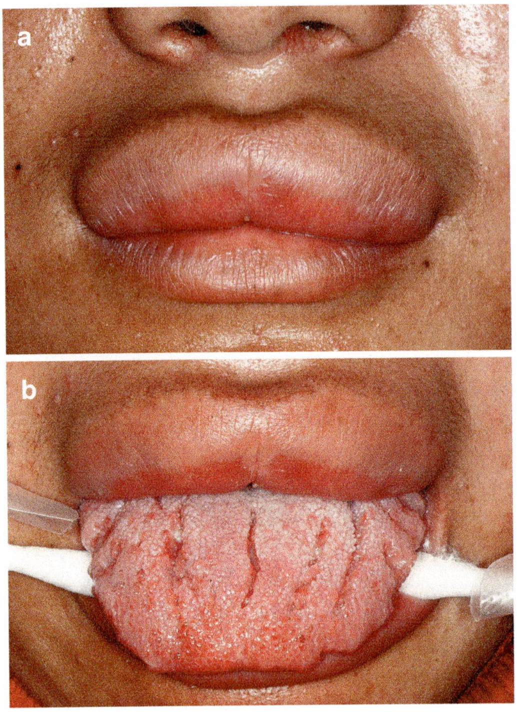

Fig. 6.4 (**a**) Edema and induration of the upper lip. (**b**) Deep grooves in dorsum of the tongue

Age: 14 years
Sex: Female
Chief Complaints:
A 14-year-old girl complained of diffusely swollen lips and cracked tongue for 3 years
History of Present Illness:
A 14-year-old girl presented to our clinic with diffuse swelling of the upper lip and nasal skin for over 3 years. She reported no obvious causes or other symptoms such as pain. In addition, she had also noted some cracks on the tongue and complained of pain while eating spicy food. The patient had taken anti-inflammatory drugs but her labial lesions did not improve.
Past Medical History: None
Allergy: None
Physical Examination:
Diffuse swelling of the upper lip with an overlying tough texture was noted (Fig. 6.4a). An oral examination revealed several grooves on the tongue (Fig. 6.4b).

Diagnosis:
Melkersson-Rosenthal syndrome (hypoplastic type)
Diagnosis Basis:

1. Diffuse swelling and decreased elasticity of the lips
2. Fissured tongue
3. Recurrent swelling of the nasal skin

Management:

1. Medication
   Rp.: Loratadine 10 mg × 12 tablets
      Sig.: 10 mg q.d. p.o.
      Multivitamin formula with minerals 60 tablets
      Sig.: 1 tablet q.d. p.o.
      2% sodium bicarbonate solution 250 ml × 1
      Sig.: rinse t.i.d.
      Dexamethasone paste 15 g × 1
      Sig.: topical use t.i.d.
      Nystatin liniment 15 g × 1
      Sig.: topical use t.i.d.
2. Triamcinolone acetonide (TA) injection 40 mg × 1
   Sig.: multipoint low-dose injection st.

[Review] Cheilitis
Cheilitis is an umbrella term for labial inflammatory diseases, and it has varied clinical manifestations. The current classifications of the cheilitis are controversial. It can be classified on the basis of progression: acute and chronic cheilitis. It may also be classified on the basis of the clinical manifestations: erosive, eczematous, and exfoliative cheilitis. In addition, it can be classified on the basis of the etiologic factors and pathology: chronic nonspecific cheilitis, cheilitis glandularis, benign lymphatic proliferative cheilitis, granulomatous cheilitis, Melkersson-Rosenthal syndrome, actinic cheilitis, and allergic cheilitis [1]. Combining our clinical and treatment experience, we divided cheilitis, except for allergic cheilitis, into the following types:

1. Eczematous cheilitis: This entity includes actinic cheilitis, cheilitis of benign lymphadenosis, and cheilitis with clinical manifesta-

tions of eczema and erosion. Actinic cheilitis is caused by an allergy to ultraviolet radiation. After exposure to sunlight, melanin deposition occurs in normal individuals, which makes their skin darker, causing the symptoms to regress spontaneously. However, individuals with sun allergy, on being exposed to an overdose of sunlight, can have changes in melanin deposition, intracellular or extracellular edema, collagen denaturation, and increased cellular proliferation; these changes may initiate pathogenesis. Cheilitis of benign lymphadenosis is related to the remnants of the primary lymphoid hyperplasia, which resulted following exposure to radiation during embryonic development.

The histopathological changes of actinic cheilitis include epithelial hyperkeratosis (or parakeratosis), intracellular or extracellular edema, bullous changes, infiltration of inflammatory cells around the blood vessels and in the submucosa, and basophilic changes in the collagen subepithelially [2]. Histopathologically, cheilitis of benign lymphadenosis is characterized by the presence of lymphoid follicle-like structures in the subepithelial connective tissue. Sometimes, there may be a focal collection of numerous lymphoid cells with less lymphoid follicles.

The main clinical features of eczematous cheilitis are erosions of the red lip, especially the lower red lip. Light yellow exudates and edema may be present on the vermilion border. If deep erosion or secondary infection occurs, an obvious swelling of the vermilion border with bleeding, ulceration, and crusting may be present. In addition, the cardinal symptom of benign lymphoproliferative cheilitis is paroxysmal severe itching.

Systemic therapies for eczematous cheilitis include administration of micronutrients and vitamin supplements. Patients are usually administered one tablet of multivitamin formula with minerals each day, for a period of 30 days. In case of more serious manifestations, the patients are administered prednisone acetate 15–25 mg once a day in the morning, or hydroxychloroquine 0.1 g twice a day, for a period of 2 weeks.

Local therapies for eczematous cheilitis mainly include hydropathic compresses with chlorhexidine solution or topical steroids, such as dexamethasone paste, prednisolone acetate injection, or triamcinolone acetonide injection (dilution, 1:5) thrice a day. Recombinant human epidermal growth factor hydrogels or solutions are also used. For cases with copious exudates, severe erosions, and thick crusts, aerosol therapy with dexamethasone sodium phosphate, gentamicin sulfate, vitamin C, and vitamin B12 injections once or twice daily for 3 days is recommended. Besides, local and multipoint low-dose injections of triamcinolone acetonide may be administered to the labial lesions once a week or every 2 weeks.

2. Exfoliative cheilitis: The etiology of exfoliative cheilitis is complicated; it may be related to dry climate; windy environment; cold weather; irritation due to tobacco, alcohol, hot food, and repeated lip licking; and fungal infection. The clinical features of exfoliative cheilitis primarily include dryness and the presence of several scales on the vermilion border. Vertical fractures, such as shallow cracks or deep fissures extending to the perioral skin, associated with bleeding, can be found in lesions of the red lip. Gray scales may be seen along the completely vermilion border. Patients with exfoliative cheilitis secondary to fungal infection complain of itching and gray scales on the vermilion border and surrounding skin. Histopathologically, the disease shows nonspecific inflammatory changes.

   Systemic therapies for exfoliative cheilitis include administration of micronutrient and vitamin supplements. Patients are administered one tablet of multivitamin formula with minerals each day, for a period of 30 days. Local therapies mainly include hydropathic compresses with chlorhexidine solution or topical steroids such as dexamethasone paste, prednisolone acetate injection, or triamcinolone acetonide injection (dilution, 1:5) thrice a day. Recombinant human epidermal growth factor hydrogels or solutions are also used. In cases with deep rhagades involving the labial lesion, local and multipoint low-dose triamcinolone acetonide and normal saline or 2% lidocaine injections may be administered into the labial lesions once a week or every 2 weeks. Besides, for exfoliative cheilitis secondary to fungal infection, nystatin liniment or ketoconazole ointment is recommended.

3. Cheilitis glandularis: The etiology of cheilitis glandularis is unknown. A recent study suggests that the function of some aquaporins (AQPs) in the minor salivary glands of the lips may be altered in cheilitis glandularis; consequently, there may be abnormalities in the water flow mechanism with possible alteration of the salivary composition [3]. The histopathological features of cheilitis glandularis include chronic sialadenitis, ectasia of the gland and the salivary ducts, and epithelial metaplasia and fibrosis of the duct. The most common site of involvement is the lower lip. Its clinical signs include macrocheilia caused by swelling and thickening of the local lesions with mucus retention and fibrosis of the dilated ducts. Many red and pinpoint-sized nodules may be seen in the medial mucosa of the lips. The use of a magnifying glass clearly revealed the enlarged ductal orifices of minor salivary glands. There is usually an intermittent discharge of a sticky clear fluid, and the lips were often stuck together on waking up in the morning.

   We recommend that the lesions should face away from the light during treatment. The drugs used for treatment are similar to those described for eczematous cheilitis although the literature reported that surgical resection of the labial lesions improved the appearance [4].

4. Cheilitis granulomatosa: The etiology and underlying mechanisms that cause cheilitis granulomatosa remain unclear. Currently, it is thought to be caused by some microbes, such as streptococcus, mycobacterium, and herpes simplex virus; allergic reactions to certain substances, such as cobalt and food additives, vasomotor disorders causing dysregulation of the autonomic nervous system, and genetic predisposition are also implicated. Literature shows that it might precede, simultaneously occur with, or give some indications as to the occurrence of intestinal Crohn's disease [5]. Besides, this study suggested that the labial lesions might be related to the adjacent teeth in the form of chronic periodontitis. The most common site of involvement of cheilitis granulomatosa is the upper lip. Its clinical features include slow and progressive swelling of the unilateral red lip with normal elasticity and color or mild redness in the early stages. Owing to considerable swelling, the patients may appear to have fissures without erosions or ulcers on the vermilion border. The swelling is usually soft and exhibits no pitting on pressure. As the disease progresses, the vermilion swelling increases to two to three times the size of a normal lip; it may even lead to the occurrence of macrocheilia with corrugated longitudinal cracks (Figs. 6.5 and 6.6). Its main histopathological features include non-caseating granulomas in the lamina propria and submucosa, accompanied by chronic inflammatory cells, such as lymphocytes and plasma cells.

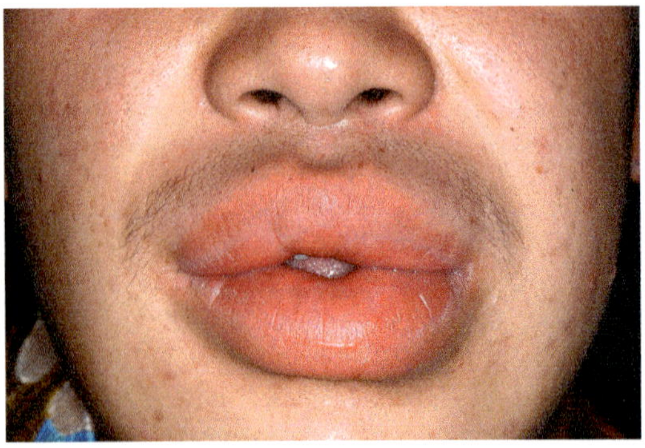

Fig. 6.5 Macrocheilia secondary to granulomatous cheilitis

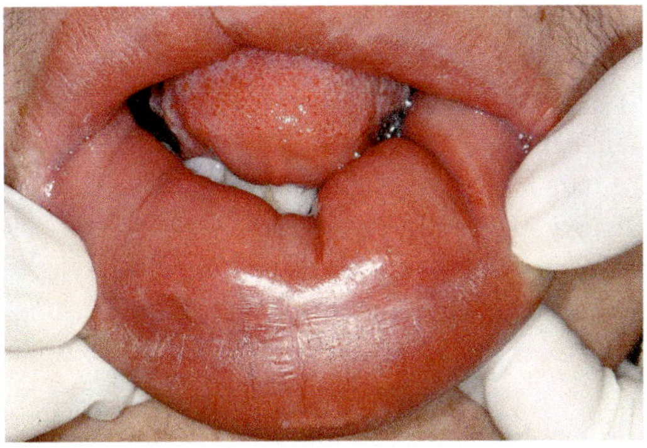

Fig. 6.6 Tile-shaped vertical fissures

Cheilitis granulomatosa is one of the main manifestations of Melkersson-Rosenthal syndrome (MRS). This entity consists of persistent or recurrent orofacial edema, relapsing facial palsy, and fissured tongue. This complete triad of symptoms is uncommon. The most frequent sign is granulomatous cheilitis [6].

The initial therapy of granulomatous cheilitis is the elimination of chronic periapical periodontitis. Current literature reports that the main treatment includes administration of corticosteroids (triamcinolone acetonide), antibiotics (minocycline and roxithromycin), or other immunomodulators (methotrexate) and even surgical resection [7]. We administer local and multipoint low-dose triamcinolone acetonide (or betamethasone) and normal saline (or 2% lidocaine) injections into the labial lesions once a week or every 2 weeks. The patients may also be administered loratadine 10 mg once a day, for a period of 2 weeks. Patients with macrocheilia may be offered surgical resection of the labial lesions for better cosmesis.

6.2 Angular Cheilitis

Case 64 Angular Cheilitis

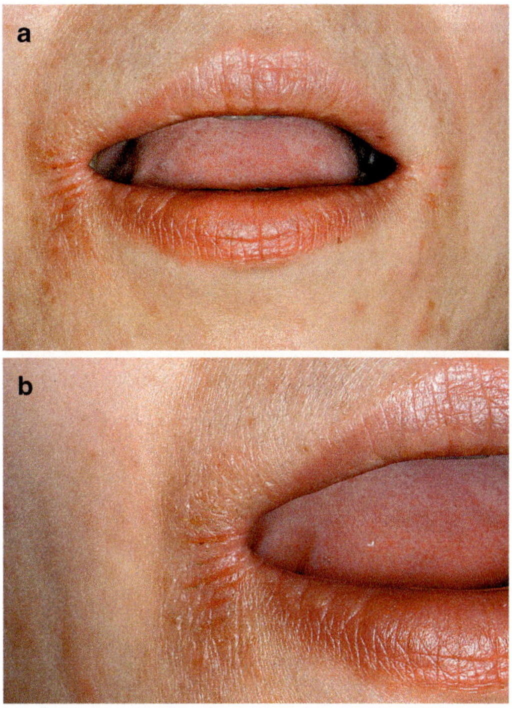

Fig. 6.7 (**a**) Bilateral angular fissuring, more severe on the right side. (**b**) Right angular fissuring

Age: 41 years
Sex: Female
Chief Complaints:
Bilateral angular rhagades for 6 months in a 41-year-old female
History of Present Illness:
A 41-year-old female presented to our clinic with rhagades of the mouth on bilateral commissures lasting for 6 months. She complained of severe pain on the right side with no itching.

Past Medical History: None
Allergy: None
Physical Examination:
Rhagades were observed on both commissures of the mouth. Additional deeper fissures were present on the right side with tenderness, and no apparent exudation was indicated (Fig. 6.7).
Diagnosis:
Angular cheilitis
Diagnosis Basis:

1. The lesion was located on both commissures of the mouth.
2. Rhagades were observed in the angular area of the mouth.

Management:

1. Medication
   Rp.: Compound vitamin B 100 tablets
   Sig.: 2 tablets t.i.d. p.o.
   Recombinant human epidermal growth factor hydrogel 20 g × 1
   Sig.: topical use q.d.
   Compound ulcer paste 15 g × 1
   Sig.: topical use t.i.d.
2. The patient was instructed not to lick the angular area of the mouth.

Case 65 Angular Cheilitis Accompanied by Perioral Dermatitis (Children)

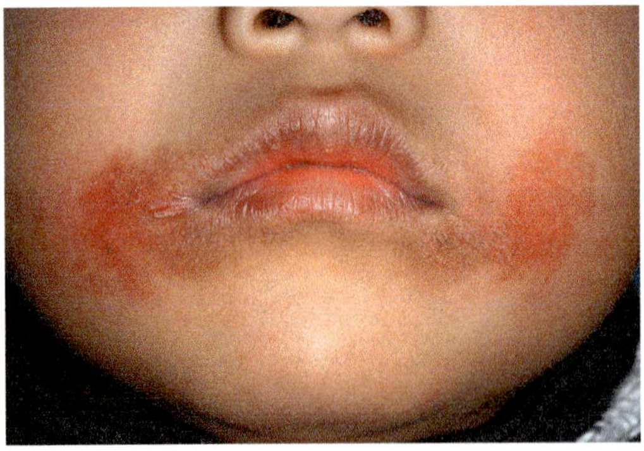

Fig. 6.8 Right angular fissuring, bilateral redness, roughness, and squamous appearance of the skin surrounding the labial angles

Age: 6 years
Sex: Male
Chief Complaints:
Red, itchy skin adjacent to the bilateral angles of the mouth for 3 weeks in a 6-year-old boy
History of Present Illness:
A 6-year-old boy visited our clinic with dryness of the bilateral commissures of the mouth lasting for 3 weeks. Fissures were observed in the right angles of the mouth, with redness and itching in adjacent areas. The child tended to lick his lips and wipe his mouth with the cuff of his clothes.
Past Medical History: None
Allergy: None.
Physical Examination:
The rhagade on the right angle of the mouth was around 6 mm in length, and the skin adjacent to both commissures of the mouth appeared to be red and rough with scales on the surface (Fig. 6.8).
Diagnosis:
Angular cheilitis accompanied by perioral dermatitis
Diagnosis Basis:

1. The lesion was located on the commissures of the mouth and perioral skin.
2. Rhagades were displayed in the angular area of the mouth.

Management:

1. Aerosol Therapy
   Rp.: Dexamethasone sodium phosphate injection 1 ml × 1
   Gentamycin sulfate injection 2 ml × 1
   Vitamin B12 injection 1 ml × 1
   Vitamin C injection 2.5 ml × 1
   Sig.: aerosol therapy b.i.d.
2. Medication
   Rp.: Compound vitamin B 100 tablets
   Sig.: 2 tablets t.i.d. p.o.
   Recombinant human epidermal growth factor hydrogel 20 g × 1
   Sig.: topical use q.d.
   Compound ulcer paste 15 g × 1
   Sig.: topical use t.i.d.
3. The child was ordered not to wipe the angular area of his mouth with the cuff of his clothes and to eat less spicy food.

Case 66 Angular Cheilitis Along with Oral Candidosis

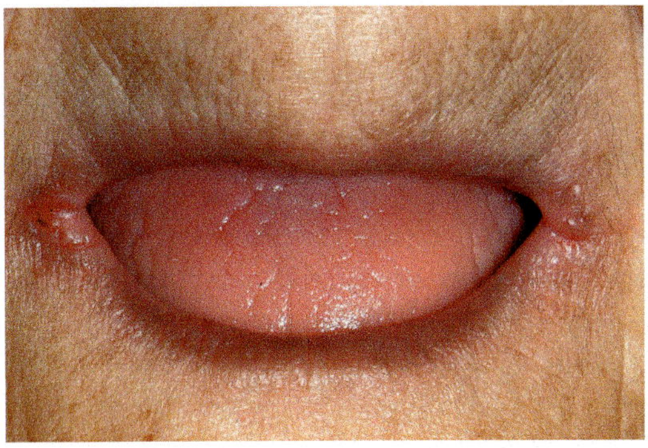

Fig. 6.9 Redness at the bilateral labial angles, obvious chapping on right side

Age: 82 years
Sex: Female
Chief Complaints:
Red lesions and rhagades in both commissures of the mouth for 6 months in an 82-year-old woman
History of Present Illness:
An 82-year-old woman visited our clinic with redness and rhagades in both commissures of the mouth lasting for 6 months, together with pain and hemorrhagic tendency when she opened her mouth to the limit.
Past Medical History: Cataract
Allergy: None
Physical Examination:
Erythematous lesions were observed in bilateral angles of the mouth, and rhagades on the right side were more obvious. Additionally, the filiform papilla on the dorsum of the tongue appeared to be slightly atrophic and erythematous, while the palate mucosa presented with congestion and redness (Fig. 6.9). The patient was toothless in both dentitions. No obvious abnormalities were observed during routine blood examination.
Clinical Impression:
Angular cheilitis
Further Examination:
No apparent results were obtained during routine blood examination and blood glucose testing. Positive results for fungal infection were obtained in the smear test of the mouth and both angular areas.

Diagnosis:
Angular cheilitis along with oral candidosis
Diagnosis Basis:

1. Redness and rhagades were visible in both commissures of the mouth, along with red mucosa on the tongue and palate.
2. Positive result for fungal infection in the smear test.

Management:

1. Medication
   Rp.: Pidotimod 0.4 g × 18 tablets
      Sig.: 0.4 g q.d. p.o.
      Folic acid 5 mg × 100 tablets
      Sig.: 10 mg t.i.d. p.o.
      Compound vitamin B 100 tablets
      Sig.: 2 tablets t.i.d. p.o.
      2% sodium bicarbonate solution 250 ml × 1
      Sig.: rinse t.i.d.
      Nystatin liniment 15 g × 1
      Sig.: topical use t.i.d.

[Review] Angular Cheilitis

Angular cheilitis is the inflammation of bilateral commissures of the upper and lower lips. The morbidity is 0.7–3.8% for adults and 0.2–15.1% for children.

Angular cheilitis, clinically characterized by erythema, moist maceration, ulceration, crusting at the corners of the mouth, and scales covering adjacent areas, is usually accompanied by various amounts of pain, burning, and itching sensation.

To date, few studies have been conducted to explore the etiology and mechanisms of angular cheilitis. However, it is generally believed to be one disease caused by multiple local and systemic factors, acting alone or in combination [8].

Angular cheilitis associated with local factors is primarily categorized as irritant, allergic, or infectious.

Irritant angular cheilitis accounts for approximately 22% of all cases. Compared with other sites, the corners of the mouth and lips are exposed to stagnant saliva for a longer period and are therefore more likely to be infused and digested by the stagnant salivin, exacerbating irritation and inflammation. Angular cheilitis is more easily induced by prolonged contact with these irritants and anatomical changes, for instance, deeper wrinkles in the skin adjacent to the corners of the mouth [9]. The reduction of vertical distance enables the formation of grooves in the skin in the corners of the mouth, which is a significant factor contributing to angular cheilitis in older people, as seen in 11% of elderly patients with angular cheilitis and 18% of denture-wearing patients with angular cheilitis. In addition, common irritant factors in the clinic include anodontia, tooth displacement, wearing orthodontic devices, destruction of elastic tissue by prolonged ultraviolet radiation and smoking, hygrostomia, and mechanical stimulation of pencils, dental floss, and oral mirror handles. All of the above factors can cause or exaggerate angular cheilitis [8, 10, 11].

Cheilitis can be induced when allergens come into contact with oral mucosa and the lips. Allergens can permeate the mucosa more easily in the presence of irritant angular cheilitis, and in turn, patients may suffer from allergic cheilitis. Several factors, namely, lipsticks, toothpastes, cosmetics, mouthwash, amalgam, and dental restoration materials, can trigger angular cheilitis [12–14].

Infectious angular cheilitis is primarily caused by *Candida albicans*, followed by *Staphylococcus aureus* [10, 15]. Recurrent herpes labialis, associated with virus infection, also classified as infectious angular cheilitis, is usually seen in the vermilion border and can resemble the symptoms of angular cheilitis when it occurs in the corners of the mouth. Pivotal clues for diagnosing herpes simplex in the corners of the mouth based on medical history are recurrence at the same site, a history of blistering, and duration of about 5–7 days [16].

Angular cheilitis is also correlated with variable systemic factors.

Angular cheilitis can sometimes predict nutritional deficiencies. About 25% of patients are lacking in iron and vitamin B, mainly vitamin B2, B6, and B12. Anemia can be found in 11.3–31.8% of patients with angular cheilitis. Additionally, the deficiency of nicotinic acid, folic acid, and zinc is related to angular cheilitis. Therefore, angular cheilitis is frequently accompanied by atrophic glossitis.

Angular cheilitis is associated with various systemic diseases, including Down's syndrome, xerostomia, inflammatory bowel disease, Sjogren syndrome, diabetes, and some systemic infectious diseases, namely, acquired immune deficiency syndrome, syphilis, and so on.

Angular cheilitis might also be caused by the adverse effects of some medicines. The conventional medicine mainly contains isotretinoin, indinavir against HIV, and narcotics like cocaine and heroin [17].

Local and systemic factors usually work together. There might be diverse causative factors for the same patient; for instance, angular cheilitis in weak elderly people is collectively caused by the reduction of vertical distance in the mouth, malnutrition, dryness of the mouth, and colonization by candida or bacteria.

Hence, it is necessary to inquire about the patients' history of angular cheilitis comprehensively, including initial site, duration, suspected allergens, exaggerated or attenuated factors, as well as whether the patient takes drugs or has malnutrition, anemia, or gastrointestinal diseases. Close attention should be paid to the presence of vertical distance reduction in the lower face, oral hygiene, and whether the patient wears denture or not, combined with the culturing results for bacteria and fungi. Topical treatment is primarily dependent on the removal of local irritant factors, including adjusting and cleaning dentures and maintaining oral hygiene. Additionally, antibiotic ointments, such as chlortetracycline eye ointment, or nystatin liniment and compound ketoconazole creams against fungi, compound ulcer pastes for rhagades, and recombinant human epidermal growth factor hydrogel or solution may be applied to target the possible causes. In addition, specifically systemic treatment should be employed to handle the possible systemic etiology.

6.3 Geographic Glossitis

Case 67 Geographic Glossitis (Adult)

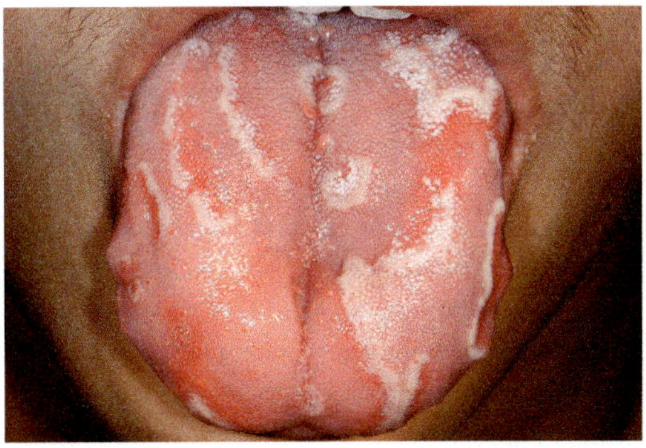

Fig. 6.10 Bilateral atrophy of filiform papillae on dorsum of the tongue, proliferation of peripheral filiform papillae, presenting as geographic tongue

Age: 24 years
Sex: Male
Chief Complaints:
Striae on the dorsum of the tongue for 1 year in a 24-year-old male
History of Present Illness:
A 24-year-old male presented to our clinic with striae on the dorsum of his tongue lasting for 1 year. The location of the striae on the dorsum changed over time, accompanied by irritant pain when eating. The patient was highly susceptible to the cold virus.
Past Medical History: None
Allergy: None
Physical Examination:
Atrophy of the filiform papillae was observed in the central area of the lesion on bilateral sides of the tongue, surrounded by hyperplasic filiform papillae in the peripheral zone. The whole area resembled a geographic map (Fig. 6.10).
Diagnosis:
Geographic glossitis
Diagnosis Basis:

1. The dorsum of the patient's tongue was covered by geographic striae.
2. The lesion was migratory.

Management:

1. Medication
   Rp.: Thymopeptide enteric-coated tablets 20 mg × 30 tablets
   Sig.: 20 mg q.d. p.o.
   Multivitamin formula with mineral tablets 30 tablets
   Sig.: 1 tablet q.d. p.o.
   Compound chlorhexidine solution 300 ml × 1
   Sig.: rinse t.i.d.
   Compound ulcer paste 15 g × 1
   Sig.: topical use t.i.d.
2. The patient was instructed to maintain a balanced diet.

Case 68 Geographic Glossitis (Children)

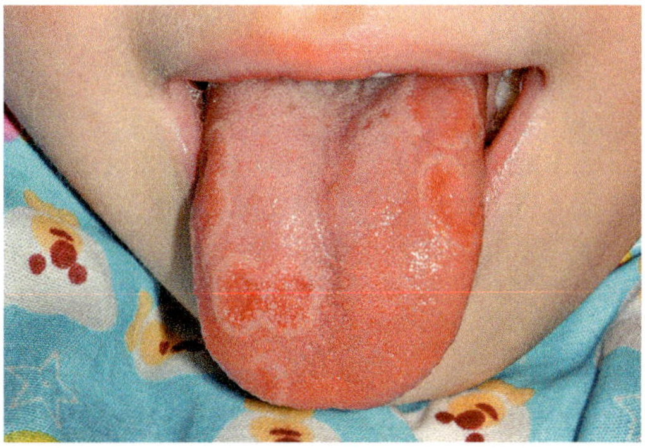

Fig. 6.11 Many scattered regions of filiform papillary atrophy on the dorsum of the tongue, proliferation of peripheral filiform papillae, presenting as geographic tongue

Age: 3.5 years
Sex: Female
Chief Complaints:
Striae on the dorsum of the tongue for 3.5 years in a 3.5-year-old girl
History of Present Illness:
A 3.5-year-old girl visited our clinic with striae on the dorsum of her tongue that had persisted since she was born. The location and shape of the striae on the dorsum changed over time, and no impact on her eating was noted. The little girl was in good condition and not selective about food.

Past Medical History: None
Allergy: None
Physical Examination:
Multiple lesions were observed on the dorsum of her tongue, characterized by atrophic filiform papillae in the central area and hyperplasic filiform papillae in the peripheral zone, appearing as a geographic map (Fig. 6.11).
Diagnosis:
Geographic glossitis
Diagnosis Basis:

1. The dorsum of the patient's tongue was partially occupied by geographic striae.
2. The lesion was migratory.

Management:
Explanation of the illness and further observation were suggested.

[Review] Geographic Glossitis
Geographic glossitis is also called migratory glossitis, named after its clinical resemblance to the winding borders of the mainland. Its prevalence is reported to be in the range of 1–14%, and a recent Malaysian study presented the prevalence as 2.2% [18, 19].

To date, the etiology of geographic glossitis remains unknown. It is, however, reported to be correlated with some systemic diseases, such as diabetes mellitus, seborrheic dermatitis, spastic bronchitis in children, gastrointestinal disorders, psoriasis, Down's syndrome, and nutritional deficiency (vitamin B, zinc). Other reports suggest a relationship with contraceptive use, allergy, and hormone level fluctuations [20, 21]. In addition, psychological factors, family heredity, endocrine factors, and an immunocompromised condition can serve as contributing factors. A large-scale study implied that young age (<30 years old), nonsmoking status, and allergies were significantly related to migratory glossitis, but there was no relationship to gender, dermatological diseases, and systemic diseases [21].

The main clinical features of geographic glossitis are the following: a smooth atrophic area of filiform papillae surrounded by a peripheral zone with white elevated filiform papillae resembling a winding border, frequent variation of location and shapes, and a migratory lesion on the dorsum of the tongue. It is usually observed on the frontal part of the dorsum of the tongue, sometimes extending to the ventral mucosa of the tongue, floor of the mouth or the buccal mucosa, termed erythema migrans [22] (Fig. 6.12). Geographic glossitis and a fissured tongue might occur simultaneously (Fig. 6.13). Most patients are asymptomatic, though some patients may experience a smarting sensation with hot and spicy food. The lesion is benign and local, and spontaneous remission may sometimes occur. The diagnosis of geographic glossitis can be performed based on medical history and physical examination.

It is not necessary to treat patients without symptoms; however, psychological guidance is suggested. When symptoms are reported, oral

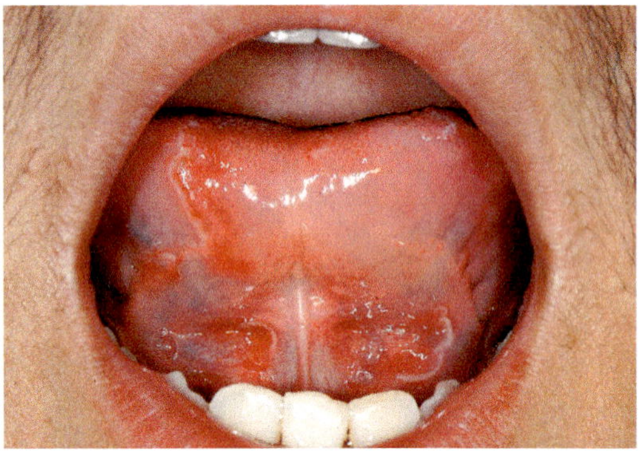

Fig. 6.12 Erythema migrans: multiple yellow and white erythematous regions visible on ventral surface of the tongue and floor of the mouth

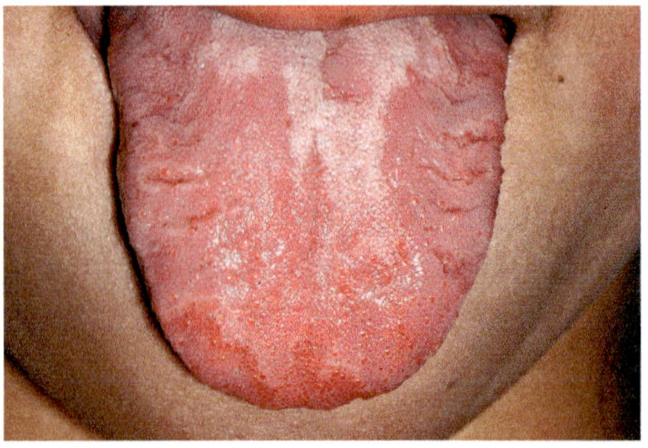

Fig. 6.13 Geographic tongue accompanied by fissured tongue

immunopotentiators may be adopted, for instance, thymopeptide enteric-coated tablets, 20 mg, q.d. or transfer factor capsules, 3–6 mg, 2–3 times/day. Multivitamin formulas with minerals tablets can also be administered, 1 tablet, q.d., for a whole month. In addition to the aforementioned, topical mouth rinses containing 4% sodium bicarbonate solution or compound chlorhexidine solution and topical use of compound ulcer pastes or corticosteroid ointments are recommended. Management of geographic glossitis aims at symptom remission rather than achieving the disappearance of striae.

6.4 Fissured Tongue

Case 69 Fissured Tongue
Age: 41 years
Sex: Female
Chief Complaints:
A 41-year-old woman presented with fissures on her tongue for thc past 6 years
History of Present Illness:
A 41-year-old woman presented to our clinic with fissures on the dorsum of her tongue for the past 6 years, accompanied by irritant pain while eating spicy food. The patient was prone to developing frequent colds.
Past Medical History: Uterus myoma
Allergy: None
Physical Examination:
Multiple fissures were present on the anterior aspect and bilateral sides of the tongue (Fig. 6.14); no other oral mucosal abnormalities were observed.

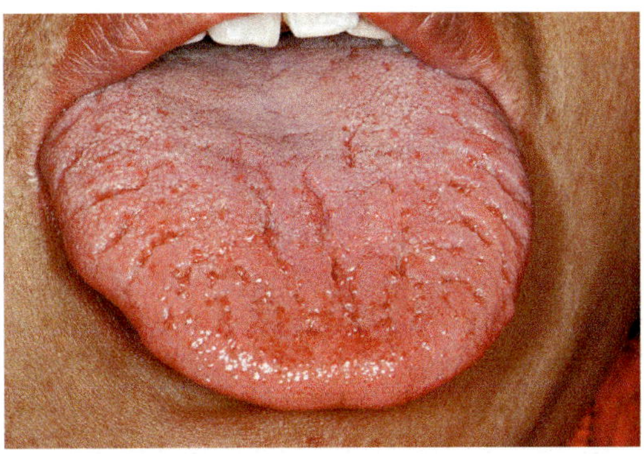

Fig. 6.14 Many fissures visible in anterior dorsum of the tongue and lateral mucosa of the tongue

Diagnosis:
Fissured tongue
Diagnosis Basis:
Fissures on the dorsum of the tongue
Management:

1. Medication
   Rp.: Thymopeptide enteric-coated tablets 20 mg × 30 tablets
   Sig.: 20 mg q.d. p.o.
   Folic acid 5 mg × 100 tablets
   Sig.: 10 mg t.i.d. p.o.
   Compound vitamin B 100 tablets
   Sig.: 2 tablets t.i.d. p.o.
   Sodium bicarbonate solution (2%) 250 ml × 1
   Sig.: rinse t.i.d.
   Compound ulcer paste 15 g × 1
   Sig.: topical use t.i.d.
2. Psychological counseling

[Review] Fissured Tongue
A fissured tongue often has fissures of various depths and alignments and presents with different shapes (mainly dendritic); its prevalence increases with age [19]. Moreover, it is usually seen in association with a geographic tongue.

The etiology of fissured tongue currently remains unknown, and it is considered hereditary by many scholars. Recent studies indicate a remarkably increased frequency of *HLA-DRB1*08*, *HLA-DRB1*14*, *HLA-DRB1*11*, and *HLA-DRB1*16* and a decreased frequency of *HLA-DRB1*03* and *HLA-DRB1*07* in patients with fissured tongue, implying its hereditary basis [23]. Furthermore, Down's syndrome, acromegaly, psoriasis, Sjogren's syndrome, Melkersson-Rosenthal syndrome, and hormonal changes are usually associated with fissured tongues [20, 24].

Fissured tongue is generally asymptomatic, and does not require treatment. Owing to the inflammation in the fissures caused by retention of food residue and bacterial or fungal infection, patients may experience pain while eating spicy or irritant food. For such symptomatic patients, cleaning the dorsum of the tongue with a toothbrush and administering folic acid (10 mg t.i.d.) along with Vitamin B (2 tablets t.i.d.) can be helpful. Besides, for patients who are immunocompromised, oral immunopotentiators are recommended, such as thymopeptide enteric-coated tablets (20 mg q.d.) or transfer factor capsules (3–6 mg, b.i.d. or t.i.d.); 2–4% sodium bicarbonate solution or chlorhexidine solution may be used for rinsing the mouth, and the ulcer paste or nystatin liniment may be administered topically.

6.5 Atrophic Glossitis

Case 70 Atrophic Glossitis
Age: 48 years
Sex: Male
Chief Complaints:
A 48-year-old man complained of a sore tongue while eating, which was persistent for the past 2 months
History of Present Illness:
A 48-year-old man presented to our clinic with a sore tongue, which was aggravated by the spicy diet he was on for the past 2 months.
Past Medical History: Chronic enteritis
Allergy: None
Physical Examination:
Atrophy of the filiform papillae on dorsum of the tongue, with punctate hemorrhages, and atrophy of the buccal mucosa were detected (Fig. 6.15).
Laboratory Studies:
Full blood count: HGB 79 g/L (110–170 g/L), RBC 1.82 × 10^{12}/L (3.5 × 10^{12}–5.5 × 10^{12} /L), MCV 120.90 fL (80–90 fL).
Diagnosis:
Atrophic glossitis (macrocytic anemia)
Diagnosis Basis:

1. Atrophy of the filiform papillae.
2. Full blood count showed macrocytic anemia.

Management:

1. Medication
   Rp.: Lusun capsules 300 mg × 54
   Sig.: 600 mg b.i.d. p.o.
   Folic acid 5 mg × 100 tablets
   Sig.: 10 mg t.i.d. p.o.
   Mecobalamin 0.5 mg × 40 tablets
   Sig.: 0.5 mg t.i.d. p.o.
   2% sodium bicarbonate solution 250 ml × 1
   Sig.: rinse t.i.d.
   Compound ulcer paste 15 g × 1
   Sig.: topical use t.i.d.
2. Advised treatment of anemia from a hematologist.

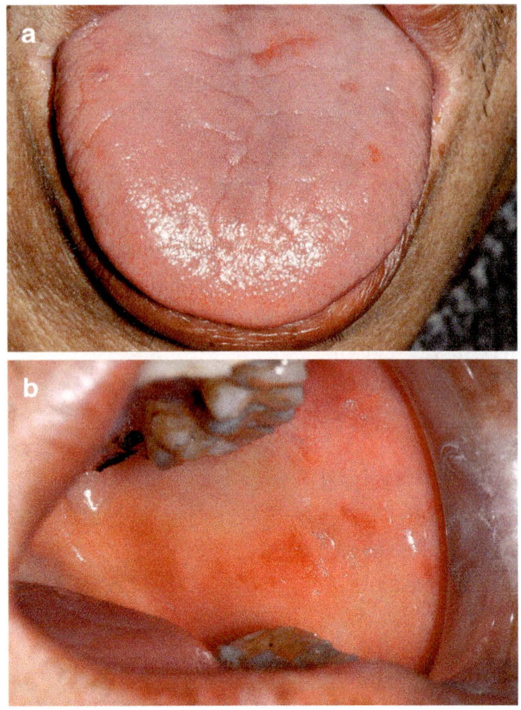

Fig. 6.15 (**a**) Atrophy of filiform papillae on dorsum of the tongue, with glossy surface and some punctate hyperemia. (**b**) Atrophy and thinning of buccal mucosa

[Review] Atrophic Glossitis
Atrophic glossitis appears as smooth, glossy tongue surface with a red or pink background. Therefore, it is also called smooth tongue. The smoothness is due to atrophy of the filiform papillae [19].

The etiology of atrophic glossitis is complex. Atrophic glossitis may be caused by infections, including localized infections (e.g., *Candida*) and systemic infections (e.g., syphilis). Atrophic glossitis may also be a primary manifestation of other underlying systemic conditions, such as anemia, nutritional deficiency (deficiencies of iron, folic acid, vitamin B12, vitamin B2, and niacin), amyloidosis, celiac disease, protein-calorie malnutrition, xerostomia (triggered by some medications), and Sjögren's syndrome [25–28]. Since anemia is the main cause of atrophic glossitis, a complete blood count is usually required for the diagnosis.

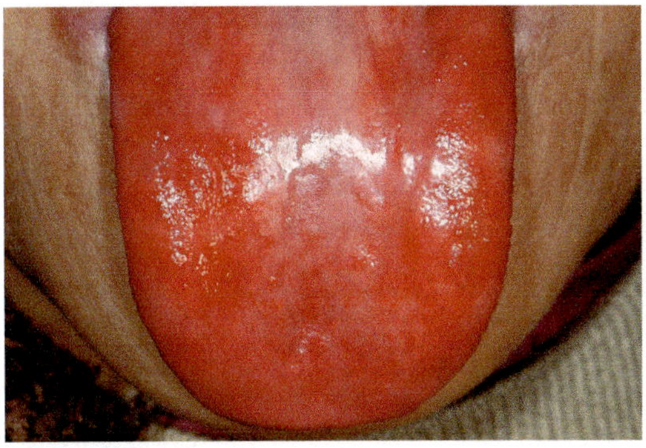

Fig. 6.16 Atrophic glossitis

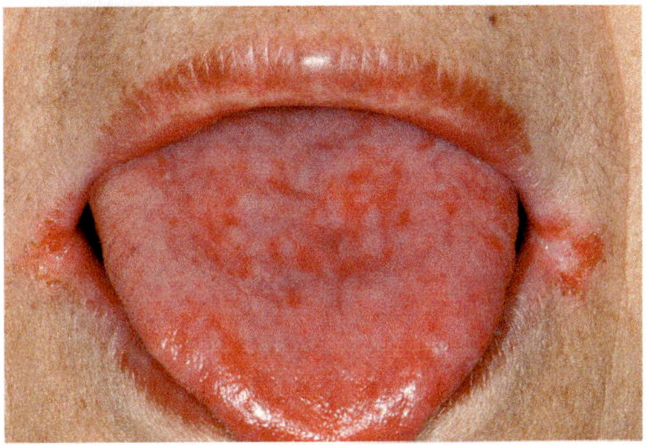

Fig. 6.17 Atrophic glossitis accompanied by angular cheilitis

Atrophic glossitis is common in aged individuals who suffer from systemic disorders. These patients complain of sore, burning tongue, and xerostomia. The major clinical manifestations include smooth, bare, red, and beefy tongue (Fig. 6.16). Atrophic glossitis is always accompanied by angular stomatitis (Fig. 6.17).

Treatment includes replacement of the missing or lacking nutrients or treatment of the underlying condition. A patient with macrocytic anemia is administered with lusun capsules, 0.3–0.6 g, 2–3 times per day; folic acid 10 mg, three times per day; mecobalamin 0.5 mg, three times per day; and vitamin B12 injection, 0.1 mg once a day, for a period of 15–30 days. If the patient has iron deficiency anemia, he/she is administered polysaccharide-iron complex capsules 150 mg once a day. Additionally, nicotinamide 100 mg is administered three times per day. Moreover, 2–4% sodium bicarbonate solution may be used for rinsing and compound ulcer paste for topical use. Nystatin liniment may also be used topically as in mycotic infections.

6.6 Median Rhomboid Glossitis

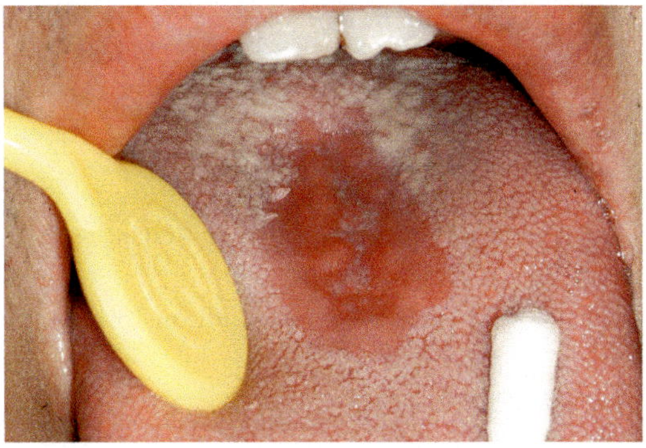

Fig. 6.18 Rhomboid regions of filiform papillary atrophy on the central and posterior dorsum of the tongue, with clear borders and glossy, red surface

Case 71 Median Rhomboid Glossitis
Age: 42 years
Sex: Male
Chief Complaints:
A 42-year-old man complained of persistent pain with partial loss of the tongue coating for the past 5 months
History of Present Illness:
A 42-year-old man presented to our clinic with a sore tongue, aggravated by the spicy diet he was on for the past 2 months.
Past Medical History: None
Allergy: None
Physical Examination:
A well-delineated erythematous area was noted, located along the dorsal midline of the posterior tongue, just anterior to the circumvallate papillae (Fig. 6.18).
Laboratory Studies:
Fungal smear was positive.
Diagnosis:
Median rhomboid glossitis
Diagnosis Basis:

1. Located along the dorsal midline of the posterior tongue
2. Rhomboid-shaped atrophy of the filiform papillae

Management:

1. Medication
   Rp.: Pidotimod 0.4 g × 24 tablets
   Sig.: 0.4 g b.i.d. p.o.
   Folic acid 5 mg × 100 tablets
   Sig.: 10 mg t.i.d. p.o.
   Compound vitamin B 100 tablets
   Sig.: 2 tablets t.i.d. p.o.
   2% sodium bicarbonate solution 250 ml × 1
   Sig.: rinse t.i.d.
   Nystatin liniment 15 g × 1
   Sig.: topical use t.i.d.

[Review] Median Rhomboid Glossitis

Median rhomboid glossitis (MRG) presents as a well-demarcated "rhomboid" area of erythema anterior to the circumvallate papillae over the mid-dorsal tongue. Most of these cases are asymptomatic. It is seen in up to 1% of the population [29, 30].

It is typically located along the dorsal midline of the posterior one-third of the tongue, anterior to the circumvallate papillae. The surface of the lesion may be smooth or lobulated. The former presents as a well-demarcated rhomboid area of erythema anterior to the circumvallate papillae over the mid-dorsal tongue. The lobulated lesion has a nodular surface, is hard on palpation, and has a soft basal bed (Fig. 8.2). MRG is more common in men. While most of these cases are asymptomatic, some patients complain of persistent pain, irritation, or pruritus [19].

The cause of MRG is unknown. Earlier, it was thought to represent a developmental anomaly. Due to the high detection rate of *Candida albicans*, antifungal therapy has proved to be effective. It is commonly believed that MRG is associated with *Candida albicans*. In a study, a tongue examination was performed on 4244 consecutive patients. The MRG frequency was 0.7%, and candida species was identified in 90.0% of the MRG patients compared with 46.6% in the controls. Results of multivariate logistic regression analysis showed that diabetes mellitus and the age group 20–39 years were significantly associated with MRG [31].

It has been suggested that the tongue is positioned against the palate at rest, during swallowing, and for the formation of certain vocal sounds. This constant irritation, coupled with a hospitable environment for candidal colonization, causes erythematous candidiasis of the palate; this is considered secondary to the intimate contact between the median rhomboid glossitis and the hard palate [32].

Asymptomatic MRG does not require any treatment. However, if the patient is symptomatic, the following medications are administered: pidotimod 0.4 g b.i.d. p.o. for 2 weeks, transfer factor capsules 6 mg t.i.d., and compound vitamin B or tablets containing multivitamin formula with minerals. Additionally, rinsing with 2% sodium bicarbonate solution and topical use of nystatin liniment may be advised. Fluconazole 50 mg q.i.d. could be administered orally for 1 week.

6.7 Lingual Papillitis

Case 72 Fungiform Papillitis

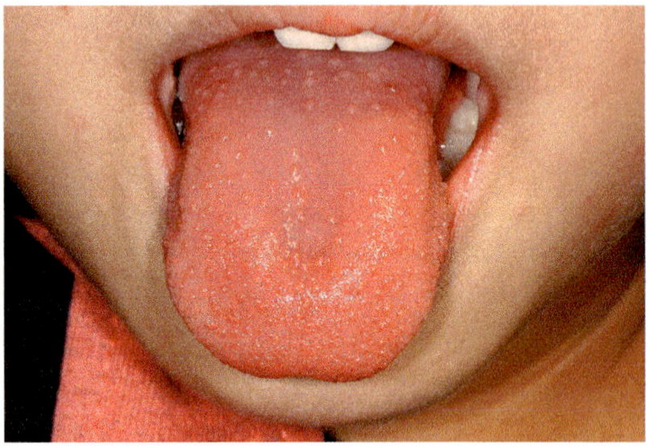

Fig. 6.19 Edema of fungiform papillae on dorsum of tongue, atrophy of filiform papillae, partial redness of tongue, no coating, dorsum of tongue exhibiting a strawberry-like appearance

Age: 5 years
Sex: Female
Chief Complaints:
A 5-year-old girl presented with a strawberry tongue for the past 3 days
History of Present Illness:
A 5-year-old girl presented to our clinic with a strawberry tongue for the past 3 days. She did not

have any pain or discomfort. She was prone to developing colds and had preferences for certain foods.

Past Medical History: None

Allergy: None

Physical Examination:

The fungiform papillae on the dorsum of the tongue were swollen, and the filiform papillae were atrophic. The tongue was reddish and without its coating, thus exhibiting the appearance of a strawberry tongue (Fig. 6.19).

Diagnosis:

Fungiform papillitis

Diagnosis Basis:

The dorsum of the tongue was swollen, and the filiform papillae were atrophic.

Management:

1. Medication
   Rp.: Compound chlorhexidine solution 300 ml × 1
   Sig.: rinse t.i.d.

Case 73 Foliate Papillitis

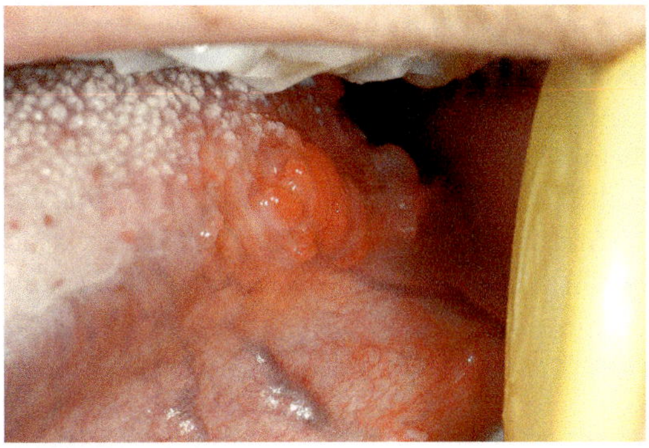

Fig. 6.20 Slight redness of foliate papillae on left tongue root

Age: 59 years

Sex: Female

Chief Complaints:

A 59-year-old woman with discomfort of the tongue root for the past 10 days

History of Present Illness:

A 59-year-old woman presented with discomfort and mild pain at the root of the tongue for the past 10 days. Several reddish vesicles were noted at the root of the tongue on the left.

Past Medical History: None

Allergy: None

Physical Examination:

The foliate papillae over the root of the tongue on the left were red and swollen (Fig. 6.20). There was no other oral mucosal involvement.

Diagnosis:

Foliate papillitis

Diagnosis Basis:

1. The patient had subjective symptoms.
2. Slight redness of foliate papillae on left tongue root.

Management:

1. Medication
   Rp.: Compound chlorhexidine solution 300 ml × 1
   Sig.: rinse t.i.d.
   Compound ulcer paste 15 g × 1
   Sig.: topical use t.i.d.
2. Psychological counseling.

[Review] Lingual Papillitis

Lingual papillae include filiform, fungiform, circumvallate, and foliate papillae. Pathologies involving the filiform papillae mainly present as atrophic lesions, and others present as nonspecific inflammation, such as congestion, swelling, and pain.

The cause of lingual papillitis is not clearly known. Filiform papillitis is related to systemic factors, such as certain anemias, blood disorders, fungal infections, antibiotic abuse, and vitamin deficiencies. Fungiform papillitis may be a presentation of the mucocutaneous lymph node syndrome (Kawasaki disease [33]) or it may present in association with some anemias. Stimulation by local factors, such as sharp teeth, dental calculi, ill-fitting prostheses, and spicy and hot food, also plays an important role in the pathogenesis of fungiform and foliate papillitis. Foliate papillitis is also related to pharyngeal inflammation.

Filiform papillitis mainly presents as atrophic glossitis with thinning of the epithelium. Additionally, the dorsum of the tongue often has shallow grooves and fissures.

Fungiform papillitis presents with swollen and congested fungiform papillae. Affected patients complain of burning sensation over the tongue and pain. The papillae are swollen, giving the appearance of a strawberry or raspberry tongue [34].

Circumvallate papillitis is very rare.

Foliate papillae are located on either side at the base of the tongue and adjacent to the pharynx. They usually appear as 5–8 vertically parallel mucosal folds at the margins of the tongue with abundant lymphoid tissue. Foliate papillitis may present with swollen foliate papillae and increased concavity of the mucosal folds. These patients often experience pain or discomfort. Moreover, the discomfort and pain may develop into a fear of cancer, which usually makes the symptoms worse [1].

Regarding treatment, if patients with lingual papillitis have evident causes such as anemia and vitamin deficiencies, they should be treated systemically by correcting the anemia and supplementing the appropriate vitamins, respectively. Local therapy includes antibacterial gargling using compound chlorhexidine solution or rinsing using compound borax solution (fivefold dilution). Adjuvant therapy includes removal of the local irritants (e.g., grinding sharp teeth and periodontal scaling).

6.8 Coated Tongue

Case 74 Coated Tongue

Age: 61 years

Sex: Male

Chief Complaints:

A 61-year-old man presented with a coated tongue for the past 4 months

History of Present Illness:

A 61-year-old man presented to our clinic with a coated and black tongue for the past 4 months. He was administered antibiotics for pneumonia and halitosis in the past; he did not complain of pain. He also reported a foreign body sensation. A recent blood glucose evaluation showed normal results. He had a history of chronic bronchitis.

Past Medical History: None

Allergy: None

Physical Examination:

The filiform papillae on his tongue were enlarged and elongated. The tongue was coated and had a brown to black coloration (Fig. 6.21).

Diagnosis:

Coated tongue

Diagnosis Basis:

The filiform papillae on the tongue were enlarged and elongated.

Management:

1. Medication
   Rp.: Pidotimod 0.4 g × 18 tablets
   Sig.: 0.4 g q.d. p.o.
   Vitamin B 100 tablets
   Sig.: 2 tablets t.i.d. p.o.
   2% sodium bicarbonate solution 250 ml × 1
   Sig.: rinse t.i.d.
   Nystatin liniment 15 g × 1
   Sig.: topical use t.i.d.
2. He was instructed to brush the dorsum of his tongue with a soft bristle toothbrush.

[Review] Coated Tongue

Coated tongue is a chronic condition in which the tiny bumps on the surface of the tongue (called filiform papillae) enlarge and elongate to form hair-like projections. The hyperplastic papillae subsequently become pigmented, taking on a black, brown, white, yellow, or green coloration; thus, the tongue is called black, brown,

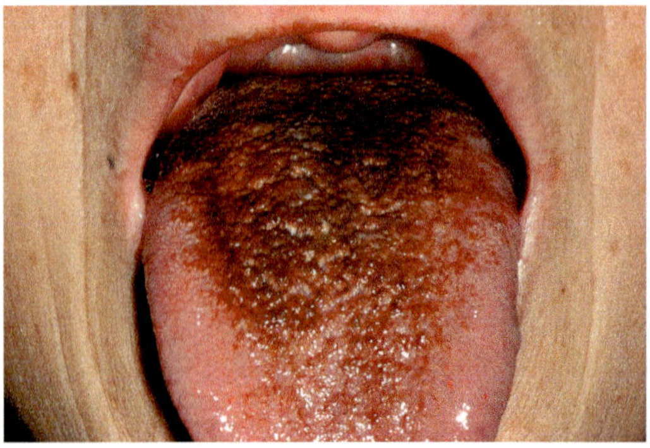

Fig. 6.21 Proliferation of filiform papillae on dorsum of the tongue, tongue coating with dark brown color

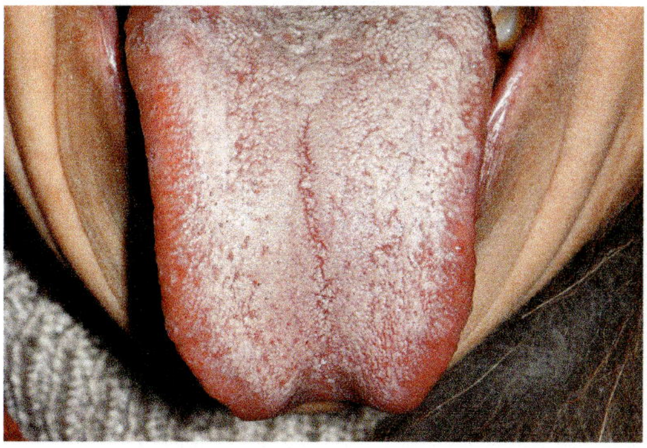

Fig. 6.22 White, hairy tongue

white (Fig. 6.22), yellow, or green hairy tongue, respectively.

Normally, the friction between the food and the mucosa of the tongue and palate causes shedding of the keratinocyte layer of the filiform papillae; subsequently, it is replaced with new basal epithelial cells. Decreased activity of the tongue due to some disease or pain may lead to impaired desquamation of the filiform papillae. Subsequently, the tongue becomes coated with bacteria and fungi, leading to the hairy clinical appearance. Long-term smoking of tobacco can stimulate epithelial hyperplasia. Long-term abuse of antibiotics can lead to oral fungal infections; infections with *Rhizopus nigricans* and *Mucor mucedo* are the most common fungal infections. Rare examples of black coated tongue include conditions with decreased immunity, such as head and neck radiotherapy and diabetes [19, 35].

Coated tongue may be seen in adults above 30 years of age, manifesting as hyperplastic and hairy filiform papillae. Elongated filiform papillae may cause nausea. These patients also have obvious halitosis without any other discomfort. A coated tongue may be seen in adults above 30 years of age, manifesting as hyperplastic and hairy filiform papillae. Elongated filiform papillae may cause nausea. These patients also have obvious halitosis without any other discomfort.

A coated tongue should be differentiated from a black coating. Filiform papillae do not become elongated in a black coating, which is caused by colored foods or drugs [36].

First, the treatment of coated tongue should target the etiological factors. These include stopping the use of a suspected drug, treating systemic diseases, and altering the acidic environment of the oral cavity. Topical therapies consist of brushing the tongue and using sterile scissors to scrape the elongated filiform papillae. Medical therapies include rinsing with sodium bicarbonate solution, topical use of nystatin liniment, and oral fluconazole, one tablet twice daily.

6.9 Lingual Tonsil Hypertrophy

Case 75 Lingual Tonsil Hypertrophy
Age: 57 years
Sex: Female
Chief Complaints:
"Vesicles" over the base of the tongue on the left for over 2 months
History of Present Illness:
A 57-year-old woman presented to our clinic with "vesicles" over the base of her tongue on the left for over 2 months; she also had oral paresthesia and slight pain while having a cold.
Past Medical History: None
Allergy: None
Physical Examination:
The lingual tonsil at the base of the tongue on the left was enlarged with limited vertical thickness; it was reddish, smooth, and soft on palpation (Fig. 6.23).

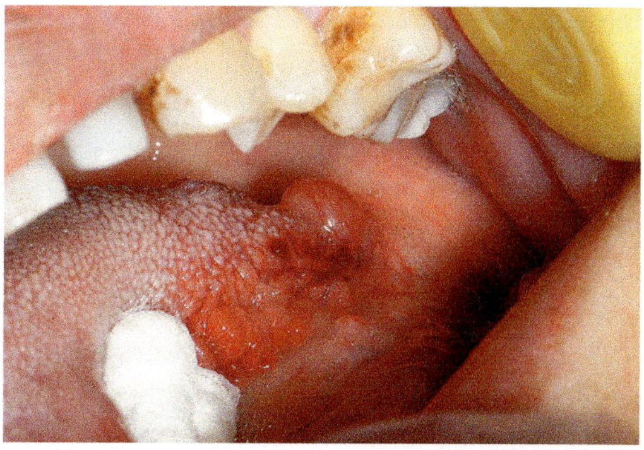

Fig. 6.23 Edema of lingual tonsil visible at the left tongue root and margin, with nodular shape, slight redness, and glossy surface

Diagnosis:
Lingual Tonsil Hypertrophy
Diagnosis Basis:

1. The lesions were located in the region of the lingual tonsils, behind the terminal sulcus.
2. The features were suggestive of hyperplasia of the lingual tonsils, which is soft on palpation.

Management:

1. Medication
   Rp.: Compound chlorhexidine solution 300 ml × 1
     Sig.: rinse t.i.d.
     Compound ulcer paste 15 g × 1
     Sig.: topical use t.i.d.
2. Psychological counseling.

[Review] Lingual Tonsil Hypertrophy
Consisting of lymphoid tissue, the lingual tonsils are located at the base of the tongue between the circumvallate papilla anteriorly and the epiglottis posteriorly. Generally, they are reddish and are waterdrop or vesicle-shaped.

Lingual tonsil hypertrophy (LTH) is essentially hyperplasia of the lingual tonsil. Multiple factors might contribute to LTH, such as infection of the upper respiratory tract and irritation arising from an ill-fitting denture. Histopathological observations have shown that there are several lymphoid follicles in the mucosa and submucosa. Some studies have reported that LTH might contribute to difficult airways [37, 38].

The clinical picture is characterized by a reddish nodular projection at the base of the tongue, which is soft on palpation. Most patients are asymptomatic, while a few have paresthesia or slight pain [39]. There is an increased prevalence of LTH in women. Patients often perform self-examination of their tongues for fear of cancer.

Explanation and psychological counseling for asymptomatic patients with LTH are effective, and medication is not necessary. Patients with upper airway infection and those with symptoms may be treated with antibiotics and collutories with anti-inflammatory effect, such as chlorhexidine solution, lysozyme hydrochloride tablets, and watermelon frost buccal tablets. Wanying capsules may also be administered on the basis of the patient's condition; a typical dosage is 0.3 g twice a day. Other therapies include removal of ill-fitting dentures, maintenance of better oral hygiene, treatment of upper respiratory tract diseases, and stopping self-examination of the tongue. Generally, the prognosis of LTH is good. Biopsy should be done in time to exclude the possibility of cancer before the lesion becomes hard or ulcerated.

6.10 Burning Mouth Syndrome

Case 76 Burning Mouth Syndrome
Age: 45 years
Sex: Female
Chief Complaints:
Tongue "herpes" with burning sensation for more than 6 months
History of Present Illness:
The patient noted blisters of different sizes on the root of his tongue more than 6 months ago, associated with burning sensation all over the dorsum of the tongue. These symptoms were less in the mornings, more in the afternoons, and alleviated while eating.
Past Medical History: None
Allergy: None
Physical Examination:
No obvious anomalies of the oral mucosa were observed (Fig. 6.24).
Diagnosis:
Burning mouth syndrome (BMS)
Diagnosis Basis:
The patient complained of a burning sensation over his tongue. However, no positive signs were found.

Management:

1. Medication
   Rp.: Oryzano 10 mg × 100 tablets
     Sig.: 20 mg p.o. t.i.d.
     Mecobalamine 0.5 mg × 40 tablets
     Sig.: 0.5 mg p.o. t.i.d.
     Vitamin E 100 mg × 60 tablets

Sig.: 100 mg p.o. q.d.
Compound chlorhexidine solution 300 ml × 1
Sig.: rinse t.i.d.
Compound ulcer paste 15 g × 1
Sig.: topical use t.i.d.

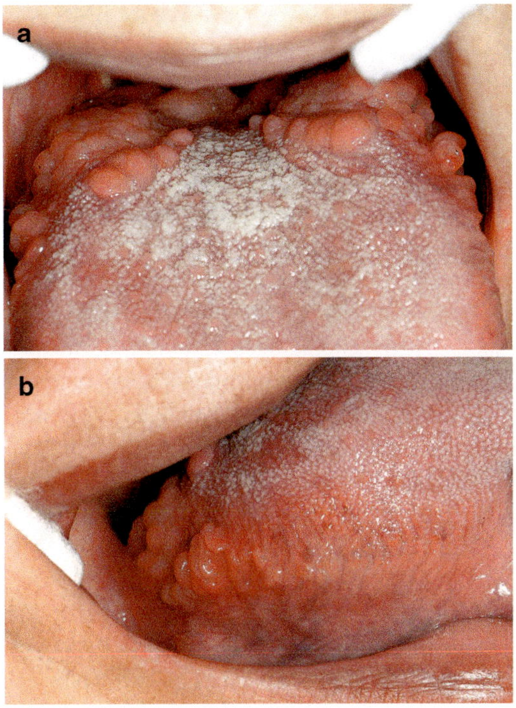

Fig. 6.24 (**a**) Normal circumvallate papillae and lingual tonsils on the posterior of the tongue. (**b**) Normal foliate papillae and lingual tonsils at the root and margins of the tongue

2. Psychological counseling involves explaining to the patient that the blisters are the circumvallate papillae, foliate papillae, and the lingual tonsil, which are normal structures on the root of the tongue.

[Review] Burning Mouth Syndrome

In BMS, burning pain over the oral mucosa is the main feature, in the absence of any physical damage. The incidence is 0.7–5%, mostly affecting women at menopause. The pathogenesis is complex; nervous and mental factors, endocrine changes, local stimulation, and systemic factors are implicated. The affected individuals have been found to have high psychological stress and a low quality of life [40, 41].

Patients with BMS often describe their symptoms as burning pain, numbness, roughness, dryness, swelling, itching, and foreign body sensation. These symptoms are usually present over the anterior two-thirds of the tongue (in 71–78% of patients with BMS). Discomfort over the lingual margin, hard palate, cheeks, and lips may be present. The pain always gets aggravated in the afternoons or evenings; it is relieved or at least unchanged while eating. More than two-thirds of the patients have concomitant dry mouth and taste abnormalities [41, 42]. The patients always mistake the normal structures of the tongue, papilla parotidea, and the teeth marks over the edge of the tongue as tumors; hence, they are very anxious, making the condition worse (Figs. 6.25,

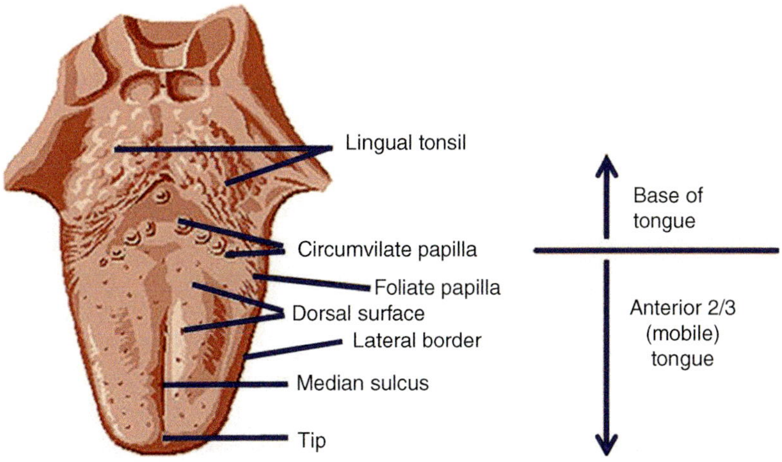

Fig. 6.25 Normal structure of the tongue

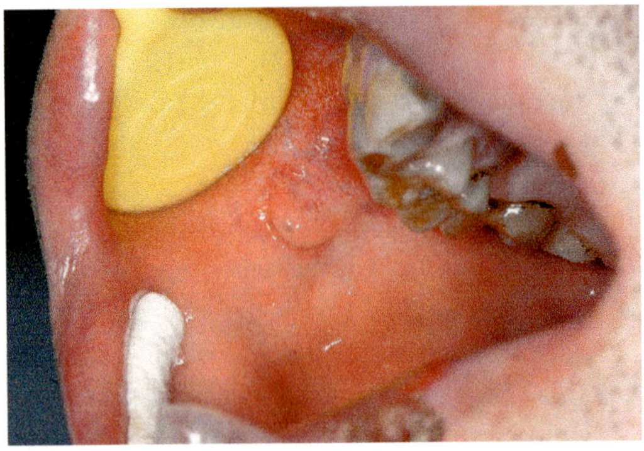

Fig. 6.26 Papilla parotidea

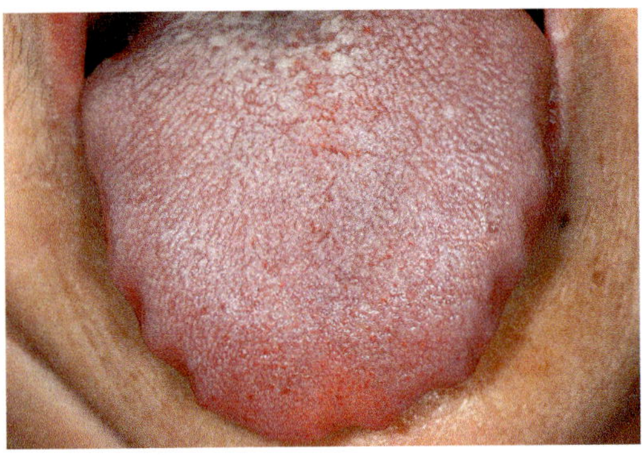

Fig. 6.27 Teeth marks over the edge of the tongue

6.26, and 6.27). In this unit, the patient in Case 76 mistakes the normal papillae and the tonsil as tumors.

It has been reported that patients with BMS and healthy controls had similar tongue mucosa with no difference in the shape, structure, integrity of the basement membrane, expression of intercellular adhesion material, desmoglein-1 and desmoglein-3, keratin-10, keratin-14, keratin-16, P3, and activated caspase-3; thus, research showed that the tongue mucosa in patients with BMS do not show any obvious abnormal changes [43].

The etiology of BMS is multifactorial; although the real etiology and pathogenesis are not yet clear, psychological factors, change in hormone levels, and nervous system disorders are considered important factors.

Depression and anxiety are common in patients with BMS, implying that BMS may be associated with mental illnesses. Mental and psychological disturbances can affect the sensation of pain, increasing or decreasing the nerve conduction function through peripheral pain receptors; after the pain threshold is reduced, even a normal stimulus may be perceived as pain. Psychological counseling and antianxiety drugs can alleviate the symptoms of BMS, further indicating that mental factors are strongly associated with BMS [44, 45]. A retrospective study involving 115 patients with BMS showed that antianxiety drug therapy had evident results [46]. However, some researchers are of the opinion that mental disorders are more likely to be the results of rather than reasons for BMS; there are several BMS patients without mental illnesses, indicating that mental disorders may not be the sole cause of BMS [47].

This condition is more common in women, especially in middle-aged individuals nearing menopause and older postmenopausal women. Age-related decrease in estrogen and progesterone can cause dry mouth, indicating that hormone level changes may affect the oral mucosal sensation, leading to discomfort [48].

There are several theories relating BMS to nervous system disorders. First, perceptual transformation, such as thermotolerance changes, hypogeusia, and increased blink reflex sensitivity, supports the view that BMS has its own biological foundation and may be accompanied by a change in the central or peripheral nervous system [49, 50].

Earlier studies have shown that chronic pain could be secondary to changes in the central nervous system. Neurons continue to accept pain signals, which activate adjacent neuron NMDA (N-methyl-D-aspartic acid) receptor, thereby increasing the neuron sensitivity; hence, even an ordinary stimulation may be considered painful. This theory can explain the pain caused by continuous automatic tongue movements in some patients secondary to continuous denture stimulation. Moreover, small changes in the diameter of nerve fibers are found on immunohistochemistry. Some patients have low levels of dopamine, indicating that dopamine system dysfunction may be associated with the pathogenesis of BMS [45].

Inflammation of the neurons is present in several diseases that are characterized by chronic pain. Hence, the pathogenesis of BMS may be associated with neuronal inflammation. Related researches mainly focus on the capsaicin receptors, which are related to neuronal adjustment and inflammation [45, 51].

Other systemic factors include metabolic and endocrine diseases, such as diabetes mellitus, hypothyroidism, and deficiencies of iron, zinc, and vitamin B.

In addition, local factors are also implicated, including dentures, smoking, morsicatio buccarum, lip biting, and tartar [42].

There is no unified standard for the diagnosis of BMS. Generally, a diagnosis cannot be made solely on the basis of complaints of burning pain and discomfort over the oral mucosa in the absence of significantly positive signs and organic pathological changes.

The therapy for BMS includes psychological counseling, followed by administration of oral medications, such as oryzano (20 mg, three times per day), appropriate use of patented Chinese medicine lusun capsules (0.3–0.6 g, 2–3 times per day), and compound danshen dripping pills (ten pills, three times per day) for 0.5–1 month. Intralesional use of compound chlorhexidine solution, 2–4% sodium bicarbonate solution, nystatin liniment, or compound ulcer paste is also advocated. Vitamin B12 and B1 injections mixed with 2% lidocaine may be used for intralesional injection into the lingual nerve.

References

1. Chen Q. Oral medicine. 4th ed. Beijing: People's Medical Publishing House; 2013.
2. Vieira RA, Minicucci EM, Marques ME, et al. Actinic cheilitis and squamous cell carcinoma of the lip: clinical, histopathological and immunogenetic aspects. An Bras Dermatol. 2012;87(1):105–14.
3. Nico MM, Melo JN, Lourenco SV. Cheilitis glandularis: immunohistochemical expression of protein water channels (aquaporins) in minor labial salivary glands. J Eur Acad Dermatol Venereol. 2014;28(3):382–7.
4. Nico MM, Melo JN, Lourenco SV. Cheilitis glandularis: a clinicopathological study in 22 patients. J Am Acard Dermatol. 2010;62(2):233–8.
5. Der Waal RI, Schulten EA, van de Scheur MR, et al. Cheilitis granulomatosa. J Eur Acad Dermatol Venereol. 2001;15(6):519–23.
6. Goncalves DU, de Castro MM, Galvao CP, et al. Cheilitis granulomatosa associated with. Melkersson-Rosenthal syndrome. Braz J Otorhinolaryngol. 2007;73(1):132–3.
7. Banks T, Gada S. A comprehensive review of current treatments for granulomatous cheilitis. Br J Dermatol. 2012;166(5):934–7.
8. Park KK, Brodell RT, Helms SE. Angular cheilitis, part 1: local etiologies. Cutis. 2011;87(6):289–95.
9. Ophaswongse S, Maibach HI. Allergic contact cheilitis. Contact Dermatitis. 1995;33(6):365–70.
10. Konstantinidis AB, Hatziotis JH. Angular cheilosis: an analysis of 156 cases. J Oral Med. 1984;39(4):199–206.
11. Garcia-Pola VMJ, Martinez DAI, Garcia MJM, et al. Risk factors for oral soft tissue lesions in an adult Spanish population. Community Dent Oral Epidemiol. 2002;30(4):277–85.
12. Strauss RM, Orton DI. Allergic contact cheilitis in the United Kingdom: a retrospective study. Am J Contact Dermat. 2003;14(2):75–7.
13. Lim SW, Goh CL. Epidemiology of eczematous cheilitis at a tertiary dermatological referral centre in Singapore. Contact Dermatitis. 2000;43(6):322–32.
14. Zoli V, Silvani S, Vincenzi C, et al. Allergic contact cheilitis. Contact Dermatitis. 2006;54(5):296–7.
15. Smith AJ, Robertson D, Tang MK, et al. *Staphylococcus aureus* in the oral cavity: a three-year retrospective analysis of clinical laboratory data. Br Dent J. 2003;195(12):701–3; discussion 694.
16. Fatahzadeh M, Schwartz RA. Human herpes simplex virus infections: epidemiology, pathogenesis, symptomatology, diagnosis, and management. J Am Acad Dermatol. 2007;57(5):737–63; quiz 764–766.
17. Park KK, Brodell RT, Helms SE. Angular cheilitis, part 2: nutritional, systemic, and drug-related causes and treatment. Cutis. 2011;88(1):27–32.
18. Koay CL, Lim JA, Siar CH. The prevalence of tongue lesions in Malaysian dental outpatients from the Klang Valley area. Oral Dis. 2011;17(2):210–6.
19. Reamy BV, Derby R, Bunt CW. Common tongue conditions in primary care. Am Fam Physician. 2010;81(5):627–34.
20. Yun SJ, Lee JB, Kim SJ, et al. Recurrent geographical tongue and fissured tongue in association with pregnancy. J Eur Acad Dermatol Venereol. 2007;21(2):287–9.
21. Miloglu O, Goregen M, Akgul HM, et al. The prevalence and risk factors associated with benign migratory glossitis lesions in 7619 Turkish dental outpatients. Oral Surg Oral Med Oral Pathol Oral Radiol Endod. 2009;107(2):e29–33.
22. Zadik Y, Drucker S, Pallmon S. Migratory stomatitis (ectopic geographic tongue) on the floor of the mouth. J Am Acad Dermatol. 2011;65(2):459–60.
23. Kalifatidis A, AlbanidouFarmaki E, Daniilidis M, et al. HLA alleles and fissured tongue. Int J Immunogenet. 2010;37(6):509–11.
24. Daneshpazhooh M, Moslehi H, Akhyani M, et al. Tongue lesions in psoriasis: a controlled study. BMC Dermatol. 2004;4(1):16.
25. Chi AC, Neville BW, Krayer JW, et al. Oral manifestations of systemic disease. Am Fam Physician. 2010;82(11):1381–8.
26. Lehman JS, Bruce AJ, Rogers RS. Atrophic glossitis from vitamin B12 deficiency: a case misdi-

agnosed as burning mouth disorder. J Periodontol. 2006;77(12):2090–2.
27. Terai H, Shimahara M. Atrophic tongue associated with Candida. J Oral Pathol Med. 2005;34(7):397–400.
28. Bohmer T, Mowe M. The association between atrophic glossitis and protein-calorie malnutrition in old age. Age Ageing. 2000;29(1):47–50.
29. Espinoza I, Rojas R, Aranda W, et al. Prevalence of oral mucosal lesions in elderly people in Santiago, Chile. J Oral Pathol Med. 2003;32(10):571–5.
30. Darwazeh AM, Almelaih AA. Tongue lesions in a Jordanian population. Prevalence, symptoms, subject's knowledge and treatment provided. Med Oral Patol Oral Cir Bucal. 2011;16(6):e745–9.
31. Goregen M, Miloglu O, Buyukkurt MC, et al. Median rhomboid glossitis: a clinical and microbiological study. Eur J Dent. 2011;5(4):367–37.
32. Noonan V, Kabani S. Median rhomboid glossitis. J Mass Dent Soc. 2011;59(4):41.
33. Grouteau E, Debuisson C, Brochard K, et al. Severe global inflammatory involvement of ocular segments and optic disc swelling in a 12-year-old girl with Kawasaki disease. Eur J Ophthalmol. 2011;21(1):112–4.
34. Brannon RB, Flaitz CM. Transient lingual papillitis: a papulokeratotic variant. Oral Surg Oral Med Oral Pathol Oral Radiol Endod. 2003;96(2):187–91.
35. Nisa L, Giger R. Black hairy tongue. Am J Med. 2011;124(9):816–7.
36. Jover-Diaz F, Cuadrado-Pastor JM, Talents-Bolos A, et al. Black tongue associated with linezolid. Am J Ther. 2010;17(4):e115–7.
37. Obata R, Obata Y, Adachi YU, et al. Successful intubation in a patient with extreme lingual tonsil hypertrophy using an intubating laryngeal mask. Acta Anaesthesiol Scand. 2008;52(7):1030.
38. Asbjornsen H, Kuwelker M, Softeland E. A case of unexpected difficult airway due to lingual tonsil hypertrophy. Acta Anaesthesiol Scand. 2008;52(2):310–2.
39. Patel AB, Davidian E, Reebye U. Complicated airway due to unexpected lingual tonsil hypertrophy. Anesth Prog. 2012;59(2):82–4.
40. Souza FT, Santos TP, Bernards VF, et al. The impact of burning mouth syndrome on health-related quality of life. Health Qual Life Outcomes. 2011;9:57.
41. Klasser GD, Epstein JB, Villines D, et al. Burning mouth syndrome: a challenge for dental practitioners and patients. Gen Dent. 2011;59(3):210–20.
42. Mock D, Chugh D. Burning mouth syndrome. Int J Oral Sci. 2010;2(1):1–4.
43. Sardella A, Gualerzi A, Lodi G, et al. Morphological evaluation of tongue mucosa in burning mouth syndrome. Arch Oral Biol. 2012;57(1):94–101.
44. Kenchadze R, Iverieli M, Okribelashvili N, et al. The psychological aspects of burning mouth syndrome. Georgian Med News. 2011;194:24–8.
45. Minguez-Sanz MP, Salort-Llorca C, Silvestre-Donat FJ. Etiology of burning mouth syndrome: a review and update. Med Oral Patol Oral Cir Bucal. 2011;16(2):e144–8.
46. Silvestre-Rangil J, Silvestre FJ, Tamarit-Santafe C, et al. Burning mouth syndrome: correlation of treatment to clinical variables of the disease. Med Oral Patol Oral Cir Bucal. 2011;16(7):e890–4.
47. Bogetto F, Maina G, Ferro G, et al. Psychiatric comorbidity in patients with burning mouth syndrome. Psychosom Med. 1998;60(3):378–85.
48. Wardrop RW, Hailes J, Burger H, et al. Oral discomfort at menopause. Oral Surg Oral Med Oral Pathol. 1989;67(5):535–40.
49. Jaaskelainen SK, Forssell H, Tenovuo O. Abnormalities of the blink reflex in burning mouth syndrome. Pain. 1997;73(3):455–60.
50. Svensson P, Kaaber S. General health factors and denture function in patients with burning mouth syndrome and matched control subjects. J Oral Rehabil. 1995;22(12):887–95.
51. Guarneri F, Guarneri C, Marini H. Contribution of neuroinflammation in burning mouth syndrome: indications from benzodiazepine use. Dermatol Ther. 2008;21(Suppl 2):S21–4.

Syphilis 7

Hongxia Dan and Xin Zeng

Keywords
Syphilis · Chancre · Syphilitic mucous patches · Syphilitic mucositis · Primary syphilis · Secondary syphilis

7.1 Primary Syphilis

Case 77 Chancre (Primary Syphilis)

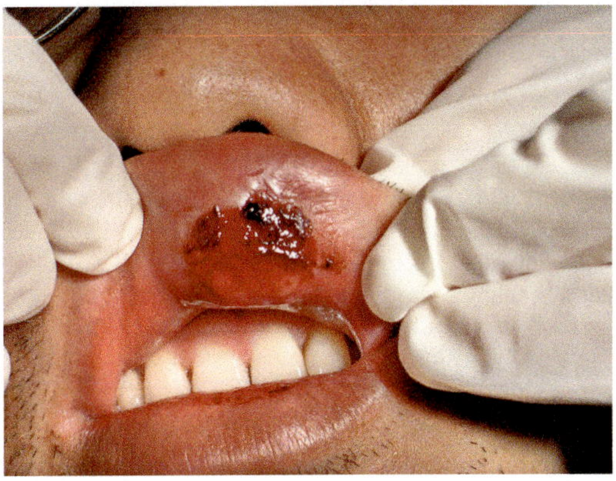

Fig. 7.1 Round ulcer with a raised edge was observed on the upper lip, covered by a little blood scab

H. Dan · X. Zeng (✉)
State Key Laboratory of Oral Diseases, National Clinical Research Center for Oral Diseases, Department of Oral Medicine, West China Hospital of Stomatology, Sichuan University, Chengdu, Sichuan, China

Age: 38 years
Sex: Male
Chief Complaints:
A 38-year-old man with an ulcer on the upper lip for 1 month
History of Present Illness:
A 38-year-old man presented to our clinic with an ulcer on the upper lip for 1 month. The ulcer was painful, with errhysis every now and then. Topical anti-inflammatory ointment was used but didn't show any significant improvement.
Past Medical History: Pulmonary tuberculosis
Allergy: None
Physical Examination:
The upper labial mucosa is slightly swollen. A round, indurated ulcer with a raised border and a diameter of 1cm was found in the middle of the upper lip. Superficial errhysis and a fine layer of blood scab were observed (Fig. 7.1).
Clinical Impression:
Labial ulcer

Laboratory Investigations:

1. Full blood count didn't show any significant abnormality.
2. Serologic tests for syphilis: rapid plasma reagin (RPR) card test (+) and anti-treponema pallidum enzyme-linked immunosorbent assay (anti-TP ELISA) test (+).
3. Human immunodeficiency virus (HIV) antibody (−).

Q. Chen, X. Zeng (eds.), *Case Based Oral Mucosal Diseases*,
https://doi.org/10.1007/978-981-13-0286-2_7

Diagnosis:
Chancre (primary syphilis)

Diagnosis Basis:
1. Single, round, indurated ulcer on the lip with a short course of disease.
2. Serologic tests for syphilis were positive.
3. Lesions disappeared after anti-syphilis therapy.

Management:

1. Medication
   Rp.: Benzathine penicillin G 2.4 × 10^6 U × 3
   Sig.: IM (on the buttocks) q.w.
   Compound chlorhexidine solution 300 ml × 1
   Sig.: rinse t.i.d.
2. In the subsequent visit after the treatment, the lesions disappeared, and result of RPR was negative.

Case 78 Chancre (Primary Syphilis)
Age: 42 years
Sex: Female
Chief Complaints:
A 42-year-old woman with painful bumps on the lips for 2 months
History of Present Illness:
A 42-year-old woman presented to our clinic with painful bumps on the lips for 2 month. She was diagnosed with herpes labialis at a local hospital. Acyclovir was prescribed for 1 week but didn't show any significant effect.
Past Medical History: None
Allergy: None
Physical Examination:
Two round, indurated bumps covered by thick blood crust were observed in the middle of the upper lip and the right side of the lower lip (Fig. 7.2a), respectively. Linear erosion could be seen around the edge of the lesions. After hydropathic compress, the blood crust was removed, and a congestive lesion with a smooth surface was revealed (Fig. 7.2b).
Clinical Impression:
Labial bumps (chancre?)

Laboratory Investigations:
1. Full blood count didn't show any significant abnormality.
2. At the first visit, tolulized red unheated serum test (TRUST) and anti-TP ELISA test were both negative. Human immunodeficiency virus (HIV) antibody was negative. After topical treatment with prednisolone for 1 week, the sizes of the lesions reduced (Fig. 7.2c). When we reviewed the history of present illness, the patient didn't deny history of unprotected sex. TRUST and anti-TP ELISA tests were carried out again, and the results were both positive.

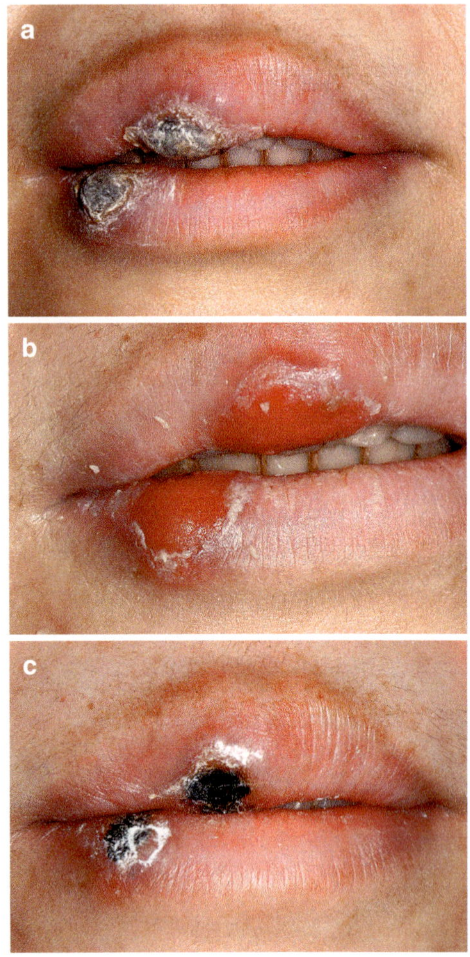

Fig. 7.2 (**a**) Two round bumps covered by thick blood crust were observed in the middle of the upper lip and the right side of the lower lip, respectively. (**b**) After hydropathic compress, the blood crust was removed and a congestive lesion with a smooth surface was revealed. (**c**) Sizes of the lesions reduced after topical treatment with anti-inflammatory agents for 1 week

Diagnosis:
Chancre (primary syphilis)

Diagnosis Basis:

1. Two isolated, round, indurated bumps on the lips.
2. Serologic tests for syphilis were positive.
3. Lesions disappeared after anti-syphilis therapy.

Management:

1. Medication
   Rp.: Benzathine penicillin G 2.4 × 10^6 U × 3
   Sig.: IM (on the buttocks) q.w.
   Compound chlorhexidine solution 300 ml × 1
   Sig.: rinse t.i.d.
2. In the subsequent visit after the treatment, the lesions disappeared, and result of TRUST was negative.

7.2 Secondary Syphilis Case 79 Syphilitic Mucous Patches (Secondary Syphilis)

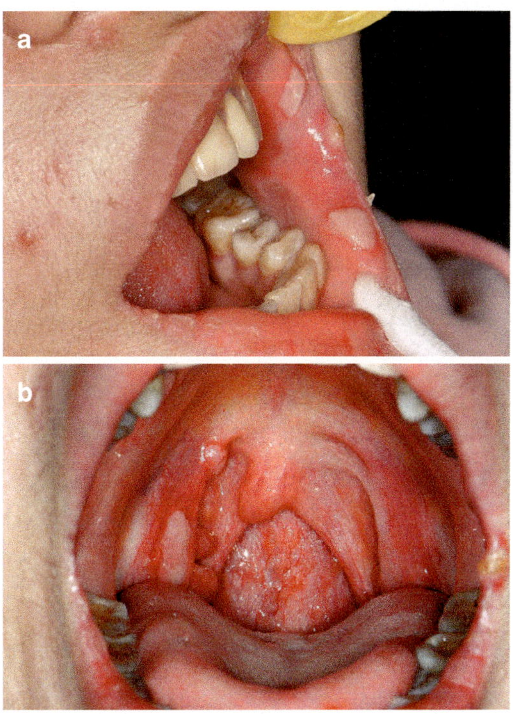

Fig. 7.3 (**a**) White oval patches with a shiny surface were observed on the mucosa of the left angle of the mouth. (**b**) White oval patches with a shiny surface were observed on the mucosa of the right palatoglossal pillar

Age: 25 years
Sex: Female
Chief Complaints:
A 25-year-old woman with white patches at the commissures of the mouth for 1 month
History of Present Illness:
A 25-year-old woman complained of white patches with mild pain at the commissures of the mouth for 1 month. The lesion became slightly firm recently. The patient denied any history of systemic diseases or allergies.
Past Medical History: None
Allergy: None
Physical Examination:
Five patches, soft, round, or oval in shape, slightly raised with sheeny surface, 3 mm × 4 mm to 6 mm × 8 mm in size, were observed on the inner surface of the commissures of the mouth and right palatoglossal pillar (Fig. 7.3a-b).
Clinical Impression:
Syphilitic mucous patches

Laboratory Investigations:

1. Serologic tests for syphilis: TRUST (+) and anti-TP ELISA (+)
2. HIV antibody test (−)

Diagnosis:
Syphilitic mucosa patches (secondary syphilis)

Diagnosis Basis:

1. Clinical manifestations: multiple, round or oval, slightly raised patches, covered with gray mucus.
2. Serologic tests for syphilis were positive.
3. Lesions disappeared after anti-syphilis therapy.

Management:

1. Medication
   Rp.: Benzathine penicillin G 2.4 × 10^6 U × 3
   Sig.: IM (on the buttocks) q.w.
   Compound chlorhexidine mouth rinse 300 ml × 1
   Sig.: rinse t.i.d.
2. In the subsequent visit after the treatment, the lesions disappeared, and result of TRUST was negative.

Case 80 Syphilitic Mucositis (Secondary Syphilis)

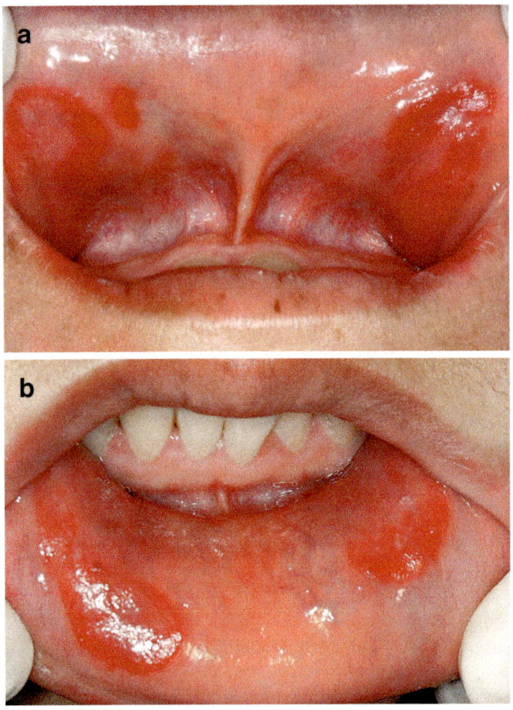

Fig. 7.4 (**a**) Multiple red oval or semilunar patches with superficial erosion were observed on the mucosa of upper lip. (**b**) Multiple red oval or semilunar patches with superficial erosion were observed on the mucosa of lower lip

Age: 32 years
Sex: Female
Chief Complaints:
A 32-year-old woman with oral ulceration for 1 month
History of Present Illness:
A 32-year-old woman complained of oral ulceration for 1 month. At first there was only one lesion, three lesions appeared recently. No skin lesion was reported. The patient denied any history of systemic diseases or allergies.
Past Medical History: None
Allergy: None
Physical Examination:
Six soft, painless red patches with erosion on the surface, oval or semilunar in shape, 0.4–1.5 cm in diameter, were observed on inner mucosa of both lips (Fig. 7.4a-b) and the right ventral surface of the tongue.
Clinical Impression:
Syphilitic mucositis

Laboratory Investigations:

1. Serologic tests for syphilis: TRUST (+) and anti-TP ELISA (+)
2. HIV antibody test (−)

Diagnosis:
Syphilitic mucositis (secondary syphilis)

Diagnosis Basis:

1. Clinical manifestation: nonspecific superficial erosion.
2. Serologic tests for syphilis were positive.
3. Lesion disappeared after anti-syphilis therapy.

Management:

1. Medication
   Rp.: Benzathine penicillin G 2.4×10^6 U × 3
   Sig.: IM (on the buttocks) q.w.
   Compound chlorhexidine mouth rinse 300 ml × 1
   Sig.: rinse t.i.d.
2. In the subsequent visit after the treatment, the lesions disappeared, and result of TRUST was negative.

Case 81 Multiple Nodular Lesions (Secondary Syphilis)

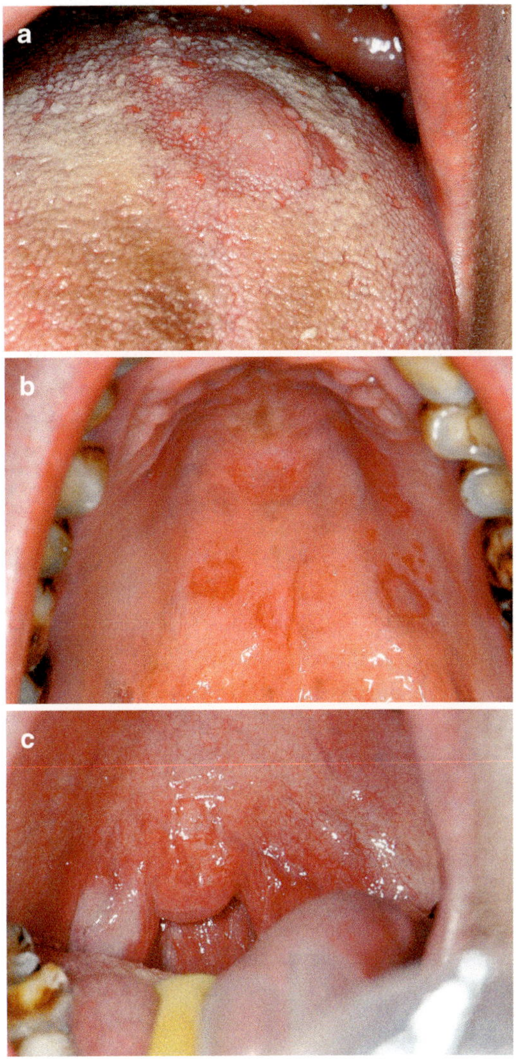

Fig. 7.5 (**a**) A well-defined nodular lump with a pink surface was observed on the dorsal surface of the tongue. (**b**) Five small bumps with an erythematous surface were seen on the palatal mucosa. (**c**) A grayish-white patch with a shiny surface was observed on the right palatoglossal pillar (Reproduced from Fu et al. (2010))

Age: 47 years
Sex: Male
Chief Complaints:
A 47-year-old man with multiple nodules in his oral cavity for 10 days
History of Present Illness:
A 47-year-old man complained of painless nodules on the palate and tongue for 10 days. No symptoms other than dryness of the pharynx were reported.
Past Medical History: Prostatitis
Allergy: Penicillin
Physical Examination:
A well-defined, soft, painless nodule with a congestive surface was found on the dorsum of the tongue (Fig. 7.5a). The size of the lesion was around 6 mm × 10 mm. Five soft, painless bumps, 2–4 mm in diameter with a congestive surface, were found on the hard palate (Fig. 7.5b). Several red maculae with diameters around 1mm were also found on the palate. Several grayish-white, slightly raised patches with sheeny surfaces were found on the palatoglossal pillars (Fig. 7.5c).

Clinical Impression:

1. Pharyngeal mucous patches (secondary syphilis)
2. Multiple nodules (probably oral manifestations of secondary syphilis)

Laboratory Investigations:

1. Full blood count test revealed no significant abnormality.
2. Serologic tests for syphilis: TRUST (+) with a titer of 1:32 and anti-TP ELISA (+).
3. HIV antibody test: (−)

Diagnosis:
Oral manifestations of secondary syphilis

Diagnosis Basis:

1. Clinical manifestations: Patch-like lesion was found on the mucosa of the pharynx.
2. Serologic tests for syphilis were positive.
3. Lesions disappeared after anti-syphilis therapy.

Management:

1. Medication
   Rp.: Tetracycline hydrochloride 250 mg × 120
   Sig.: 500 mg q.i.d. p.o.
   Compound chlorhexidine mouth rinse 300 ml × 1
   Sig.: rinse t.i.d.
2. At the subsequent appointment after the treatment, the lesion disappeared, and result of TRUST was negative.

[Review] Syphilis

Syphilis is a well-known sexually transmitted disease (STD) that has been discovered for centuries. The pathogen of this disease is *Treponema pallidum*. In the past few decades, the morbidity of syphilis has significantly increased, probably due to the prevalence of unprotected sex. The number of reported new cases each year is about 10–12 million. Syphilis itself can cause a series of conditions affecting various systems of the body, some of which can be fatal. Moreover, it can increase individual's susceptibility to HIV infection. Therefore, prevention and treatment of syphilis are still in urgent need [1]. Oral lesions are mostly seen at the stage of secondary syphilis, although they may be present in all stages. Due to the prevalence of sexual transmission, the incidence of congenital syphilis has also increased significantly, which mostly affect teeth, bone, skin, and facial nerve.

Syphilis spirochete, also known as *Treponema pallidum* (*T. pallidum*), is slender and curly in shape. When observed under a dark field microscope, it moves in a way like a working corkscrew. Human is the only natural host of *T. pallidum*. As it can't synthesize nutrients to support its own metabolism, it is difficult for *T. pallidum* to survive outside the human body or be cultured in vitro. Syphilis is mainly transmitted by sexual intercourse. After *T. pallidum* penetrates the skin or mucosa of the genitals, it enters the vascular and lymphatic circulation and then moves to other parts of the body. Other ways of syphilis transmission include oral sex, kiss, intimate contact of lesions, blood transfusion, mother-to-child transmission, etc. The length of window period depends on the number of *T. pallidum* transmitted to the host when the inoculation happens. It may vary from 3 to 90 days.

When exposed to a source of infection, the possibility of developing syphilis is about 50%. *T. pallidum* has a talent of escaping from immune system of human. Its outer membrane contains very few integral proteins that can be recognized by the immune system. Due to its lack of immunogenicity, the body is not able to activate immune response that is strong enough to eradicate the infection. Antibodies to *T. pallidum* can be detected in the early primary stage and remain detectable during the infection. Serological tests of these antibodies are useful for monitoring patient's response to therapy. The symptoms of primary and secondary syphilis can dissolve with the aid of the immune system, but *T. pallidum* will survive in the body of the host for years if no treatment is given [2–4].

Syphilis can be classified into acquired and congenital syphilis according to the way of transmission. Acquired syphilis can be classified into early and late syphilis based on the disease progression. The former can be divided into primary, secondary, and early latent syphilis, while the latter can be further divided into tertiary and late latent syphilis. Oral lesions are often the first clinical manifestation of syphilis at all stages. Acquired syphilis, particularly secondary syphilis, is called "the great imitator" because it can masquerade as many other diseases. Clinicians should be aware of this disease and be able to differentiate this disease from other diseases with white patches or ulcerative lesions in the oral cavity [5].

The characteristic manifestation of primary syphilis is syphilis chancre. It can affect any site of the body, especially the genital area. Chancre appears as a nodule or papule that may develop into a painless, indurated ulcer with a well-defined border ulcer. The size of ulcer usually varies between 0.3 cm and 3 cm. Chancre lesions can be single or multiple. If untreated, they usually disappear in 2–8 weeks spontaneously. Up to 80% patients will suffer from adenitis of reginal lymph nodes, which usually occurs about 7–10 days after the onset of chancre lesion Adenitis of regional lymph nodes happens [6].

Of all the patients with primary syphilis, about 4–12% have oral chancres. The lesion usually appears on the lips, gingiva, tongue, and soft palate. Both upper and lower lips can be affected, but usually not simultaneously. Lip chancre usually has a smooth surface which may be covered with a yellowish crust. It can develop into an ulcerative lesion with an irregular raised border. Submandibular and cervical lymphadenectasis may be observed. The lesion of lip chancre is usually single and symptomless. It usually disappears within 3–7 weeks. Since the duration of this period is short, chancre is often ignored by patients and clinicians and may be difficult to be differentiated from other cutaneous or mucosal disorders, such as traumatic ulcer, recurrent aphthous ulcer, and oral squamous cell carcinoma. Since results of nontreponemal tests are usually negative at this stage, early diagnosis of primary syphilis can be difficult. Inquiries about history of unprotected sex may be helpful. *T. pallidum*-specific IgG antibody is usually detectable at an early stage. If nontreponemal tests are negative but the diagnosis of primary syphilis is highly suspected, treponemal tests should be used. *T. pallidum* in the lesions of primary syphilis can also be observed under dark field microscope; however, this test is now considered unsuitable as it may increase the risk of iatrogenic transmission. Due to the lack of specific histopathological features, biopsy is usually not recommended [2, 7]. However, some researchers still suggest that biopsy should be conducted to eliminate the possibility of other disorders.

Secondary syphilis occurs in 2–12 weeks after patient's primary contact with the pathogen. During this stage, *T. pallidum* colonize in various organs and tissues, leading to appearance of mucosal and/or cutaneous lesions. The most common lesions are various types of skin rashes, often on the arms, palms, and soles. The rashes usually do not itch. Most rashes are pink or red, with diameters from 3 to 10 mm. The rashes may become popular or pustular (Figs. 7.6 and 7.7). They usually heal within several weeks without complications. Skin rashes of secondary syphilis should be differentiated from other cutaneous disorders such as eczema, psoriasis, drug eruption, and lichen planus. The prevalence of condylomata lata is 5–22%, and the lesion is mainly observed on the genitals and anal area. Five to six percent of the patients have patchy hair loss. Antiaditis, as well as conditions involving the kidney, eye, liver, bone, and joints, may also be present. Meningitis occurs when the central nervous system is affected.

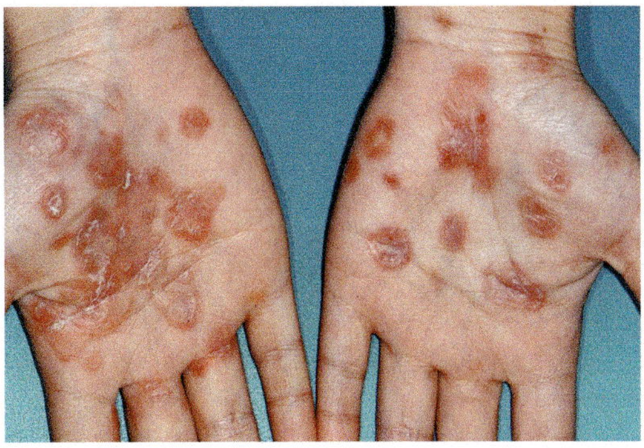

Fig. 7.6 Syphilitic rashes (secondary syphilis)

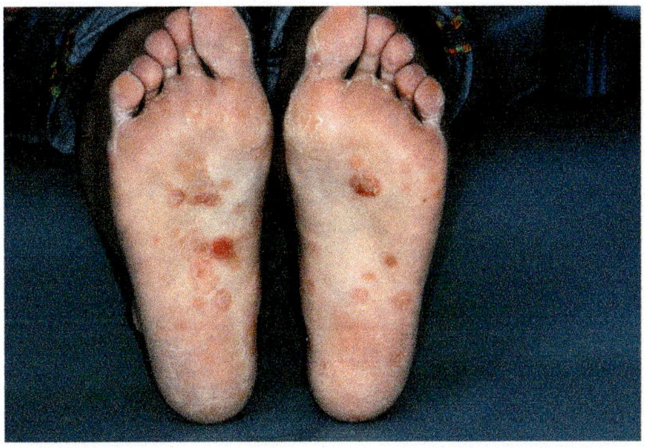

Fig. 7.7 Syphilitic rashes (secondary syphilis)

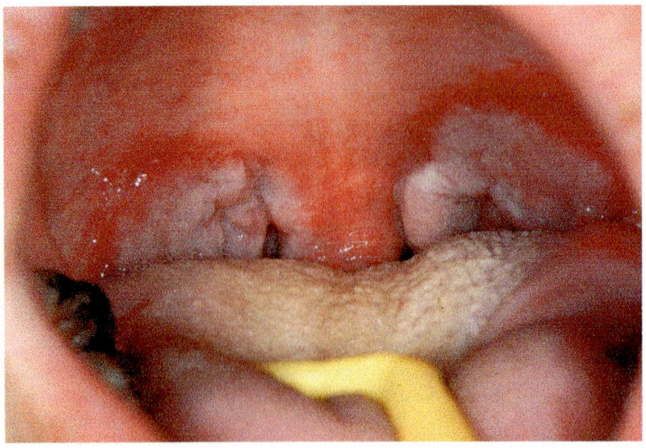

Fig. 7.8 Syphilitic mucous patches on the soft palate (secondary syphilis)

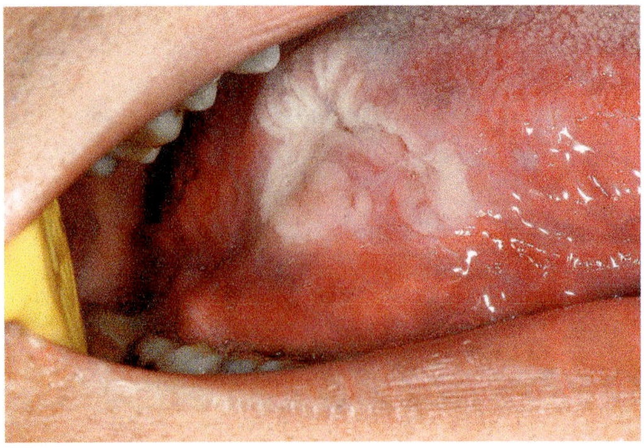

Fig. 7.9 Syphilitic mucous patches on the lateral surface of the tongue (secondary syphilis)

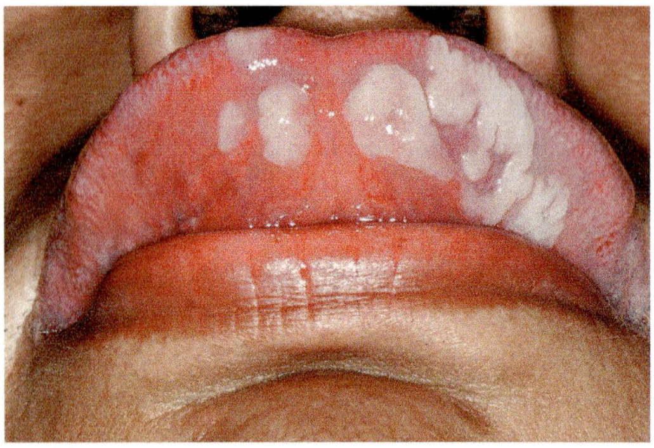

Fig. 7.10 Syphilitic mucous patches on the ventral surface of the tongue (secondary syphilis)

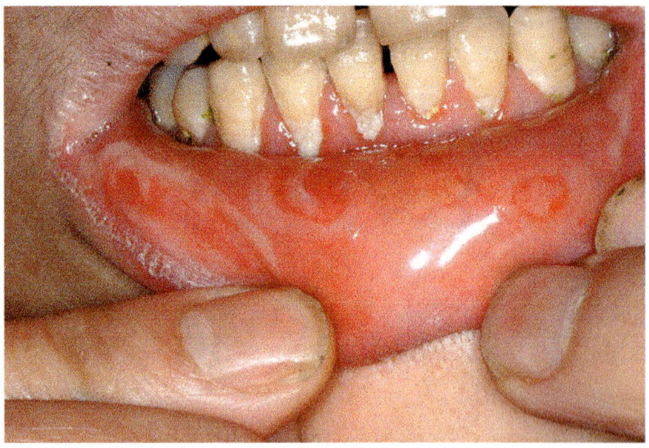

Fig. 7.11 Snail-track lesions on the inner surface of the lower lip (secondary syphilis)

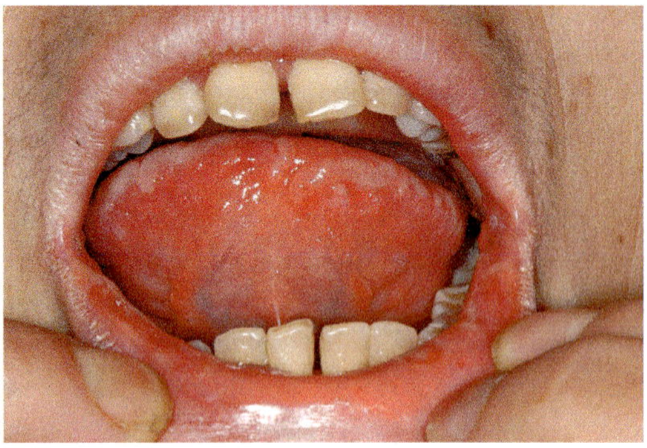

Fig. 7.12 Snail-track lesions on the tip and ventral surface of the tongue (secondary syphilis)

At least 30% of patients with secondary syphilis have oral lesions. The lesions are quite variable and nonspecific. Mucous patches and mucositis are the common oral lesions that are associated with secondary syphilis. Maculopapular lesions can also be observed, while nodular lesions are rare.

Mucous patches, usually observed on the mucosa of palate and tongue, are the most characteristic oral lesions of secondary syphilis. Syphilitic mucous patches are round or oval patches with diameters between 0.3 and 1 cm (or even bigger), covered by grayish mucous exudate (Figs. 7.8, 7.9, and 7.10). The lesions are usually multiple, which can get in touch with each other to form lesions called "snail track" ulcers (Figs. 7.11 and 7.12). Cervical lymphadenopathy is usually present, with unspecific pharyngitis and antiaditis. Notably, mucous patch on the mucosa of palatoglossal pillar is extremely common in secondary syphilis, which may be an important implication of syphilis when other manifestations are quite confusing.

Syphilitic mucositis appears as extensive mucosal congestion with or without erosion.

Macular syphilitic eruptions usually affect the hard palate and appear as red, firm lesions that are flat to slightly raised (Fig. 7.13). Papular

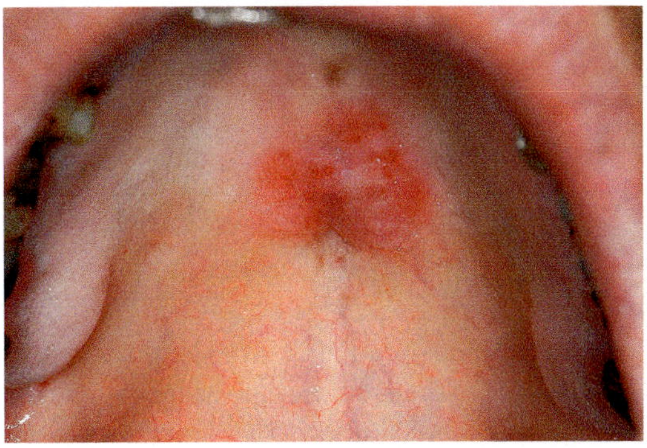

Fig. 7.13 Macular syphilitic eruptions (secondary syphilis)

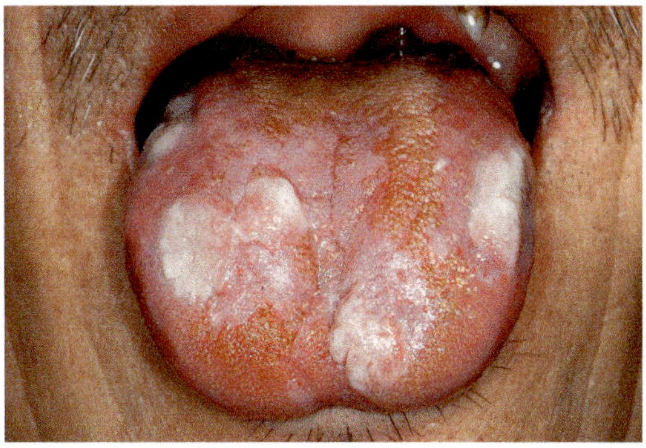

Fig. 7.14 Leukoplakia-like lesions (secondary syphilis)

syphilitic eruptions are rare. They usually affect the buccal mucosa or the angles of the mouth and appear as red papules that are firm, raised, and round in shape, with or without ulcer in the center. Nodular syphilitic lesions are rare. They are usually observed on the face, palms, and soles. When lesions appear on the vermillion, they may masquerade as squamous cell carcinoma or keratoacanthoma.

Moreover, oral lesions associated with secondary syphilis could be diverse and nonspecific, often clinically and histologically mimicking other oral diseases, such as multiple oral nodules [8], leukoplakia [5] (Fig. 7.14), and pemphigus vulgaris [9].

The results of non-treponemic and treponemic tests are usually positive in patients with secondary syphilis. The lesions of secondary syphilis will resolve in 3–12 weeks spontaneously. If the disease is untreated, recurrence of secondary syphilis will occur in 25% of the patients [2, 5, 7, 10–12].

After secondary stage of syphilis, there is a period of latent syphilis, during which patients have no symptoms. The first 12 months of latent syphilis is called early latency; the carrier has strong infectivity. After that, it is called late latent syphilis, and the infectivity is decreased. Latent syphilis can be diagnosed by serologic tests.

Tertiary syphilis occurred in 1/3 patients without treatment. It is progressive and may affect multiple organs, leading to a series of complications. The characteristic skin lesion of tertiary syphilis is the "gumma," a painless brownish-red lump which usually infiltrates the surrounding tissue. Ulceration and necrosis may occur in the center of the gumma, leading to scar formation after healing.

Gummas on the hard palate, tongue, and lips are the common oral manifestations of tertiary syphilis. The gummas may initially appear as single or multiple painless lumps which may develop into ulcerations or even destruction of bone underneath. When the palate is involved, perforation of the palate may occur, leading to communication between the oral and nasal cavity. X-ray shows radiolucency with unclear border that resembles malignant lesions.

A less common oral manifestation of tertiary syphilis is syphilitic leukoplakia. It usually affects the dorsal surface of the tongue and carries a high risk of malignant transformation [5].

Neurosyphilis can cause unilateral or bilateral trigeminal neuropathy and facial nerve paralysis. Cardiovascular syphilis is rare and mainly manifest as inflammation of the aorta.

The characteristic pathological change of syphilis is endovasculitis, which can be seen in all stages. Chancre is characterized by inflammatory infiltration of lymphocytes and macrophages, with large amount of *T. pallidum*. Gumma is a granulomatous lesion, with necrosis in the center, accompanied by endovasculitis and perivasculitis. *T. pallidum* is rarely detected.

Congenital syphilis has its particular manifestations. *T. pallidum* get through the placenta after the 16th week of pregnancy; due to the schedule of fetal organ development, it mainly affects facial structures. Congenital syphilis can be divided into two stages: early and late. Infants with early congenital syphilis can be asymptomatic or with manifestations such as skin rashes, rhinitis, hepatosplenomegaly, and meningitis. If left untreated, late congenital syphilis may occur, at least 24 months after birth. Common signs of late congenital syphilis include Hutchinson's teeth, interstitial keratitis, and deafness. The incisal edges of the incisors, more often the maxillary ones, are usually notched and narrower than the cervical area of the teeth. The first molar can be bud-shaped, and even smaller than the second molar hypoplasia of the dental enamel is often observed. Other manifestations, such as hard palate defect and saddle nose, can also be observed in some cases [13].

Serologic tests are necessary for diagnosis of syphilis. Nontreponemal tests, including rapid plasma reagin (RPR), venereal disease research laboratory (VDRL), unheated serum reagin (USR), and toluidine red unheated serum test (TRUST), are used to detect nonspecific antibodies which react to cardiolipin-cholesterol-lecithin antigens. These tests are used for screening of syphilis and follow-up of patients after treatment. Treponemal tests, including fluorescent treponemal antibody absorption (FTA-ABS), *T. pallidum* hemagglutination test (TPHA), *T. pallidum* particle agglutination (TPPA), and enzyme-linked immunosorbent assay (TP-ELISA), are used to confirm the infection if the results of the nontreponemal tests are positive [14]. Treponemal tests detect treponema-specific IgG antibodies in the serum, which usually persist for a long time or even lifetime after the infection has been successfully treated. They can't be used for evaluation of treatments.

Coinfection of *T. pallidum* and HIV is usually caused by sexual transmission. Syphilitic ulcers of the genital area increase the risk of HIV infection. HIV can also be transmitted by oro-genital contact. Oral syphilis with ulceration may facilitate transmission of HIV through oral sex. It was also reported that non-ulcerative syphilis could promote HIV infection.

HIV may have a significant effect on the clinical process of syphilis. Due to the immunodeficiency induced by HIV, coinfection is more aggressive than single one. Some studies indicated that HIV might not significantly affect manifestation of syphilis, except for an increasing incidence of genital ulcers in the secondary stage. Some researchers found that HIV infection might extend the duration of primary and secondary syphilis, accelerate progression of neurosyphilis, and increase the incidence of nodular-ulcerative lesions [15, 16].

Once the diagnosis of syphilis is confirmed, patients can be referred to the department of dermatology and STD. The treatment of syphilis depends on the stage of the disease.

Early syphilis: benzathine penicillin G, 2.4×10^6 U, IM (on the buttocks), q.w., three times in total. Procaine penicillin G, 8×10^5 U, IM, q.d., consecutively for 10–15 days, $8{\sim}12 \times 10^6$ U in total. For patients allergic to penicillin, ceftriaxone sodium can be used. 1.0 g ceftriaxone sodium IV, consecutively for 10–14 days, or tetracycline hydrochloride 500 mg p.o., q.i.d., consecutively for 15 days, or doxycycline 100 mg p.o., b.i.d., consecutively for 15 days.

Late syphilis: benzathine penicillin G, 2.4×10^6 U, IM (on the buttocks), q.w., three times in total. Procaine penicillin G, 8×10^5 U, IM, q.d., consecutively for 20 days. For patients allergic to penicillin, ceftriaxone sodium can be used. 1.0 g ceftriaxone sodium IV, consecutively for 30 days, or doxycycline 100 mg p.o., bid, consecutively for 30 days.

After regular treatment, patients should make return visits and repeat nontreponemal antibody serologic tests to rule out possible relapse. Follow-up of 2–3 years is recommended. Examination, including clinical examination and serologic tests (nontreponemal antibody serologic test), should be scheduled every 3 months during the first year and every 6 months after that. Patients with active or latent syphilis can resist repeated infection of *T. pallidum*. Though the disease can be cured, patients with a history of syphilis are still susceptible to *T. pallidum* [17].

References

1. French P. Syphilis. BMJ. 2007;334(7585):143–7.
2. Ficarra G, Carlos R. Syphilis: the renaissance of an old disease with oral implications. Head Neck Pathol. 2009;3(3):195–206.
3. Peeling RW, Hook EW 3rd. The pathogenesis of syphilis: the Great Mimicker, revisited. J Pathol. 2006;208(2):224–32.
4. Lukehart SA. Scientific monogamy: thirty years dancing with the same bug: 2007 Thomas Parran Award Lecture. Sex Transm Dis. 2008;35(1):2–7.
5. Compilato D, Amato S, Campisi G. Resurgence of syphilis: a diagnosis based on unusual oral mucosa lesions. Oral Surg Oral Med Oral Pathol Oral Radiol Endod. 2009;108(3):e45–9.
6. Mullooly C, Higgins SP. Secondary syphilis: the classical triad of skin rash, mucosal ulceration and lymphadenopathy. Int J STD AIDS. 2010;21(8):537–45.
7. Scott CM, Flint SR. Oral syphilis – re-emergence of an old disease with oral manifestations. Int J Oral Maxillofac Surg. 2005;34(1):58–63.
8. Wang F, Fu J, Zhu X, Chen Q, Zeng X. Case report: Multiple nodules as the oral manifestations of secondary syphilis. Chin J Stomatol. 2010;45(10):640.
9. Mignogna MD, Fortuna G, Leuci S, Mignogna C, Delfino M. Secondary syphilis mimicking pemphigus vulgaris. J Eur Acad Dermatol Venereol. 2009;23(4):479–80.
10. Baughn RE, Musher DM. Secondary syphilitic lesions. Clin Microbiol Rev. 2005;18(1):205–16.
11. Singh AE, Romanowski B. Syphilis: review with emphasis on clinical, epidemiologic, and some biologic features. Clin Microbiol Rev. 1999;12(2):187–209.
12. Domantay-Apostol GP, Handog EB, Gabriel MT. Syphilis: the international challenge of the great imitator. Dermatol Clin. 2008;26(2):191–202, v.
13. Follett T, Clarke DF. Resurgence of congenital syphilis: diagnosis and treatment. Neonatal Netw. 2011;30(5):320–8.
14. Vinals-Iglesias H, Chimenos-Kustner E. The reappearance of a forgotten disease in the oral cavity: syphilis. Med Oral Patol Oral Cir Bucal. 2009;14(9):e416–20.
15. Johns DR, Tierney M, Felsenstein D. Alteration in the natural history of neurosyphilis by concurrent infection with the human immunodeficiency virus. N Engl J Med. 1987;316(25):1569–72.
16. Kumar B, Gupta S, Muralidhar S. Mucocutaneous manifestations of secondary syphilis in north Indian patients: a changing scenario. J Dermatol. 2001;28(3):137–44.
17. Leao JC, Gueiros LA, Porter SR. Oral manifestations of syphilis. Clinics (Sao Paulo). 2006;61(2):161 6.

8 Acquired Immune Deficiency Syndrome

Lu Jiang, Xin Jin, and Qianming Chen

Keywords
Acquired Immune Deficiency Syndrome · Kaposi sarcoma · hairy leukoplakia

L. Jiang
State Key Laboratory of Oral Diseases, National Clinical Research Center for Oral Diseases, Department of Oral Medicine, West China Hospital of Stomatology, Sichuan University, Chengdu, Sichuan, China

X. Jin
College of Stomatology, Chongqing Medical University, Chongqing Key Laboratory of Oral Diseases and Biomedical Sciences, Chongqing, China

Q. Chen (✉)
Changjiang Scholars Program, Ministry of Education, Beijing, China

State Key Laboratory of Oral Diseases, National Clinical Research Center for Oral Diseases, Department of Oral Medicine, West China Hospital of Stomatology, Sichuan University, Chengdu, Sichuan, China
e-mail: qmchen@scu.edu.cn

8.1 Acquired Immune Deficiency Syndrome

Case 82 HIV-Associated Pseudomembranous Candidiasis

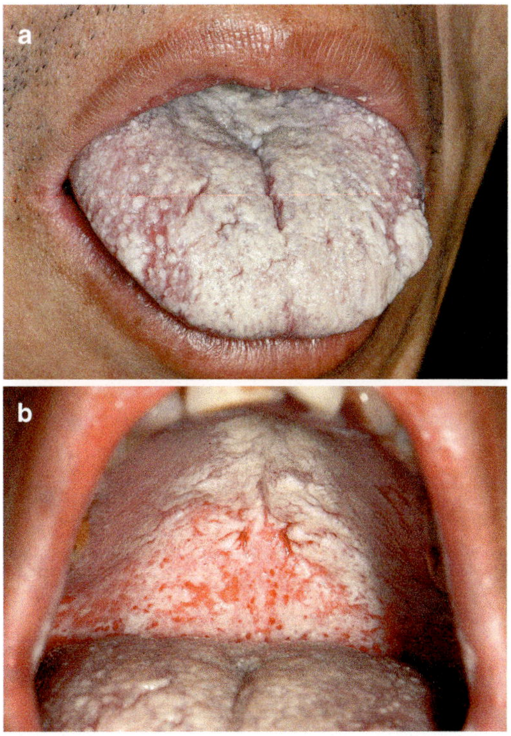

Fig. 8.1 (**a**) Widespread, thick, white pseudomembrane visible on the dorsum of tongue. (**b**) Widespread, thick, white pseudomembrane visible on the palate

Q. Chen, X. Zeng (eds.), *Case Based Oral Mucosal Diseases*,
https://doi.org/10.1007/978-981-13-0286-2_8

Age: 49 years
Sex: Male
Chief Complaints:
A 49-year-old man presented with whitish oral mucosa for the past 6 months
History of Present Illness:
The patient reported that the whitish discoloration of the tongue was noticed 6 months ago, which was followed by the appearance of a markedly white pseudomembrane in the oral cavity, associated with pain. He reportedly lost 10 kg during those 6 months and complained of recent diarrhea. He did not have fever or take long-term medication before the skin lesions appeared.
Past Medical History: None
Allergy: None
Physical Examination:
White and thick pseudomembranes were seen widely distributed on the palate, buccal mucosa, and dorsum of the tongue, which could be forcibly wiped away. There was hyperemia on the posterior aspect of the soft palate and pharynx (Fig. 8.1).

Laboratories and Imaging Studies:

1. Complete blood count was normal; blood glucose was 5 mmol/L.
2. HIV antibody testing was positive; syphilis serology testing was negative.

Diagnosis:
HIV-associated pseudomembranous candidiasis

Diagnosis Basis:

1. Oral manifestations are suggestive of pseudomembranous candidiasis.
2. Young men with significant weight loss with no past medical history, and no long-term use of antibacterial drugs or glucocorticoids.
3. HIV antibody testing confirmed.

Management:

1. Medication
   Rp.: 2% sodium bicarbonate solution 250 ml × 4
   Sig.: rinse t.i.d.
   Nystatin liniment 15 g × 2
   Sig.: topical use t.i.d.
2. He was referred to the Department of Infectious Diseases or the Center for Disease Control.

Case 83 HIV-Associated Median Rhomboid Glossitis

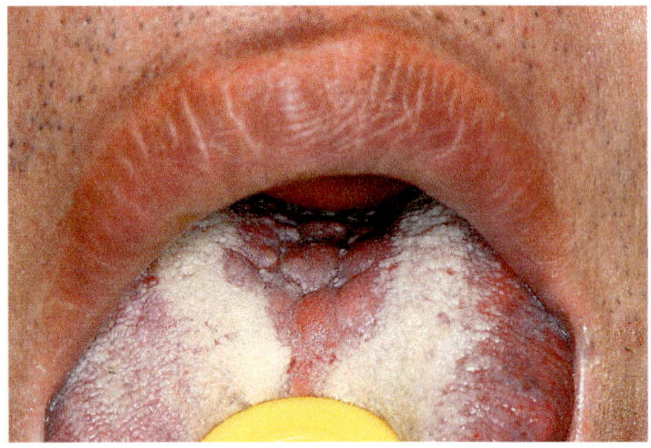

Fig. 8.2 Rhomboid regions of lingual papillary atrophy visible on the central and posterior dorsum of the tongue, with some nodular processes

Age: 44 years
Sex: Male
Chief Complaints:
Pain involving the tongue and exfoliation of the coating on the tongue for the past 5 months
History of Present Illness:
A 44-year-old man presented to our clinic with pain involving his tongue for the past 5 months; hot and spicy food aggravated the pain. Exfoliation of the coating of the tongue was observed during self-examination. The lesions were recurrent. In the past 6 months, he had frequent fever and lost 5 kg.
Past Medical History: None
Allergy: None
Physical Examination:
An erythematous lesion measuring approximately 2.5 cm × 1.3 cm with atrophy of the filiform papillae in the central posterior part of the dorsum of the tongue and a few nodular bumps on its surface were noted. It was firm on palpation, and a thick coating over the tongue was present surrounding the lesion; there was no haphalgesia (Fig. 8.2).

Laboratories Studies:

1. Complete blood count was normal; blood glucose was 5.6 mmol/L.
2. HIV antibody testing was positive; syphilis serology testing was negative.

Diagnosis:
HIV-associated median rhomboid glossitis

Diagnosis Basis:

1. Oral manifestations were suggestive of median rhomboid glossitis.
2. Young men with significant weight loss and frequent fevers and no significant past medical history.
3. HIV antibody testing positive.

Management:

1. Medication
   Rp.: 2% sodium bicarbonate solution 250 ml × 4
   Sig.: rinse t.i.d.
   Nystatin liniment 15 g × 2
   Sig.: topical use t.i.d.
2. He was referred to the Department of Infectious Diseases or the Center for Disease Control.

[Review] Acquired Immune Deficiency Syndrome

Acquired immune deficiency syndrome, short for AIDS, is a human disease caused by the human immunodeficiency virus (HIV), leading to a series of opportunistic infections and cancers. So far, AIDS has become one of the most significant infectious diseases all over the world. AIDS has been prevalent in human for more than 30 years. The figures of global HIV epidemiological survey from 1990 to 2009 show that the number of HIV carriers was nearly 350,000,000, and the number of deaths and infected people increased. In Asia, especially in China, Indonesia, and Vietnam, AIDS has been noted to spread rapidly, and the number of infected individuals is approximately 5,000,000. With an increase in the treatment funding and global attention to this disease, the number of newly infected individuals has declined since 1994. In 2011, there were approximately 780 (620–940) thousand adults and children living with HIV in China, which included approximately 48 (41–54) thousand new HIV infections; the number of AIDS-related deaths among adults and children was approximately 28 (25–31) thousand (UNAIDS, 2012).

HIV, an enveloped retrovirus, appears spherical with several spikes on its surface, is approximately 120 nm in diameter. The viral structure is composed of a core, a protein capsid, and a lipid bilayer. The HIV genome consists of two linear RNA molecules; long terminal repeats (LTR) are present at the end of the RNA. Structural genes located in the middle of the LTR encode at least nine kinds of proteins, including structural, regulatory, and aid proteins. HIV includes HIV-1 and HIV-2, and the homology of their nucleotide sequences is 40%. In China, HIV-1 is mainly epidemic. HIV is sensitive to heat and a variety of disinfectants, but it has a strong resistance to ultraviolet rays and γ radiation.

After entering the host's body, HIV selectively invades the $CD4^+$ cells. $CD4^+$ cells include Th lymphocytes, monocytes, and dendritic cells. HIV has a high-affinity interaction with the CD4 present on the surface of the cell, followed by fusion and destruction of the cell. Owing to the key role of CD4+ T cell in immune response, the immune function of patients decline. Several opportunistic infections and cancers may occur, leading to death.

The way of HIV infection is definite. HIV can be spread through unprotected sexual intercourse with a HIV-infected partner, sharing injector, blood or blood products polluted by HIV, artificial insemination, skin and organ transplantation, and maternal-fetal transmission (pregnancy, production, breastfeeding). Occupational infection of healthcare workers may occur, although it is not frequent [1].

The success of HIV transmission is dependent on the dynamic balance between the viral and host vulnerabilities, similar to other viral infections. The course of the disease from HIV infection to AIDS is complex and long.

Acute infection refers to the period from the onset of infection to antibody production; the clinical manifestations during this stage are usually similar to mononucleosis, such as fever, diarrhea, and lymphadenopathy. These may occur within a few days to weeks of the HIV infection; however, not all infected patients show clinical manifestations [2].

After the stage of acute infection, the balance between the viral replication and host immune response is reached. Many clinical manifestations of HIV infection may not appear in infected individuals for several years. This period of clinical latency may last 8–10 years or more [3]. However, the term "latency period" may be misleading. In fact, the amount of the virus is incredibly much, and the destruction of CD4+T cells is relentless at this time. At the end of the latency period, there may occur several symptoms or illnesses that do not fulfill the definition of AIDS, including mild immunological, dermatological, hematological, neurological, or orofacial signs [4, 5].

Oral lesions are among the earliest and most important signs of HIV infection [6]. Oral manifestations of HIV disease include oral candidiasis, oral hairy leukoplakia, Kaposi's sarcoma, non-Hodgkin's lymphoma, linear gingival erythema, and necrotizing (ulcerative) gingivitis. Besides, it also includes atypical ulcers, viral infections (cytomegalovirus, human papilloma virus, varicella zoster virus, and herpes simplex virus), and salivary gland diseases [7].

Most patients present initially with oral candidiasis, Kaposi's sarcoma, oral hairy leukoplakia, and ulcerative periodontitis. The indications that the CD4+ T cell count is less than 200 and the plasma viral loads more than 3000 copies/ml are related with most symptoms. Oral lesions not only indicate HIV infection but also are the sign of assessing the efficacy of highly active antiretroviral therapy [8, 9]. It is of great significance to acknowledge the oral manifestations of HIV infection in early diagnosis and treatment, preventing further spread of infection.

The incidence of oral candidiasis in individuals infected with HIV is high. Especially, oral pseudomembranous candidiasis is the most common manifestation of fungal infection, it has been connected with a further progression of HIV infection to AIDS, and it has also been regarded as a clinical marker to estimate the severity of HIV infection [10]. The prevalence of candida infections in HIV-infected people varies from 1.5 to 56%. Pseudomembranous candidiasis, the most prevalent clinical presentation of all Candida infection, accounts for 55.8–69.7%, followed by erythematous candidiasis (25.7–50%) (Fig. 8.3), angular cheilitis (13.7–27.1%) (Fig. 8.4), and hyperplastic candidiasis (0–1.7%). Among children the prevalence rates of oral candidiasis range from 22.5% to 83.3%. Pseudomembranous candidiasis infection is the most common form in children followed by erythematous candidiasis and angular cheilitis. The frequency of oral candidiasis usually associates with a decreasing CD4+ T lymphocyte count and an increasing HIV viral load. Other susceptible factors are age below 35 years, intravenous drug abuse, and smoking more than 20 cigarettes a day [1].

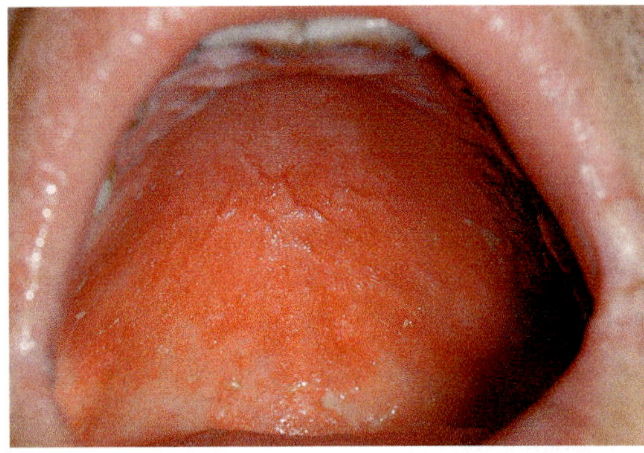

Fig. 8.3 AIDS-related erythematous candidiasis

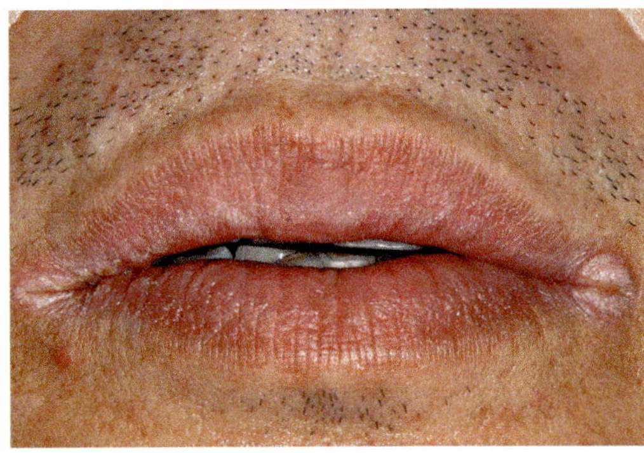

Fig. 8.4 AIDS-related angular cheilitis

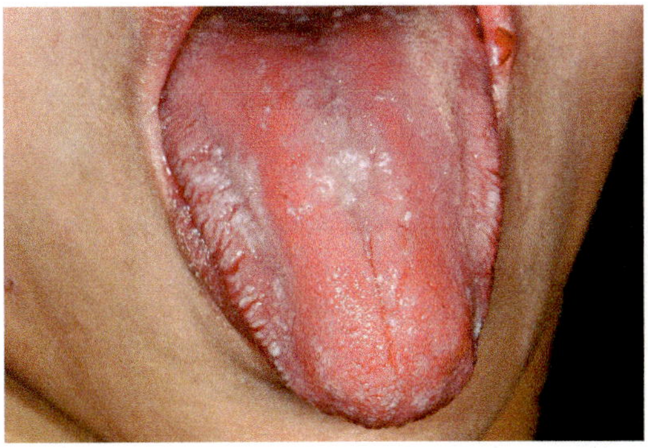

Fig. 8.5 AIDS-related hairy leukoplakia (dorsum of the tongue)

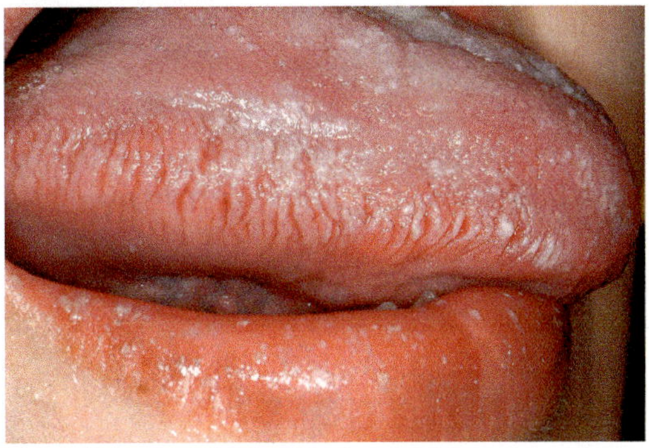

Fig. 8.6 AIDS-related hairy leukoplakia lateral tongue

Oral hairy leukoplakia (OHL) caused by Epstein-Barr virus (EBV) infection is almost exclusively found in patients with untreated AIDS and typically occurs on the margin of the tongue, sometimes spreading to the back and the abdomen of the tongue (Figs. 8.5 and 8.6). The prevalence of OHL involving HIV-infected adults is 0.42–38% [11–13]. The increased prevalence of OHL might be associated with a higher exposure to EBV, the decrease of CD4+ count, and a higher HIV viral load.

Kaposi's sarcoma (KS) is a malignant, multifocal systemic disease that originates from the vascular endothelium. Currently, it is thought to be caused by human herpesvirus 8 (HHV-8), being transmitted sexually or via blood or saliva [14]. The most frequently involved site is the skin; in addition, mucous membranes, the lymphatic system, and viscera, particularly the lung and gastrointestinal tract, can also be involved [15]. In HIV disease, 20% of the KS was initially found in the oral cavity. Oral KS manifests as red to purple macules, papules, or nodules that may ulcerate and cause local tissue destruction. The palate and gingiva are the most frequently affected intraoral sites (Figs. 8.7, 8.8, 8.9, 8.10, 8.11, and 8.12) [16].

HIV-infected individuals may be more likely to carry human papillomavirus (HPV) in the mouth

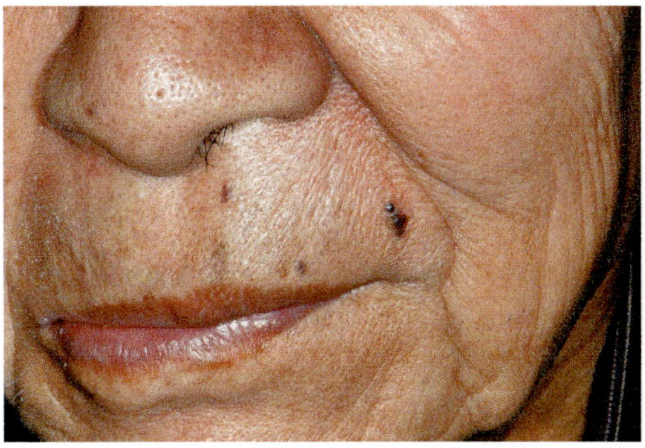

Fig. 8.7 AIDS-related Kaposi sarcoma (skin)

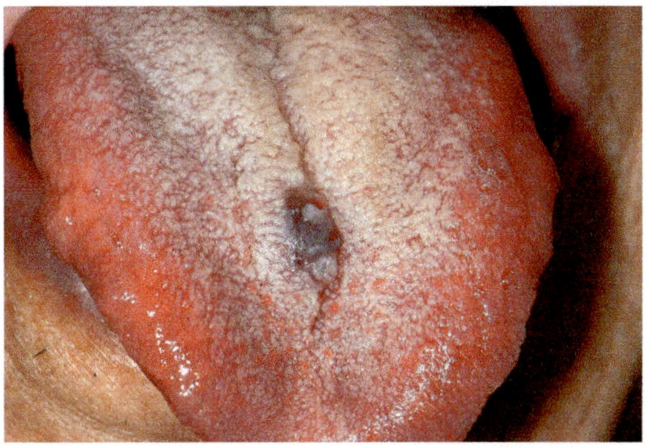

Fig. 8.8 AIDS-related Kaposi sarcoma (tongue mucosa)

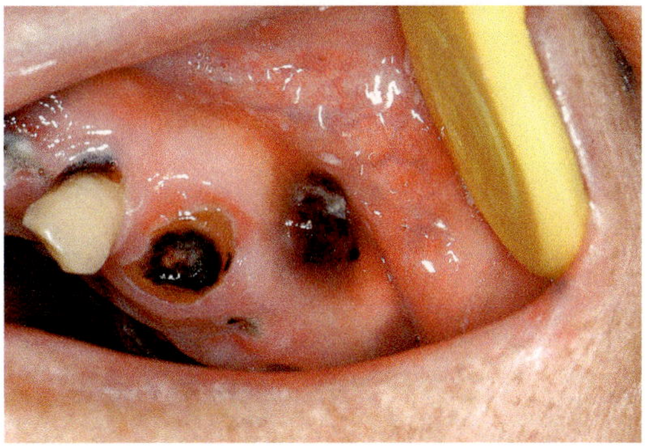

Fig. 8.9 AIDS-related Kaposi sarcoma (posterior gums)

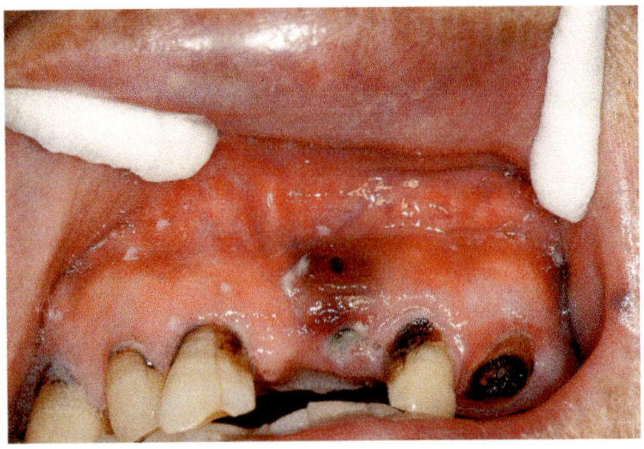

Fig. 8.10 AIDS-related Kaposi sarcoma (anterior gums)

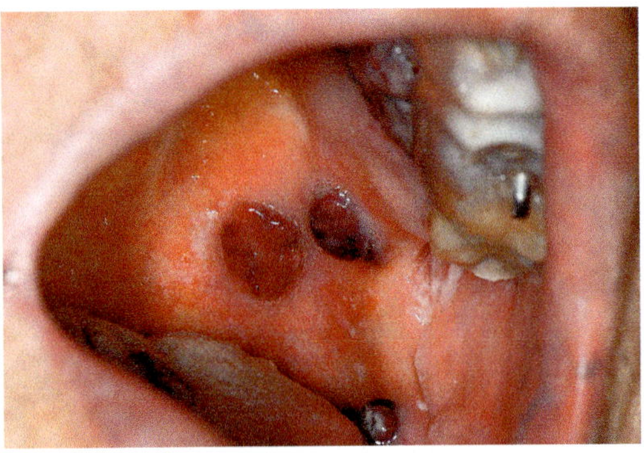

Fig. 8.11 AIDS-related Kaposi sarcoma (soft palate mucosa)

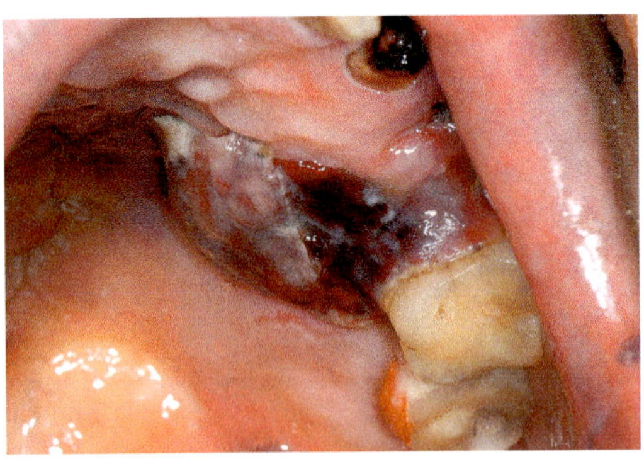

Fig. 8.12 AIDS-related Kaposi sarcoma (hard palate mucosa)

than immunocompetent individuals. The HPV infection rate of the HIV-infected individuals is 25.3%, while that of the immunocompetent individuals is 7.6% HIV-infected individuals are also more likely to be infected by more than one HPV genotype and carry a high-risk genotype, such as HPV-16 [17]. In HIV-infected populations, the risk factors for oral HPV infection mainly include male sex and human herpes simplex virus 2 (HSV-2) seropositivity, the strongest association being with oral-genital contact [18]. Up till now, the etiology of the high prevalence of oral HPV infection in HIV-infected individuals is unclear [19].

Gingival and periodontal disease, including linear gingival erythema, necrotizing (ulcerative) gingivitis, necrotizing (ulcerative) periodontitis, and necrotizing stomatitis, is more common in HIV patients from developing countries. Gingival linear erythema is characterized with a clear red line along the free gingival margin and easy bleeding. Initial periodontal treatments are often ineffective. Nevertheless, the most common gingival and periodontal features of HIV-infected individuals are plaques related to gingivitis and chronic periodontitis. The HIV-specific periodontal disease has not been observed in all groups of HIV-infected patients, indicating that HIV infection alone does not lead to pocketing, attachment loss, or bleeding on probing. HIV-positive patients often have other relevant risk factors, such as tobacco smoking and poor oral hygiene [1, 7].

HIV-associated salivary gland disease is characterized by unilateral or bilateral salivary gland swelling with or without xerostomia. Xerostomia, a common symptom in AIDS individuals, has many potential causes, such as salivary gland diseases and side effects of drugs.

Non-Hodgkin's lymphoma (NHL) is the second most common HIV-associated tumor. The initial clinical manifestations are enlarged lymph nodes in the neck and painless supraclavicular swelling. The oral manifestations of NHL present as red or purple soft tissue masses with or without ulceration and tissue necrosis, usually found on the gingival, palatal, and alveolar mucosa [20].

The oral manifestations of children infected by HIV are generally similar to those of adults. However, diseases like KS, NHL, and OHL, which are usually seen in HIV-positive adult patients, are rarely seen in children. Oral candidiasis, salivary gland enlargement, recurrent aphthous ulcers, and periodontal diseases are the most common oral manifestation of HIV-positive children. Accelerated eruption of permanent teeth and over-retention of primary teeth have also been observed in some HIV-infected children, owing to HIV-associated xerostomia [21].

HIV infection should be considered in young adults with these mentioned oral lesions, especially accompanied by recent (3–6 months) weight loss (>10%), chronic diarrhea/cough for more than 1 month, or intermittent/persistent fever for more than 1 month.

The gold standard for the clinical diagnosis of HIV is HIV antibody testing. The most widely used serological methods with high sensitivity and specificity are enzyme-linked immunosorbent assay (ELISA) and Western blotting (WB). ELISA with the appropriate sensitivity and specificity can be used as the primary screening test; furthermore, twice positive reactions should be regarded as indicative of HIV infection. WB tests the structural proteins of the virus, including protein capsid p24, glycoprotein (gp) 41, and gp120/160; it has a high specificity and is used as a confirmatory test.

A patient with HIV antibody-positive with any of the following may be diagnosed as a patient with AIDS:

1. Recent (3–6 months) weight loss (>10%) and persistent fever (exceeding 38 °C) for more than 1 month
2. Recent (3–6 months) weight loss (>10%) and persistent diarrhea (more than 3–5 times per day) for more than 1 month
3. Pneumocystis carinii pneumonia (PCP)
4. Kaposi's sarcoma (KS)
5. Significant fungal and other opportunistic infections

Infectious disease practitioners usually administer antiviral drugs to treat patients with AIDS. Dentists treat oral lesions in HIV-positive patients symptomatically.

Oral candidiasis may be treated by rinsing with sodium bicarbonate solution (2–4%) and administering topical nystatin liniment. In severe cases, itraconazole (200 mg per day orally for 10–14 days) may be used.

As OHL is asymptomatic and has no malignant potential, it rarely needs to be treated. Although acyclovir and valacyclovir have been used to treat OHL, unfortunately, acyclovir resistance may prevent the clinical resolution of OHL [22].

At present, there is no effective vaccine or antiviral agent to treat AIDS-related KS. Consequently, the aim of the treatment is the elimination or at least reduction of cosmetically unacceptable lesions, relief of pain, or unsightly edema and lymphadenopathy. Local therapy may be effective for limited disease, while systemic therapy is required for disseminated KS. Treatment approaches for oral KS include local radiation, laser therapy, surgical excision, and cytotoxic therapy with vinca alkaloids (vinblastine, vincristine, and vinorelbine) and bleomycin. However, only five agents are approved by the Food and Drug Administration (FDA) for the treatment of KS alitretinoin gel for topical therapy, liposomal daunorubicin, liposomal doxorubicin, paclitaxel, and interferon-alpha for systemic therapy [1, 23].

Up till now, systemic therapy with intensive, high-dose chemotherapy and autologous stem cell transplantation are utilized to treat oral NHL; however, these therapies do not cure NHL.

References

1. Leao JC, Ribeiro CM, Carvalho AA, Frezzini C, Porter S. Oral complications of HIV disease. Clinics (Sao Paulo). 2009;64(5):459–70.
2. Miro JM, Sued O, Plana M, Pumarola T, Gallart T. Advances in the diagnosis and treatment of acute human immunodeficiency virus type 1 (HIV-1) infection. Enferm Infecc Microbiol Clin. 2004;22(10):643–59.
3. Jeeninga RE, Westerhout EM, van Gerven ML, Berkhout B. HIV-1 latency in actively dividing human T cell lines. Retrovirology. 2008;5:37.
4. Han Y, Wind-Rotolo M, Yang HC, Siliciano JD, Siliciano RF. Experimental approaches to the study of HIV-1 latency. Nat Rev Microbiol. 2007;5(2):95–106.
5. Kahn JO, Walker BD. Acute human immunodeficiency virus type 1 infection. N Engl J Med. 1998;339(1):33–9.
6. Greenspan D, Komaroff E, Redford M, et al. Oral mucosal lesions and HIV viral load in the Women's Interagency HIV Study (WIHS). J Acquir Immune Defic Syndr. 2000;25(1):44–50.
7. Nokta M. Oral manifestations associated with HIV infection. Curr HIV/AIDS Rep. 2008;5(1):5–12.

8. Coogan MM, Greenspan J, Challacombe SJ. Oral lesions in infection with human immunodeficiency virus. Bull World Health Organ. 2005;83(9):700–6.
9. Hodgson TA, Naidoo S, Chidzonga M, Ramos-Gomez F, Shiboski C. (A1) Identification of oral health care needs in children and adults, management of oral diseases. Adv Dent Res. 2006;19(1):106–17.
10. Ranganathan K, Hemalatha R. Oral lesions in HIV infection in developing countries: an overview. Adv Dent Res. 2006;19(1):63–8.
11. Arendorf T, Holmes H. Oral manifestations associated with human immunodeficiency virus (HIV) infection in developing countries – are there differences from developed countries. Oral Dis. 2000;6(3):133–5.
12. Greenspan JS, Greenspan D. The epidemiology of the oral lesions of HIV infection in the developed world. Oral Dis. 2002;8(Suppl 2):34–9.
13. Patton LL. Sensitivity, specificity, and positive predictive value of oral opportunistic infections in adults with HIV/AIDS as markers of immune suppression and viral burden. Oral Surg Oral Med Oral Pathol Oral Radiol Endod. 2000;90(2):182–8.
14. Martro E, Esteve A, Schulz TF, et al. Risk factors for human Herpesvirus 8 infection and AIDS-associated Kaposi's sarcoma among men who have sex with men in a European multicentre study. Int J Cancer. 2007;120(5):1129–35.
15. Leao JC, Hinrichsen SL, de Freitas BL, Porter SR. Human herpes virus 8 and Kaposi's sarcoma. Rev Assoc Med Bras. 1999;45(1):55–62.
16. Feller L, Masipa J, Wood N, Raubenheimer E, Lemmer J. The prognostic significance of facial lymphoedema in HIV-seropositive subjects with Kaposi sarcoma. AIDS Res Ther. 2008;5:2.
17. Coutlee F, Trottier AM, Ghattas G, et al. Risk factors for oral human papillomavirus in adults infected and not infected with human immunodeficiency virus. Sex Transm Dis. 1997;24(1):23–31.
18. Kreimer AR, Alberg AJ, Daniel R, et al. Oral human papillomavirus infection in adults is associated with sexual behavior and HIV serostatus. J Infect Dis. 2004;189(4):686–98.
19. Arora A, Chiao E, Tyring SK. AIDS malignancies. Cancer Treat Res. 2007;133:21–67.
20. Navarro CM, Shibli JA, Ferrari RB, d'Avila S, Sposto MR. Gingival primary extranodal non-Hodgkin's lymphoma as the first manifestation of acquired immunodeficiency syndrome. J Periodontol. 2008;79(3):562–6.
21. Yengopal V, Bhayat A, Coogan M. Pediatric oral HIV research in the developing world. Adv Dent Res. 2011;23(1):61–6.
22. Walling DM, Flaitz CM, Nichols CM, Hudnall SD, Adler-Storthz K. Persistent productive Epstein-Barr virus replication in normal epithelial cells in vivo. J Infect Dis. 2001;184(12):1499–507.
23. Dezube BJ. Management of AIDS-related Kaposi's sarcoma: advances in target discovery and treatment. Expert Rev Anticancer Ther. 2002;2(2):193–200.

Human Papillomavirus Infections of Oral Mucosa

9

Xin Jin and Xin Zeng

Keywords
Human Papillomavirus · HPV · Focal Epithelial Hyperplasia · Oral Condyloma Acuminatum · Papilloma

X. Jin
College of Stomatology, Chongqing Medical University, Chongqing Key Laboratory of Oral Diseases and Biomedical Sciences, Chongqing, China

X. Zeng (✉)
State Key Laboratory of Oral Diseases, National Clinical Research Center for Oral Diseases, Department of Oral Medicine, West China Hospital of Stomatology, Sichuan University, Chengdu, Sichuan, China

9.1 Human Papillomavirus Infections of Oral Mucosa

Case 84 Focal Epithelial Hyperplasia (Lips and Buccal Mucosa of Children)

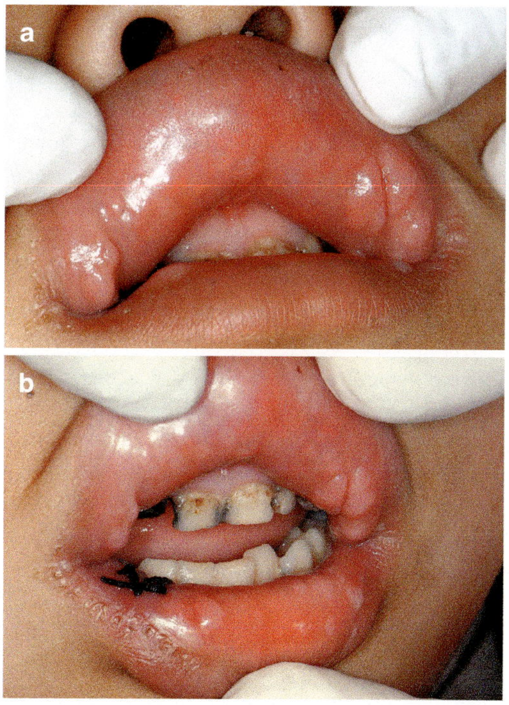

Fig. 9.1 (**a**) Multiple soft, protruding nodules on the upper labial mucosa. (**b**) Multiple soft, protruding nodules on the upper and lower labial mucosa (Reproduced from Liu et al. 2012)

Q. Chen, X. Zeng (eds.), *Case Based Oral Mucosal Diseases*,
https://doi.org/10.1007/978-981-13-0286-2_9

Age: 7 years
Sex: Female
Chief Complaints:
7-year-old girl with "vesicating lips" for 1 year
History of Present Illness:
A 7-year-old girl presented to our clinic with "vesicating lips" for 1 month. There was no pain or other discomfort. The lesions first appeared on upper lip a year ago and gradually increased, without family history.
Past Medical History: None
Allergy: None
Physical Examination:
Multiple soft and slightly raised nodules were inside the lips. They were round with 3–10 mm in diameter. The color was consistent with the surrounding mucosa or a little whiter. A few similar lesions were detected on the buccal mucosa (Fig. 9.1).
Laboratories Studies:

1. Hematological examination: Full blood count (normal, serologic tests for syphilis (−), HIV (−)).
2. Hematoxylin and eosin staining of the lower lip biopsy revealed significant acanthosis and widened epithelial pegs, without epithelial dysplasia. Mitotic-like cells characterized by enlarged and hyperchromatic nuclei are visible in the suprabasal layer of the epithelium, which indicated virus infections.
3. Amplification of HPV DNA was performed from formalin-fixed, paraffin-embedded biopsies, showing HPV 6/11/16/18 (−), HPV 13 (+).

Diagnosis:
Focal epithelial hyperplasia
Diagnostic Basis:

1. Multiple soft circumscribed sessile nodular elevations of oral mucosa.
2. The histopathologic examination of biopsy indicated virus infection.
3. Amplification of HPV DNA from biopsies showed HPV 13 (+).

Management:
Regular follow-up visit and observation was suggested.

Case 85 Focal Epithelial Hyperplasia (Gingiva of Adult)

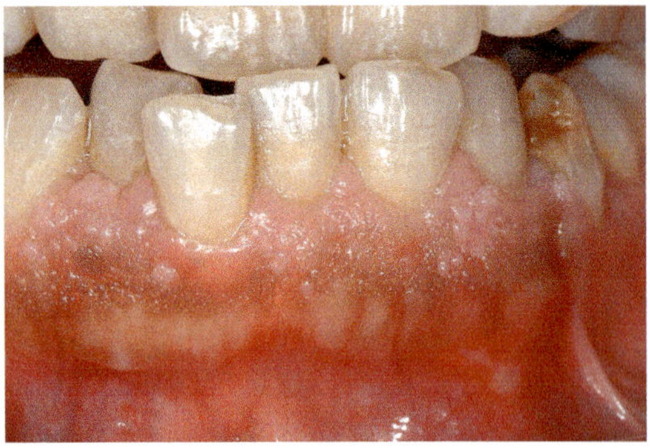

Fig. 9.2 Multiple pale, protruded, soft papules on the anterior labial gingiva (Reproduced from Liu et al. 2012)

Age: 33 years
Sex: Female
Chief Complaints:
33-year-old woman with spots on the gums for 1 month
History of Present Illness:
A 33-year-old woman presented to our clinic with spots on the gums for 1 month, with no apparent discomfort. The family history was unremarkable.
Past Medical History: None
Allergy: None
Physical Examination:
Plenty of pale, raised, asymptomatic papules of 1–3 mm in diameter were located on the anterior labial gingiva. The lesions were soft or firm on palpation, covered by normal-looking mucosa (Fig. 9.2).
Laboratories Studies:

1. Hematological examination: Full blood count (normal, serologic tests for syphilis (−), HIV (−)).
2. Histological analyses revealed parakeratosis and severe acanthosis with elongated and widened rete ridges. Cellular edema and perinuclear vacuoles were detected in the upper layers of the epithelium, indicating virus infection.
3. HPV 6, 11, 16, and 18 were detected when polymerase chain reaction (PCR) is

performed, and all results were negative. HPV 32 was positive in DNA samples extracted from the paraffin-embedded block of the specimen.

Diagnosis:
Focal epithelial hyperplasia
Diagnosis Basis:

1. Multiple soft circumscribed sessile nodular elevations of oral mucosa.
2. The histopathologic examination of biopsy indicated virus infection.
3. Amplification of HPV DNA from biopsies showed HPV 32 (+).

Management:
Regular follow-up visit and observation was suggested.

Case 86 Oral Condyloma Acuminatum

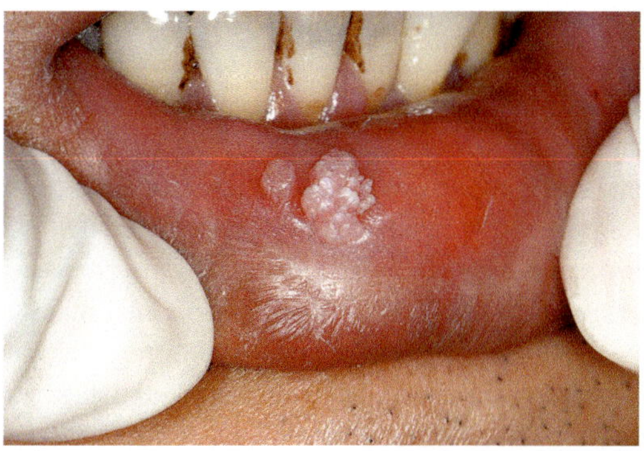

Fig. 9.3 Two growths with the surface covered by cauliflower-like protuberances on the labial mucosa

Age: 42 years
Sex: Male
Chief Complaints:
42-year-old man with masses on the lower lip for 2 months
History of Present Illness:
A 42-year-old man presented to our clinic with masses on the lower lip for 2 month. The masses were painless and easily got bitten. The sizes of the lesions were stable. He had feculent sexual intercourse history recently.
Past Medical History: None
Allergy: None
Physical Examination:
Two growths were detected on the labial mucosa with diameters of 3 mm and 9 mm, respectively. The color of the right one was normal-appearing. The left one was whitish with rough surface, and tiny cauliflower-like protuberances were detected, which was not painful (Fig. 9.3).
Laboratories Studies:

1. HPV 6 and 11 were positive in DNA samples extracted from the paraffin-embedded specimen.
2. Hematoxylin and eosin staining of lesions revealed epithelial parakeratosis, thickened stratum spinosum, and elongated epithelial pegs like papillomatosis. Upper epithelial cell showed swelling, edema, and vacuolar degeneration along with inflammatory cell infiltration.

Diagnosis:
Oral condyloma acuminatum
Diagnosis Basis:

1. Nodular protuberances with cauliflower-like surface.
2. Feculent sexual intercourse history.
3. Amplification of HPV DNA from biopsies showed HPV 6/11 (+).

Management:
Excisional biopsy and subsequent visit was suggested.

Case 87 Papilloma

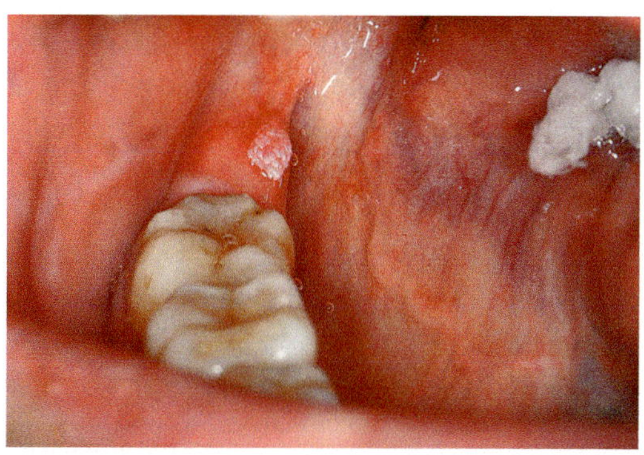

Fig. 9.4 Whitish and soft masses with burrlike surface on the right retromolar region

Age: 45 years
Sex: Female
Chief Complaints:
45-year-old woman with "foreign matter in mouth" for 20 days
History of Present Illness:
A 45-year-old woman presented to our clinic with foreign matter at the right back side of mouth for 20 days, without any discomfort.
Past Medical History: None
Allergy: None
Physical Examination:
Whitish and soft hyperplastic lesion was seen on the right retromolar region. The lesion was 3 mm in diameter, with burrlike protuberances on its surface (Fig. 9.4).
Laboratories Studies:
Hematoxylin and eosin staining of the excised lesion biopsy revealed oral mucosa squamous papillary hyperplasia.
Diagnosis:
Oral squamous cell papilloma
Diagnosis Basis:

1. Single hyperplastic lesion with burrlike surface.
2. Oral lesions biopsy confirmed oral squamous cell papilloma.

Management:
The lesion was completely excised for biopsy and observation was suggested.

[Review] Human Papillomavirus Infections of Oral Mucosa

Human papillomavirus (HPV) is one of the most common virus groups, and the infection rate of HPV tends to increase year by year. HPV affects the human skin and mucosa, leading to epithelial hyperplasia, which could cause verrucous damage, even involved in tumor formation.

HPV are small double-stranded DNA viruses, containing about 7900 nucleotide base pairs. Human can be infected only by HPV, not papillomavirus from animals. The HPV genome includes eight open reading frames (ORFs), which are coding sites of six early proteins (E1, E2, E4, E5, E6, E7) involved in viral gene regulation and two late proteins (L1, L2) which form the shell of the virus. The L1 is the most conserved OFR and can be used to identify new HPV types. If the L1 ORFs DNA sequence differ more than 10% from the known HPV types, it can be defined as a new HPV genotype. HPV has been described as more than 120 types according to its different gene sequences. According to the target site of the infection, HPV has been classified as cutaneous or mucosal types. High-risk and low-risk subtypes could also be defined according to the malignant degree. To date, there are 30 HPV genotypes: 15 high-risk types, 3 types that probably are high risk, and 12 low-risk types have been identified [1–3]. HPV 6 and HPV 11 are the most common low-risk types, and the most common high-risk types are HPV 16 and HPV 18 [4].

Life cycle of HPV is closely related to the differentiation program of the host keratinocytes. HPV entry into the epithelial basal layer requires epithelial wounding, and the HPV receptors include alpha 6 integrin, extracellular laminin 5, and heparan sulfate proteoglycans [5–7]. After entry, HPV establishes itself in nucleus as an episome. At this stage, the viral proteins E1, E2, E6, and E7 are lower expressed, and no virus is productive. After cell division, the infected cells migrate toward the suprabasal layer and begin to differentiate, which activate the transcriptional cascade of viral genome. Viral proteins, mainly E6 and E7, can delay or terminate differentiation through inducing cell proliferation and lead to high-level amplification of the viral genome through interfering with and preventing the expression of cell cycle regulators. Viral proteins E1, E2, E4, and E5 are essential for replication, which are increased in upper layers of the epithelium. Capsid proteins, such as L1 and L2, are also produced. In terminally differentiated cells, the viral DNA is packaged in viral capsids and shed from the epithelium surface [5, 8].

HPV affects most of the cutaneous and mucosal area, such as the anogenital tract, urethra, skin, larynx, tracheobronchial mucosa, nasal cavity, and oral mucosa. Oral HPV infection may be associated with a variety of oral diseases, but the specific mode of transmission is still unclear. HPV can lead to latent subclinical infection, which probably from cervical infected mother when they delivered. However, horizontal transmission is common, such as sexual contact (orogenital contact), nonsexual transmitted (wet towel sharing, etc.), and autoinoculation. A systematic review showed that 4.5% of 4070 individuals were positive for any type of HPV, and HPV16 accounted for 28% of HPV detected in the oral cavity [9]. Another meta-analysis of the relationship between HPV and oral cancer revealed that 12% of control group were HPV positive [10], which indicated that HPV may be detected on normal oral mucosa.

Oral HPV infection can lead to different clinical manifestations. Low-risk HPV types often cause benign oral lesions, such as common wart, condyloma acuminatum, focal epithelial hyperplasia, and oral papilloma. The most common low-risk types are HPV 6 and HPV 11 and also the HPV 13 and HPV 32 mentioned in this unit. The cutaneous HPV types, such as HPV 2 and HPV 4, have also been detected in oral verrucous lesions [2].

Focal epithelial hyperplasia (FEH) is a benign disorder caused by HPV, which is characterized by multiple soft well-demarcated sessile nodules on the oral mucosa. Histologically, koilocytes, virions, and HPV antigens can be detected in FEH lesions, which suggest the etiology of the disease related to virus. HPV 1, 6, 13, and 32 have been reported in many studies. People with human leukocyte antigen beta chain 1 × 0404 allele are at an increased risk of developing it. No treatment is necessary in view of the benign nature of the disease.

Oral squamous cell papilloma is a benign lesion which is commonly seen in patients of 30–40 years. HPV etiology is considered as HPV virus particles are detected in the lesions. HPV 6 and HPV 11 are the most common types. The lesions are prone to be single and palate is the predilection site. It usually presents with circumscribed pedunculated papillary growths, which appear as whitish and hairlike lesions. Surgical removal of the elevations is the preferred treatment.

Oral condyloma acuminatum is often characterized by lots of small white or pink nodules, which could proliferate and coalesce to soft growths. They are rare seen in oral cavity, with cauliflower-like surface. Patients often had a history of feculent sexual intercourse. Histopathologic examination shows koilocytes. Intranuclear viral inclusions have been demonstrated by electron microscope. HPV 6 and 11 have often been isolated from these lesions. Surgical resection or laser treatment could be performed. Close observation during follow-up is needed as it is easy to relapse. It is hard to be differentiated from oral squamous cell papilloma if the lesion is single, so the medical history should be considered.

Verruca vulgaris occasionally observed on the oral mucosa. They manifests as firm, whitish, sessile well-defined lesions. Pathological examination show significant hyperkeratosis of the upper epithelia and thickening of stratum spinosum. The mucosal HPV types (HPV 6, 11, 16) and cutaneous HPV types (HPV 1, 2, 4, 7) have been reported in oral verruca. Surgical resection is often applied.

Oncogenic HPV have a well-established association with uterine cervical carcinoma. Their relationship to oral premalignant conditions and OSCC, however, is less well defined. Our understanding of the role of HPV in oncogenic development of OSCC remains limited, and its prevalence varies widely in different studies. Researches about relationship between HPV and oral premalignant diseases mainly concentrated on oral leukoplakia. The likelihood of detecting HPV in benign leukoplakia (22.2%) was significantly more than of detecting normal oral mucosa (10.0%) [11]. HPV 6 and HPV 11 were found in 55.8% of HPV-positive leukoplakia compared with HPV 16 and HPV 18 (28.8%) [12]. These findings provided evidence for the HPV etiology of oral leukoplakia.

Some studies suggested that during oral carcinogenesis, massive episomes can lead to viral integration into the host genome. The viral E2 gene is interrupted, leading to the loss control of E6 and E7 mRNA expression. By inhibition of the protein p53 and pRb, they could stimulate the host gene mutation, and change the DNA repair mechanisms, leading to get involved in the regulation of cell cycle. Continuous and abnormal expression of E6 and E7 genes of high-risk HPV type can lead to genomic instability of the host cells, accumulation of mutational events, and finally malignant transformation. Malignant transformation of epithelial cells requires several stepwise processes with other cofactors and carcinogens such as smoking, radiation, etc. Therefore, HPV-associated malignancy is a rare event when compared with the frequency of infection in persons [13].

HPV 16 and 18 are associated with oral cancer. Recently, a meta-analysis about oral cavity and oropharyngeal dysplasia (OOPD) showed that the overall prevalence of HPV 16/18 in OOPD lesions was 24.5%, while the prevalence for HPV 16 alone was 24.4%. HPV 16/18 were 3 times more common in dysplastic lesions and invasive cancers. There was no significant difference in HPV-16/18 infection ratio between dysplastic lesions and cancers [14]. Some researchers found pooled prevalence of HPV DNA in OSCC was 38.1%, and PCR-based studies reported a higher prevalence rate than ISH-based rates [15]. Study examined 66 OSCCs for HPV-16 infection to assess the prognostic significance. Cox regression analysis of 5-year survival indicated that patients with HPV 16 inside the tumor showed better prognosis compared with their counterpart, perhaps because HPV-positive exophytic tumors are easily found and could be completely excised leading to better prognosis [16]. Low-risk HPV types can also be detected in OSCC, not only the benign lesions [17]. Oral verrucous carcinoma (OVC) is a rare variant of SCC, with an exogenous cauliflower-like warty appearance. Recently, the association between HPV 6/11/16/18 and OVC has been confirmed [18].

HPV cannot be cultured in vitro, and detection of HPV infections mainly depends on the molecular biology techniques, including dot blotting, in situ hybridization (ISH), Southern blotting, polymerase chain reaction (PCR), hybrid capture, etc. ISH and PCR methods are of high sensitivity. PCR has limited specificity and higher false-positive rate, while ISH is too complicated to be used in large-scale clinical application. At present, hybrid capture II (HC-II) assay with sensitivity and specificity has been granted US FDA approval in detection of HPV DNA [2]. But at this stage in China, PCR is still the most commonly performed to detect HPV DNAs of lesions.

References

1. Rautava J, Syrjänen S. Human papillomavirus infections in the oral mucosa. J Am Dent Assoc. 2011;142(8):905–14.
2. Kumaraswamy KL, Vidhya M. Human papillomavirus and oral infections: an update. J Cancer Res Ther. 2011;7(2):120–7.
3. Lacour DE, Trimble C. Human papillomavirus in infants: transmission, prevalence, and persistence. J Pediatr Adolesc Gynecol. 2012;25(2):93–7.
4. Syrjänen S. Human papillomavirus infection and its association with HIV. Adv Dent Res. 2011;23(1):84–9.
5. Joyce JG, Tung JS, Przysiecki CT, et al. The L1 major capsid protein of human papillomavirus type 11 recombinant virus-like particles interacts with heparin and cell-surface glycosaminoglycans on human keratinocytes. J Biol Chem. 1999;274(9):5810–22.
6. Giroglou T, Florin L, Schäfer F, Streeck RE, Sapp M. Human papillomavirus infection requires cell surface heparan sulfate. J Virol. 2001;75(3):1565–70.
7. Yoon CS, Kim KD, Park SN, et al. Alpha (6) integrin is the main receptor of human papillomavirus type 16 VLP. Biochem Biophys Res Commun. 2001;283(3):668–73.
8. Doorbar J, Griffin H. Intrabody strategies for the treatment of human papillomavirus associated disease. Expert Opin Biol Ther. 2007;7(5):677–89.
9. Kreimer AR, Bhatia RK, Messeguer AL, González P, Herrero R, Giuliano AR. Oral human papillomavirus in healthy individuals: a systematic review of the literature. Sex Transm Dis. 2010;37(6):386–91.
10. Syrjänen S, Lodi G, von BI, et al. Human papillomaviruses in oral carcinoma and oral potentially malignant disorders: a systematic review. Oral Dis. 2011;17(Suppl 1):58–72.
11. Miller CS, Johnstone BM. Human papillomavirus as a risk factor for oral squamous cell carcinoma: a meta-analysis, 1982-1997. Oral Surg Oral Med Oral Pathol Oral Radiol Endod. 2001;91(6):622–35.
12. Miller CS, White DK. Human papillomavirus expression in oral mucosa, premalignant conditions, and squamous cell carcinoma: a retrospective review of the literature. Oral Surg Oral Med Oral Pathol Oral Radiol Endod. 1996;82(1):57–68.
13. Sinal SH, Woods CR. Human papillomavirus infections of the genital and respiratory tracts

in young children. Semin Pediatr Infect Dis. 2005;14(4):306–16.
14. Jayaprakash V, Reid M, Hatton E, et al. Human papillomavirus types 16 and 18 in epithelial dysplasia of oral cavity and oropharynx: a meta-analysis, 1985-2010. Oral Oncol. 2011;47(11):1048–54.
15. Termine N, Panzarella V, Falaschini S, et al. HPV in oral squamous cell carcinoma vs head and neck squamous cell carcinoma biopsies: a mata-analysis (1988-2007). Ann Oncol. 2008;19(10):1681–90.
16. Sugiyama M, Bhawal UK, Kawamura M, et al. Human papillomavirus-16 in oral squamous cell carcinoma: clinical correlates and 5-year survival. Br J Oral Maxillofac Surg. 2007;45(2):116–22.
17. Mendelsohn AH, Lai CK, Shintaku IP, et al. Histopathologic findings of HPV and p16 positive HNSCC. Laryngoscope. 2010;120(9):1788–94.
18. Walvekar RR, Chaukar DA, Deshpande MS, et al. Verrucous carcinoma of the oral cavity: a clinical and pathological study of 101 cases. Oral Oncol. 2009;45(1):47–51.

10 Oral Mucosal Lesions of Systemic Diseases

Xin Jin, Xin Zeng, and Lanyan Wu

Keywords
Thrombocytopenic Purpura · Leukemia · Acute Monocytic Leukemia · Myeloid Sarcoma · Lymphoma · NK-/T-Cell Lymphoma · Langerhans Cell Histiocytosis · Amyloidosis · Florid Papillomatosis · Acanthosis Nigricans Maligna · Focal Dermal Hypoplasia

X. Jin
College of Stomatology, Chongqing Medical University, Chongqing Key Laboratory of Oral Diseases and Biomedical Sciences, Chongqing, China

X. Zeng (✉)
State Key Laboratory of Oral Diseases, National Clinical Research Center for Oral Diseases, Department of Oral Medicine, West China Hospital of Stomatology, Sichuan University, Chengdu, Sichuan, China

L. Wu
Department of Oral Pathology, West China Hospital of Stomatology, Sichuan University, Chengdu, Sichuan, China

Q. Chen, X. Zeng (eds.), *Case Based Oral Mucosal Diseases*,
https://doi.org/10.1007/978-981-13-0286-2_10

10.1 Thrombocytopenic Purpura

Case 88 Thrombocytopenic Purpura

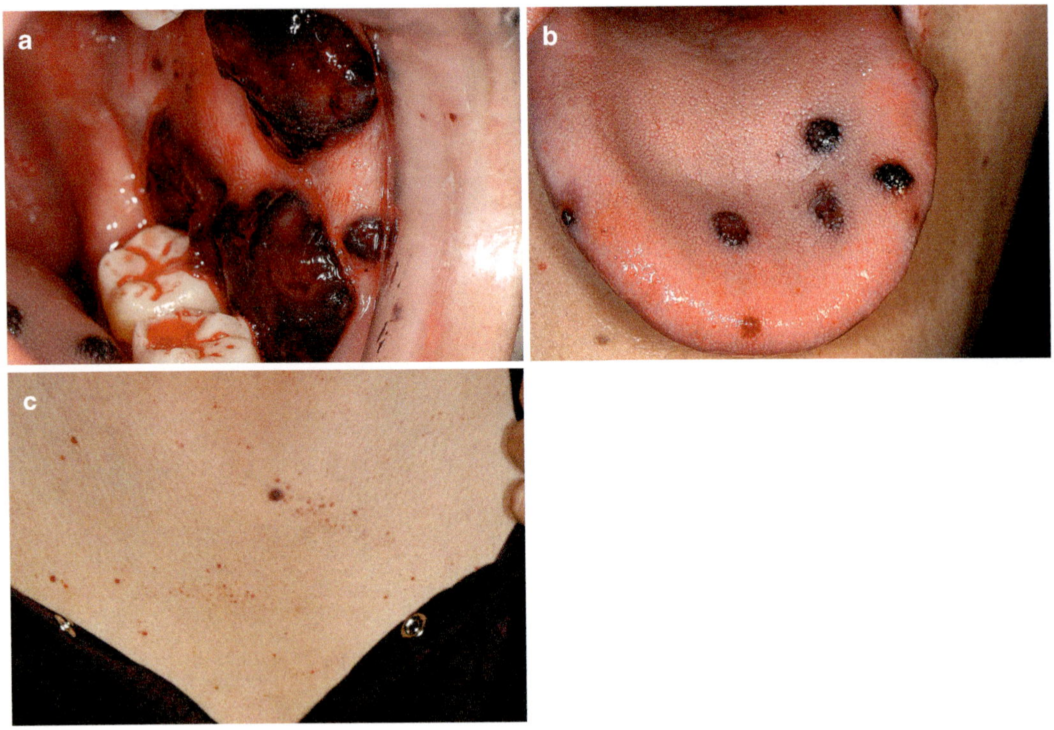

Fig. 10.1 (**a**) Multiple blood blisters of different sizes on the left buccal mucosa. (**b**) Multiple blood blisters of different sizes on the dorsum of the tongue. (**c**) Dozens of pinhead-size petechiae and small blood blisters on the chest skin

Age: 29 years
Sex: Female
Chief Complaints:
29-year-old woman with *hemophysallis* on the oral mucosa and skin for half a day
History of Present Illness:
A 29-year-old woman presented to our clinic with painless blood blisters on the oral mucosa and skin of the upper body for half a day. The lesions had no obvious causes.
Past Medical History: None
Allergy: None
Physical Examination:
Multiple blood blisters with 0.1–2.5 cm in diameter were observed on the buccal mucosa, dorsum, and ventral surface of the tongue. Dozens of pinhead-size petechiae and small blood blisters with 1–4 mm in diameter were also noticed on the chest skin (Fig. 10.1).
Clinical Impression:
Hemorrhagic disease
Laboratories Studies:

1. Full blood count: PLT $0 \times 10^9/L$ (100×10^9–$300 \times 10^9/L$).

2. Clotting check: prothrombin time (PT) and activated partial thromboplastin time (APTT) are normal.

Diagnosis:
Thrombocytopenic purpura
Management:
She was transferred to the hematology department for further treatment promptly.

[Review] Thrombocytopenic Purpura
Thrombocytic purpura is a hemorrhagic disease caused by platelet disorder, leading to oral, cutaneous, and visceral hemorrhage. It could be divided into two categories: thrombocytopenic purpura and purpura caused by platelet dysfunction. Thrombocytopenic purpura includes immune thrombocytopenic purpura, thrombotic thrombocytopenic purpura, drug-related thrombocytopenia, thrombocytopenic purpura secondary to some primary diseases, etc. The reasons of platelet dysfunction include thrombopathy, Glanzmann's thrombasthenia, uremia, abnormal globulinemia, drugs, etc. Symptoms of drug-induced thrombocytopenia range from no bleeding to intracranial hemorrhage causing death. The physician should be especially alert to this kind of adverse drug reaction. The most common drugs which can lead to thrombocytopenia include anti-infective drugs (ampicillin, aspirin, cephalosporins, azithromycin, levofloxacin, moxifloxacin, compound sulfamethoxazole, rifampicin, chloramphenicol, sulfanilamide, etc.), antipyretic analgesics (aspirin, acetaminophen, diclofenac, etc.), antimetabolic agents, cytotoxic drugs, and heparin [1]. Primary diseases which can cause thrombocytopenia consist of chronic lymphocytic leukemia, acute leukemia, lymphoma, systemic lupus erythematosus, rheumatoid arthritis, hyperthyroidism, liver diseases, and so on. In addition, bacterial, fungal, or viral infection (rubella, Epstein-Barr virus, cytomegalovirus, and hepatitis A), hypersplenism, and disseminated intravascular coagulation may also be related to thrombocytopenia [2].

Oral manifestations include spontaneous gingival bleeding which can be aggravated by mild stimulus like teeth-brushing and sucking. Oral lesions manifest as multiple petechiae, ecchymoses, and hematomas of different sizes, especially on the buccal mucosa and tongue. The hematomas rupture easily, leaving round or oval erosions with clear borders.

Skin lesions are mainly presented by purpura, ecchymoses, blood blisters, or hematomas, accompanied with nasal bleeding and menorrhagia. Rare visceral hemorrhage such as hemoptysis, hematemesis, and hematuria can be noticed in severe cases, with potentially fatal consequences.

Diagnosis could be made according to the clinical manifestations and blood routine examination. The patients should be transferred to the hematology department for further checks and treatment promptly.

Patients with secondary thrombocytopenia should stop taking suspected drugs or get active treatment of primary disease. Systemic treatment for thrombocytopenic purpura should be conducted by hematologist; and glucocorticoid is the priority. Keep the mouth clean, and oral rinse with 1–3% hydrogen peroxide could be prescribed.

Pressure hemostasis (periodontal dressing, gelatin sponge, or gauze) and hemostatics (adrenaline, thrombin, Yunnan Baiyao, injection of vitamin K1 or K3) can be applied to stop gingival bleeding, while suture hemostasis can be used in severe cases. Local application of anti-inflammatory and antiseptic drugs can be helpful for erosions or secondary infection of oral mucosa.

10.2 Leukemia

Case 89 Acute Monocytic Leukemia

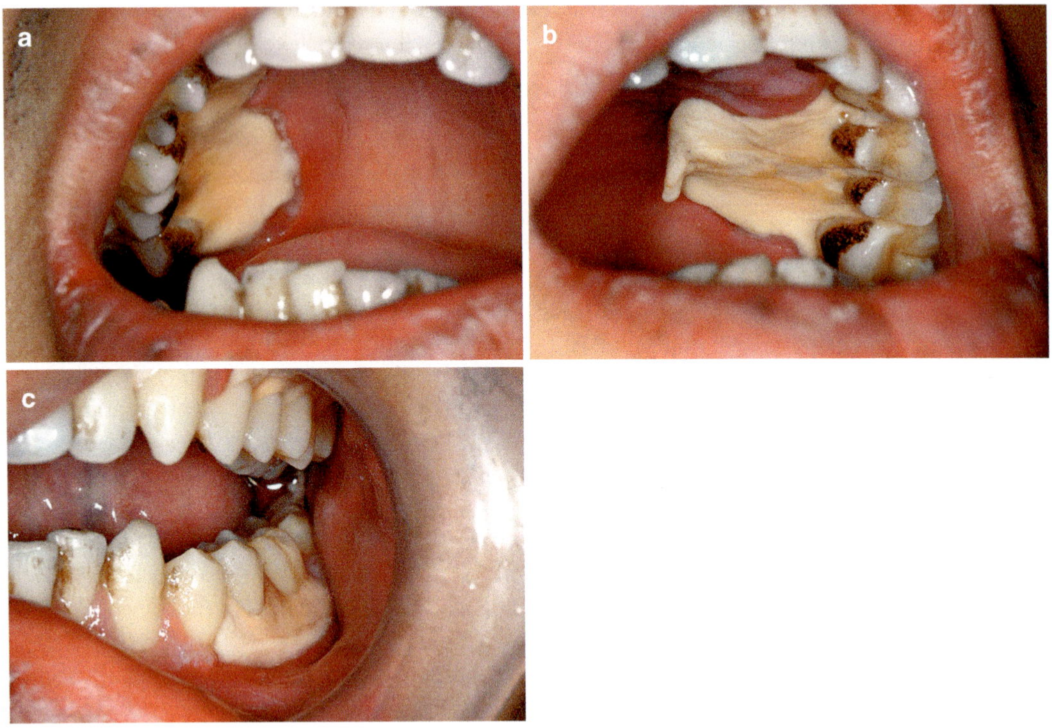

Fig. 10.2 (**a**) Widespread necrotic ulcers on the right maxillary gingiva, extending to the hard palate, with smooth and thick yellowish-white pseudomembrane. (**b**) Widespread necrotic ulcers on the left maxillary gingiva, extending to the hard palate, with smooth and thick yellowish-white pseudomembrane. (**c**) Widespread necrotic ulcers on the left mandibular gingiva, with smooth and thick yellowish-white pseudomembrane

Age: 22 years
Sex: Male
Chief Complaints:
22-year-old man with oral ulcers for 3 days
History of Present Illness:
A 22-year-old man complained of painful ulcers with unknown cause for 3 days. He had a high fever (39.8 °C) 8 days ago, which had been subdued after anti-infectious treatment.
Past Medical History: None
Allergy: None
Physical Examination:
Widespread necrotic ulcers were distributed on the maxillary and left mandibular gingival mucosa, extending to the hard palate. The ulcers were covered by a yellowish-white pseudomembrane, which is dense, smooth, and thick. The surrounding mucosa appeared normal color and morphology (Fig. 10.2).
Clinical Impression:
Gingival ulcer
Laboratories Studies:

1. Routine blood test: RBC, HGB, and PLT were normal. The percentage of neutrophilic segmented granulocytes decreased significantly (2.0%), while the ratio of monocytes increased (10%), and the proportion of abnormal white blood cells was 44%.
2. Serological tests for syphilis and HIV were normal.

3. The bone marrow biopsy and immunotyping of the cells revealed acute monocytic leukemia, type M5.

Diagnosis:
Oral manifestations of acute monocytic leukemia

Management:

1. He was advised to the hematology department for further therapy.
2. Topical use of compound chlorhexidine solution, oral rinse, 3 times daily.

Case 90 Hematopoietic Malignancy (Myeloid Sarcoma or Leukemia?)

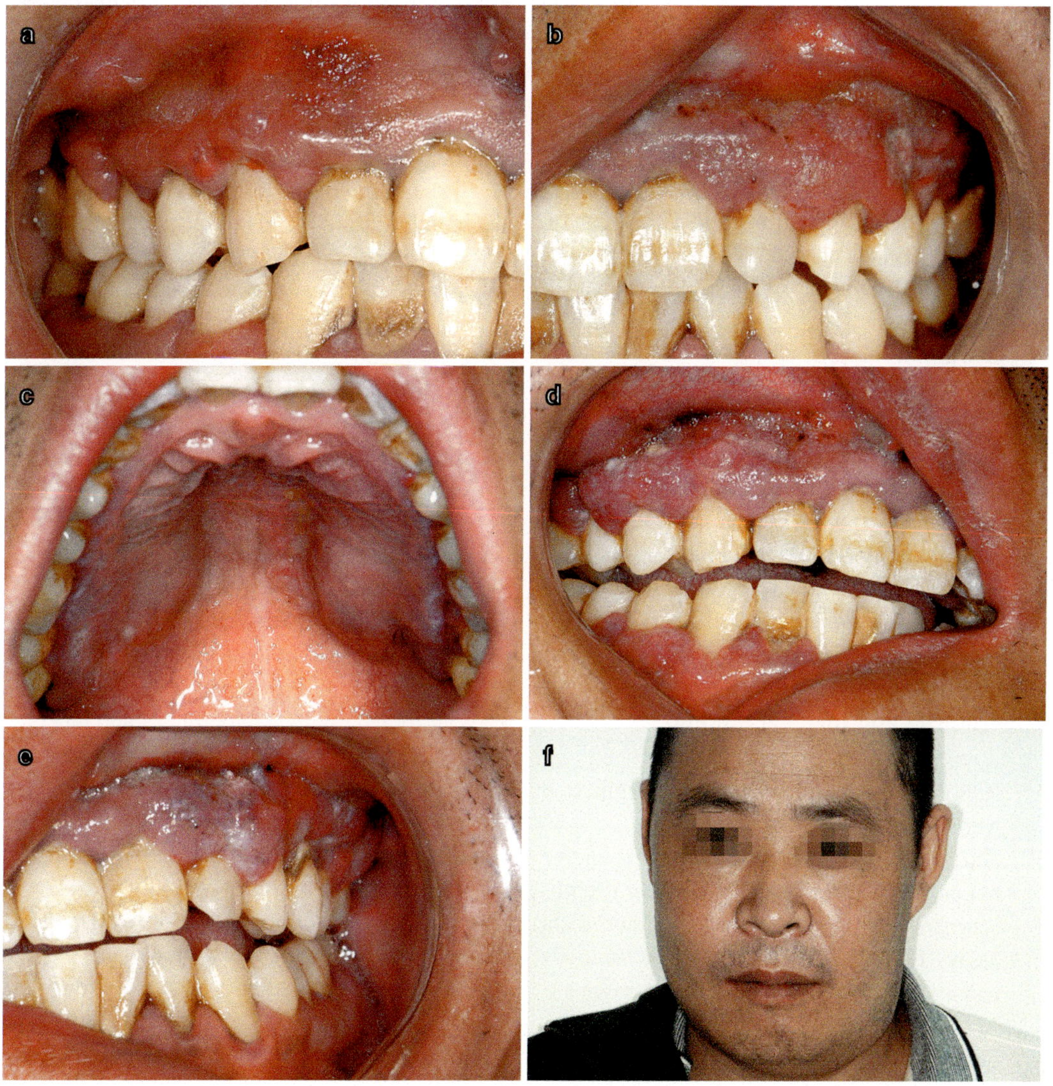

Fig. 10.3 (**a**) Diffuse enlargement of the right maxillary gingiva, with fine granular appearance changes. (**b**) Diffuse enlargement of the left maxillary gingiva, with fine granular appearance and irregular superficial ulcers. (**c**) Hemispheric enlargement of the posterior maxillary palatal mucosa. (**d**) Two weeks later, widespread enlargement of the right maxillary and mandibular gingiva with fine granular appearance. (**e**) Two weeks later, more severe enlargement of the left maxillary gingiva with fine granular appearance. (**f**) Two weeks later, more severe swelling of the left submandibular region

Age: 47 years
Sex: Male
Chief Complaints:
47-year-old man with swelling jaw for 1 month and painful gingiva for 20 days
History of Present Illness:
He had a sudden feeling of swelling in the mandibular area 1 month ago, with size of the table tennis and severe pain. After infusion of antibiotic drugs (unknown details), the mass reduced to pigeon egg in size, but it was easy to relapse. Twenty days ago, the painful gingiva and swollen palate occurred, with a feeling of numbness. Routine blood test performed 4 days ago showed increased WBC (15.2×10^9/L), decreased lymphocyte proportion (16.4%), and PLT (82×10^9/L). The liver and kidney function showed elevation of ALT (110U/L), with normal blood glucose.
Past Medical History: None
Allergy: None
Physical Examination:
Diffuse enlargement was observed on the gingival mucosa, with fine granular appearance changes. Irregular superficial ulcers were located on the surface of left maxillary gums. A physical examination revealed firm, non-tender enlarged lymph nodes in the bilateral submandibular region (the left side with 2 cm in diameter and the right side with 1 cm × 2 cm in size) (Fig. 10.3a–c).
Clinical Impression:
Gingival hyperplasia and ulcer
Laboratories and Imaging Studies:

1. Routine blood test and blood coagulation were normal.
2. Serological test for HIV was normal. Toluidine red unheated serum test (TRUST) for syphilis is negative, but enzyme-linked immunosorbent assay (ELISA) used to screen the antibody against *Treponema pallidum* was positive.
3. Maxillofacial X-ray showed no bony destruction.
4. Chest X-ray showed normal heart and lungs.
5. Abdominal ultrasound showed slight strong hypoechoic nodules (hepatic hemangioma?); cholesterol deposits in the wall of gallbladder.
6. Hematoxylin and eosin staining of the maxillary gingival biopsy indicated malignancy, and it was considered as myeloid sarcoma or leukemia, so bone marrow inspection was suggested. Immunohistochemical studies of the specimen showed positive staining with myeloperoxidase (MPO), leukocyte common antigen (LCA), CD56, and Ki67 (80%). But the tumor cells were negative for melanoma-associated antigen (HMB45), melanoma differentiation antigen (MART1), pan cytokeratin (PCK), epithelial membrane antigen (EMA), nonspecific esterase (NSE), and S-100.
7. The result of bone marrow aspiration smear was normal.
8. The score of bone marrow aspiration smear analyzed by alkaline phosphatase staining was 2 (normal reference value is 13–80).
9. The condition of the patient has progressed rapidly during the above inspection process. Two weeks later, oral examination revealed more fine-grained appearance changes and irregular superficial ulcers located on the gingival mucosa, with more severe swelling of the left submandibular region (Fig. 10.3d–f).
10. He was advised to the hematology department for further examination and treatment, but he died without definite diagnosis.

Diagnosis:
Oral manifestations of hematopoietic malignancy (myeloid sarcoma or leukemia?)
Diagnosis Basis:

1. Widespread gingival hyperplasia and ulcers
2. Results of HE staining and immunohistochemical studies of the gingival biopsy
3. Decreased score of alkaline phosphatase staining of bone marrow aspiration smear

[Review] Leukemia

Leukemia is a hematological malignancy which is characterized by marked proliferation of abnormal and immature white blood cells of the bone marrow or blood cell-forming tissues and tends to accumulate in various tissues of the body. The clinical features include anemia, fever, bleeding, hepatosplenomegaly, lymphadenopathy, and changes in the quantity and quality of peripheral blood leukocytes [3].

According to its clinical behavior, leukemia is classified as acute or chronic type. Patients with acute leukemia generally present fever as the early symptoms, and bleeding may occur at each part of the body. Leukemic cells may also infiltrate the spleen and lymph nodes, causing lymphadenopathy, hepatosplenomegaly, and other lesions. Chronic leukemia is usually slow progression; patients mainly suffer from low-grade fever, profuse sweating, weight loss, anemia, bleeding, and splenomegaly [4, 5].

Gingival infiltration of leukemic cells is one of the most common clinical signs and symptoms, especially in the acute phase; thereby many timely diagnoses are made by dentists. Some diagnoses are further confirmed because of unremitting bleeding after teeth extraction, subgingival scaling, and root planing. Gingival overgrowth, hyperplasia, and edema are typical oral features. As a result of direct infiltration by malignant leukocytes, the height of the hyperplastic gingiva could be close to the occlusal surface, with irregular shape and flabby texture. Spontaneous bleeding is always seen in the oral mucosa and gums; blood clots, petechiae, ecchymosis, and hematoma are also noted. The patients sometimes present with mucosal pallor and irregular superficial ulcers which are not easy to heal. Gingival inflammation, necrosis, pyorrhea, and loosening of the teeth could be identified [6–10].

Diagnosis of leukemia relies on clinical features, characteristic of hemogram, and bone marrow. Dentists and physicians should be vigilant about the diffuse hyperplasia, erosion, and ulcers of oral mucosa, especially gingiva. Furthermore, biopsy should be avoided without clear systemic condition.

Myeloid sarcoma mentioned in Case 90 is a solid malignant tumor consisting of immature myeloid cells and occurring at an extramedullary site, mostly infiltrated by acute leukemia blasts. It could be identified as the precursor of acute myeloid leukemia; however, a few patients will not progress to acute leukemia [11].

In some cases, due to the myeloperoxidase, green color is observed in the fresh tumor tissue, which is defined as chloroma. Myeloid sarcoma typically appears as localized mass or the compression symptoms, which can often be misdiagnosed mainly as lymphoma [12]. Intraoral MS is extremely rare, and gingival and palatal enlargement with superficial ulcerations has been reported [13, 14]. The diagnosis and immunophenotyping of MS rely mainly on immunohistochemical staining. MPO-positive staining is very informative for diagnosis of MS. The following markers are also the useful: CD43, CD56, CD15 (a marker for the granulocytic series), and CD 68 (the accepted marker for cells from the monocytic series despite its absence of specificity) [12].

Treatments of leukemia or MS need combination chemotherapy and other comprehensive treatment measures. Keep oral cavity clean, and use compound chlorhexidine acetate solution to prevent secondary infection [15].

10.3 Lymphoma

Case 91 NK/T-Cell Lymphoma (Palatal Ulcer)

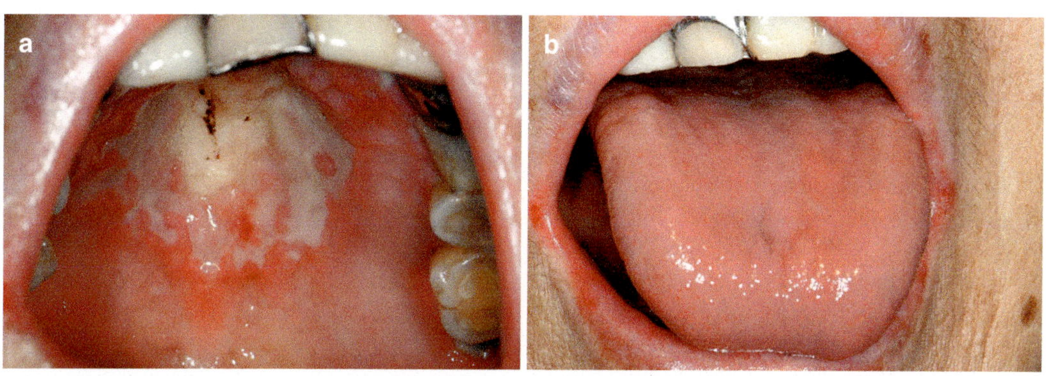

Fig. 10.4 (**a**) Ulcer and necrosis on the hard palate with an area of 4 × 5 cm (Reproduced from [16]). (**b**) Atrophic tongue with smooth surface

Age: 63 years
Sex: Female
Chief Complaints:
63-year-old woman with serious palatal ulceration for 1 month
History of Present Illness:
A 63-year-old presented to our clinic with painful palatal ulceration for about a month. Pathologic findings revealed ulceration and necrosis in a local hospital. After the topical and systemic anti-inflammatory treatment, the palatal ulcer did not heal. Spike fevers and fatigue occurred for 3 weeks, accompanied by five times of intermittent hematemesis before admission.
Past Medical History: Gastric ulcer
Allergy: None
Physical Examination:
Severe ulcer with an area of 4 × 5 cm was located on the anterior palate, with no bone damage or perforation by systemic examination. Atrophic tongue can also be detected (Fig. 10.4).
Clinical Impression:
Palatal ulcer with atrophic glossitis
Laboratories and Imaging Studies:

1. The routine blood test showed asphaerinia (HGB, 90 g/L; RBC, 3.23 × 10^{12}/L), leukopenia (WBC, 2.12 × 10^9/L), and thrombocytopenia (PLT, 81 × 10^9/L).
2. Serum alanine aminotransferase was 99 IU/L, aspartate aminotransferase 218 IU/L, lactate dehydrogenase 573 IU/L, and hydroxybutyric acid dehydrogenase 480 IU/L.
3. Gastroscopy showed chronic moderate atrophic gastritis.
4. Chest CT and abdominal ultrasound showed normal results.
5. Both aerobic and anaerobic bacteria in blood culture for 5 consecutive days were negative.
6. No obvious change was found among granulocyte series of the bone marrow aspirate, but more pale cytoplasm in erythrocytes.
7. No necrotic debris was detected after a complete endoscopic examination of the nasal cavity. A corona CT of the nasal part revealed a soft tissue mass in the walls of maxillary sinus, ethmoid sinus, frontal sinus, and right sphenoid sinus. Then the nasal malignant lymphomas or nasal-type NK-/T-cell lymphoma on the palate was suspected.
8. The second biopsy was performed in our clinic after platelet transfusion to normal range. HE staining showed a widespread infiltration of large- and medium-sized lymphoma cells with unconspicuous nucleoli and clear cytoplasm, as well as normal-appearing lymphocytes, plasma cells, and eosinophils.
9. Immunohistochemical staining was conducted on the right nasal vestibule and the palatal lesion. Both of the biopsy specimens revealed the same results. Ki67, as a cell proliferation marker, was positive in almost all cells (80–90%). High levels of cytoplasmic poly-CD3ε, cytoplasmic and membranous CD56, as well as granzyme B were detected but negative for CD20. Strong expression of EBER-ISH was also detected in the tumor cells by in situ hybridization. Given the above, final diagnosis as nasal-type extranodal NK-/T-cell lymphoma (invasive, WHO) was made.

Diagnosis:
Nasal-type extranodal NK-/T-cell lymphoma
Diagnosis Basis:

1. Oral lesion manifested as palatal ulcer, which was unresponsive to anti-inflammation treatment.
2. Results of HE staining and immunohistochemical studies of the second biopsy confirmed the diagnosis.

Management:

1. He was transferred to the hematology department for further therapy.
2. Topical use of compound chlorhexidine solution, oral rinse, 3 times daily.

Case 92 NK-/T-Cell Lymphoma (Gingival, Palatal, and Labial Ulcers)

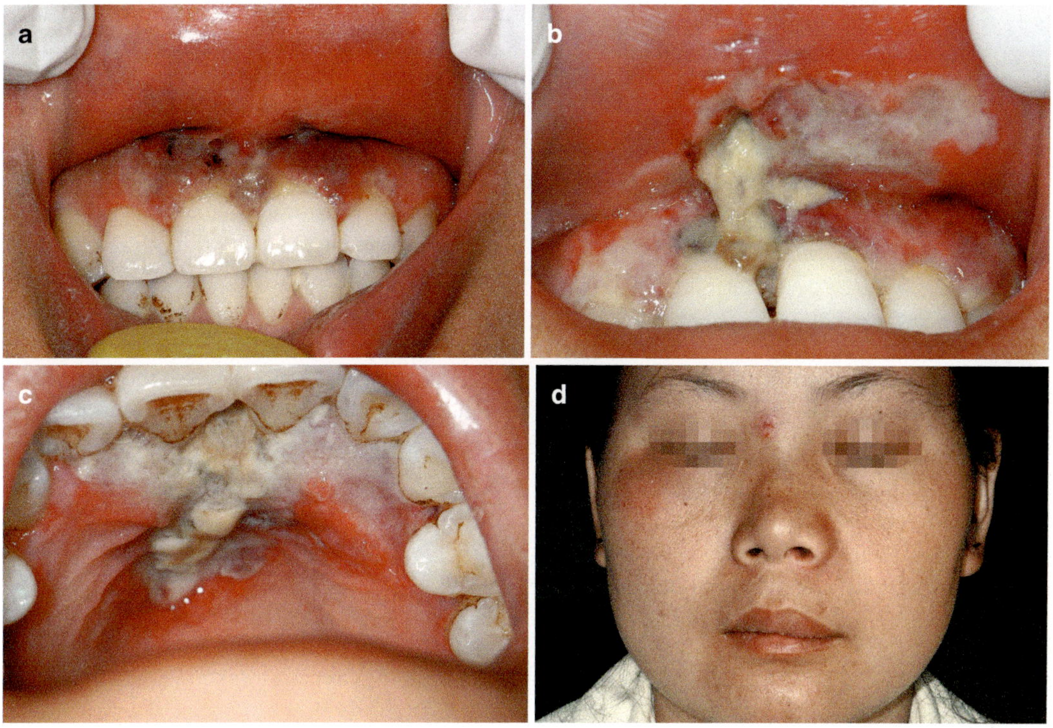

Fig. 10.5 (**a**) Serious erosion and congestion on the labial aspect of anterior maxillary gingiva covered by yellowish-white pseudomembrane, with partial necrosis. (**b**) Half a month later, diffuse ulcer and necrosis of anterior maxillary gingiva, extending to the upper labial mucosa covered by yellowish-white pseudomembrane. (**c**) Half a month later, widespread ulcer and necrosis of maxillary palatal gingiva, extending to the palate covered by yellowish-white pseudomembrane. (**d**) Half a month later, obvious swelling of the left face

Age: 28 years
Sex: Female
Chief Complaints:
28-year-old woman with swollen gingiva for 1 month and facial swelling for 15 days
History of Present Illness:
A 28-year-old lady presented to our clinic with swollen maxillary anterior gingiva for 1 month, with slow disease progression to the left maxillary gingiva. Fifteen days ago, painful facial swelling occurred which impaired eating. The blood test, chest X-ray, and abdominal ultrasound showed normal results in a local hospital. Dacryocystorhinostomy was performed 8 months ago before admission.
Past Medical History: None
Allergy: None
Physical Examination:
Serious erosion and congestion was located on the labial aspect of anterior maxillary gingiva. The erosions were covered by a yellowish-white pseudomembrane, with partial necrosis. The vestibule was involved, extending to the upper labial mucosa. Mild swelling of upper lip and left face were noticed (Fig. 10.5a).
Clinical Impression:
Gingival erosion
Laboratories and Imaging Studies:

1. The routine blood test showed WBC (3.2×10^9/L). Liver and kidney function was normal. Serological test for HIV was normal.
2. Local anti-infective therapy (compound chlorhexidine solution, oral rinse) and biopsy simultaneously were suggested.

3. Hematoxylin and eosin staining of the gingival biopsy revealed gingival inflammatory ulcer. Swelling of the left face was obvious. Oral examination showed widespread ulcers on the labial and lingual aspect of maxillary anterior gingiva, the corresponding labial vestibule, and mucous membrane inside the upper lip and the palate, which were covered by a yellowish-white pseudomembrane, with increased necrosis (Fig. 10.5b–d).
4. Maxillofacial contrast-enhanced CT revealed increased density of the soft tissue in bilateral nasal cavity, nasolabial fold, left wing of the nose, and the upper lip, and inflammation was considered.
5. The second biopsy was suggested, and results of HE staining and immunohistochemical studies supported the diagnosis of nasal-type extranodal NK-/T-cell lymphoma.

Diagnosis:
Nasal-type extranodal NK-/T-cell lymphoma
Diagnosis Basis:

1. Oral lesion manifested as gingival and palatal ulcer, which was unresponsive to regular anti-inflammation treatment.
2. Results of HE staining and immunohistochemical studies of the second biopsy confirmed the diagnosis.

Management:

1. She was transferred to the hematology department for further therapy.
2. Topical use of compound chlorhexidine solution, oral rinse, 3 times daily.

[Review] Lymphoma
Lymphoma is a group of malignancies that develop from lymph nodes or extranodal lymphoid tissues. In 2008, the World Health Organization (WHO) classification includes two main categories as types of lymphoma: Hodgkin's lymphomas and non-Hodgkin's lymphomas. The latter category is comprised of precursor lymphoid neoplasms, mature B-cell lymphomas, and mature T-cell and NK-cell lymphomas [17].

The data from the Chinese Anti-Cancer Association estimated 84,000 new patients of lymphoma and more than 47,000 deaths each year, which indicate that the mortality of lymphoma in China is rising by 5%. Lymphoma incidence is gradually approaching the crowd of young people and middle-aged. Because of the active period of lymphatic system, high sensitivity makes the young adults at high risk of lymphoma (Chinese Center for Disease Control and Prevention, 2013). The constituent ratio of lymphoma is ranked second in oral and maxillofacial malignancies after oral squamous cell carcinoma, with increasing morbidity.

The etiology remains unknown. It's generally accepted that it is closely associated with Epstein-Barr virus (EBV) and HIV infection, far greater risk of lymphoma in HIV patients than general populations. Moreover, abnormal immunity, autoimmune diseases, repeated infection, and xenogenic organ transplantation can cause reactive lymphoid hyperplasia stimulated by host antigens. Loss or dysfunction of T-cell lymphocytes results in lack of self-adjusting feedback control and unlimited proliferation of lymphoid tissues, which lead to lymphoma finally. In addition, environmental pollution solvent dyes, heavy traffc fumes, great work and psychological pressure, psychentonia, irregular life and fatigue, could reduce immune function, inducing lymphoma [18, 19].

Oral involvement of extranodal natural killer/T-cell lymphoma (ENKTL) is more common. ENKTL belongs to a group of mature NK-/T-cell lymphoma, which often present at extranodal sites with a broad morphological spectrum. It is designated as an "NK-/T-cell" lymphoma because, although most of the cases are believed to be of "true" natural killer (NK)-cell origin, "some" of the cases are known to demonstrate a T-cell phenotype. The actual proportion of cells is not well established. NK-/T-cell lymphomas that originate from the nasal cavity/nasopharynx may manifest similar signs and symptoms, clinical features, and immunophenotype; therefore, the diagnosis of ENKTL covers these kinds of malignancies [20].

ENKTL often present intranasally characteristic of septal perforation and destruction. But some extranodal sites can be affected, such as the hard palate, orbital cavity, gastrointestinal tract, lung, and skin, and even the spine is involved. Most (80–90%) patients present with stuffy or runny noses, hemorrhinia, sore throat, and dysphagia. The major sign presents as ulcerative neoplasms, with dry and puric crust covered on the ulcer. Some patients also have local bone destruction, presented by perforation of nasal septum or hard palate, and bridge collapse, even involving the midline facial tissues [16, 21]. Oral cases are often manifested as palatal necrotic ulcers; bone destruction on the palate could be found.

The typical pathological findings are diffusely infiltrating lymphoma cells, large- or medium-sized. The nuclear contours are irregular. Tumor cells infiltrated in the area of necrosis mixed with abundant lymphocytes, plasma cells, eosinophils, and histiocytes, which may be easily misdiagnosed as chronic inflammation.

The immunohistochemistry demonstrated a characteristic phenotype expressing CD2, CD56, and CD3 epsilon and cytotoxic granule-associated protein, such as TIA-1, granzyme B, and perforin. In situ hybridization with a specific RNA probe demonstrated strong EBER-1(EBV-encoded small nuclear RNA) expression in neoplastic cells. Strong positive Ki-67 and negative CD3 can be observed. According to the typical morphological features, with immunophenotypic and in situ hybridization profiling, we could make an early and actual diagnosis [16, 19].

The disease may be easily misdiagnosed. First, it is hard to make the accurate impressions at the early stage, because low incidence of the disease, unawareness of the doctor, and atypical symptoms and signs, especially primary, present at extranodal sites. Second, the necrotic lesion is the main clinical signs, so it is relatively difficult to choose the biopsy site. Repeated biopsy is considered, if necessary. In addition, it is difficult to distinguish from chronic inflammation due to neoplastic cell infiltration with diffused inflammatory cells.

Cases 91 and 92 showed atypical clinical symptoms and signs at first visit. Anti-inflammatory therapeutic response could not be qualified for a diagnosis of common ulcerative diseases. Therefore, repeated biopsy, combined with nasal endoscopy, was suggested. The definite diagnosis was made by multidisciplinary consultation. As a consequence, oral medicine specialists should pay attention to the repeated biopsy in the diagnostic process, as well as close collaboration with pathology department, otorhinolaryngological department, and oral surgery. We also highlight the honest and patient communications with the sufferers, in order to gain the understanding and support of complex diagnostic process from them.

The patients would be transferred to the hematology or oncology department for further treatment by chemoradiotherapy. Median survival was 4.2 years, and 5-year overall survival was 46% (median follow-up, 3.8 years). Extranasal type of ENKTL correlated with poorer prognosis [22]. The two patients described above were transferred to the hematology department immediately after diagnosis; unfortunately, they both died 6 months later.

10.4 Langerhans Cell Histiocytosis

Case 93 Langerhans Cell Histiocytosis

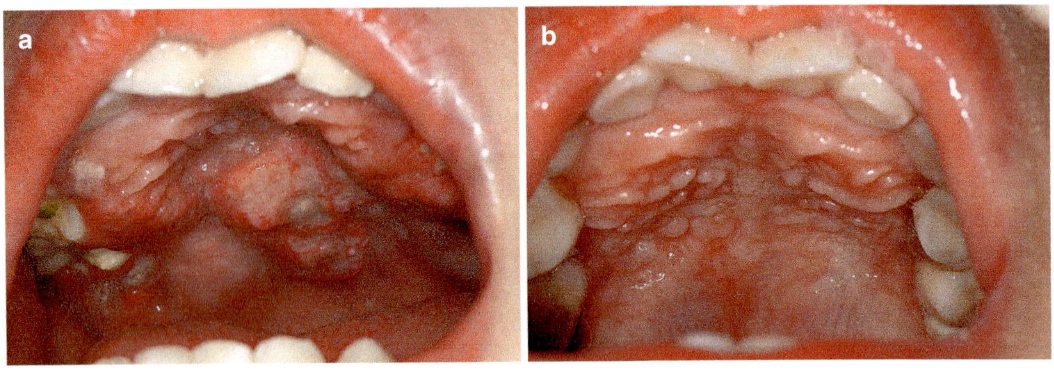

Fig. 10.6 (**a**) Widespread swelling and masses on the palate and maxillary palatal gingiva. (**b**) Ulcers and masses gradually normalized after chemotherapy (Reproduced from Jin et al. 2014)

Age: 21 months
Sex: Female
Chief Complaints:
21-month-old girl with an ulcerated palate for 1 month
History of Present Illness:
A 21-month-old girl presented to our clinic with an ulcerated palate for 1 month. She did not have any fever or hypothermia, reduced intake of food, or disturbed sleep. The lesions first appeared as pustules. An incision and drainage was performed at a local hospital. Her parents sought a second opinion as the ulcers showed no sign of healing. The ulcer was found to have enlarged in size and almost the entire palate was involved.
Past Medical History: None
Allergy: None
Physical Examination:
Widespread ulcers and masses were observed on the palate and maxillary palatal gingiva without detectable teeth mobility and lymphadenopathy (Fig. 10.6a). There was no cutaneous involvement.
Laboratories and Imaging Studies:

1. The routine blood test showed WBC 7.05×10^9/L (11×10^9–12×10^9/L), MONO% 18.2% (1–8%).
2. Maxillofacial cone-beam computed tomography (CBCT) showed bony destruction of the left orbital plate and maxilla in a pattern suggestive of Langerhans cell histiocytosis.
3. HE staining of the palate biopsy revealed a diffusely infiltration of round and oval cells with kidney-shaped nuclei. Immunohistochemical studies of the specimen showed positive staining with CD1a, S100, and langerin, supporting the diagnosis of Langerhans cell histiocytosis.

Diagnosis:
Langerhans cell histiocytosis
Diagnosis Basis:

1. Young children with ulcers and masses on the palate that cannot be characterized clinically as any other disease.
2. The diagnosis was confirmed by CT examination and HE and IHC staining.

Management:

1. Medication
   Rp.: Compound chlorhexidine solution 300 ml × 1
   Sig.: 1:1 dilution rinse t.i.d.
2. She was transferred to the hematology department immediately. The ulcers healed, and masses in the palate gradually resolved after chemotherapy with vincristine (0.9 mg, once a week, intravenously) and prednisone (12.5 mg, (twice a day, orally for 4 months) (Fig. 10.6b).

[Review] Langerhans Cell Histiocytosis

Langerhans cell histiocytosis (LCH) is characterized by anomalous proliferation of bone marrow-derived Langerhans cells, as well as lots of leucocytes, eosinophils, neutrophils, lymphocytes, plasma cells, and giant multinucleated cells, leading to tissue damage. It is a group of neoplastic disorders with widespread violation of multiple systems and organs. The bone, skin, internal organs, and mucocutaneous system may be involved. LCH is a rare disease, which is estimated at approximately 2–5 cases per million inhabitants per year. It is more common in children [23–25].

The etiology of LCH remains unclear. It may be caused by immune dysfunction, manifesting as a hypersensitive response to an unknown stimulation of the histiocyte-macrophage system [26, 27]. Failure of suppressor lymphocytes, altered autoantibodies, abnormal lymphocytic reactions to multiple mitogens, and structural modification in the thymus have been observed in all the advanced forms of LCH individuals [28]. The origin of inflammation or bacteriology is also suspected [26, 27]. It is also associated with virus infection, such as human herpesvirus 6, Epstein-Barr virus, and herpes simplex virus. Moreover, accumulation of Langerhans cell infiltrate could produce different systemic alterations depending on the location [29].

LCH was classified into four clinical forms depending on the first-onset age and their distribution sites, including chronic focal LCH (eosinophilic granuloma), chronic diffuse LCH (Hand-Schüller-Christian disease), acute disseminated LCH (Letterer-Siwe disease), and congenital reticulohistiocytosis (Hashimoto-Pritzker syndrome) [23–25].

Chronic focal LCH (eosinophilic granuloma) is the most common form. It appears as a unifocal or multifocal lesion in a single or occasionally various bones. Long bones and skulls are mainly affected, as well as the mandible. The soft tissue could be involved, without systemic manifestations [25]. Swelling and pain could be found in local lesions. X-ray shows localized bone destruction, presenting as a round or oval shape with clear border. No bone sequestration could be seen and has a good prognosis.

Chronic diffuse LCH (Hand-Schüller-Christian disease) usually appears in children or young adults, with slow onset. Hospital admissions are mainly due to skull soft tissue mass or teeth loose and loss. The bone is damaged by numerous proliferated Langerhans cells and granulation tissues. It often affects the skull, dura mater, and adjacent bone tissue; the skull base, sella turcica, and orbital cavity are also involved. Moreover, hyperplasia of the tissue may press on neurohypophysis and hypothalamus, which can lead to diabetes insipidus; and pressure on eyeballs could result in exophthalmos. The common clinical manifestation was triad of exophthalmos, osteolysis of the cranium, and diabetes insipidus. Other manifestations may also occur, such as petechiae, purpura, seborrheic dermatitis, and lung dysfunction [25, 30].

Acute disseminated LCH (Letterer-Siwe disease) generally affects children under 3 years old and progresses rapidly. It manifests in multiple organs and systems, such as the liver, lung, lymph nodes, skin, bone marrow, and bone, presenting clinically with eczema, hepatosplenomegaly, otitis media, anemia, hemorrhages, lymphadenopathies, and osteolytic lesions. Therefore, it has a poor prognosis, and death usually occurred within few months.

Congenital reticulohistiocytosis (Hashimoto-Pritzker syndrome) is characterized by the clinical features of dark nodules on the trunk, face, and scalp. The mucosa and skin are always involved, without implication of other organs [31].

For the case of this unit, we could not confirm the subtype based on the present results. Because it should also be determined in consultation with an oncologist to make a typing diagnosis, other than examinations mentioned, which can be helpful for predicting prognosis.

Oral lesions may be the initial manifestation of LCH, and sometimes the only location involved [29]. There are 77% of the LCH patients who suffered from oral lesions, which often occur in the bone, mucosa, and periodontal tissue [28].

The cranium, maxilla, and mandible are the most affected bones, usually infiltrating together. Mandibular lesions are the most frequent in all three forms of LCH. Studies have found that posterior zone and ramus of mandible were the most sites for bone lesions [24]. Solitary intra-bony lesions always appeared in the initial phases, localized outside the alveolar process. Multiple alveolar lesions, "scooped-out" alveolar lesions, alveolar lesions with bone sclerosis, and alveolar lesions with bone neoformation were noted.

Oral mucosal involvement tends to manifest as round and painful ulceration, with surrounding hyperemia. They are always limited to the buccal mucosa and hard palate. Red and white lesions on anterior mandibular vestibule were also shown in other studies [32].

Skin lesions such as the typical eczematoid rash are mainly presented, which could be confused with sebaceous dermatitis. Subcutaneous nodules are detected occasionally; therefore careful checkups should be considered [33]. In addition, enlarged lymph nodes are found.

Periodontal lesions are usually caused by underlying alveolar bone destruction, accompanying gingival ulceration, gingivitis, periodontal pocket formation, and teeth mobility.

The diagnosis is made by pathological observation combined with clinical and radiographic examinations. Histologic appearance reveals large atypical histiocytic cells with round shape. The kidney-shaped nuclei and a moderate number of eosinophilic cytoplasm can be detected, as well as abundant eosinophils, lymphocytes, and mononuclear phagocytes. Immunohistochemical results show S-100 and/or CD1a protein positivity of lesional cells.

LCH in most patients is self-limited, with alternate period of relapse and remission. The prognosis is unpredictable. Firstly, the outcome is poor if internal organs are involved (liver, lung, bone marrow). Secondly, the mortality rises to 50% in case of the age less than 2 years at the first admission. Thirdly, the disease spreading to various bones or soft tissues may worsen the prognosis [23, 25].

Diverse therapeutic options are available, including antibiotic treatment, chemotherapy, radiotherapy, surgery, adrenocorticotropic hormone (ACTH), and glucocorticoids (both systemic and intralesional) performed either individually or in combination. Correct mucosal and periodontal treatment involves tartar removal and subgingival scaling and planing, as well as rigorous hygiene and maintenance to conserve both teeth and periodontal tissue. Systemic chemotherapy could participate in accelerating oral ulcer healing. In mucosal forms, complete resolution of a palatal lesion after the perilesional infiltration of triamcinolone acetonide (eight sessions over a 6-month period, for a total dose of 200 mg) has been reported. Another patient was treated successfully with radiotherapy to the oral lesions [31].

10.5 Amyloidosis

Case 94 Amyloidosis (Macroglossia, Yellowish-White Nodular Lesions)

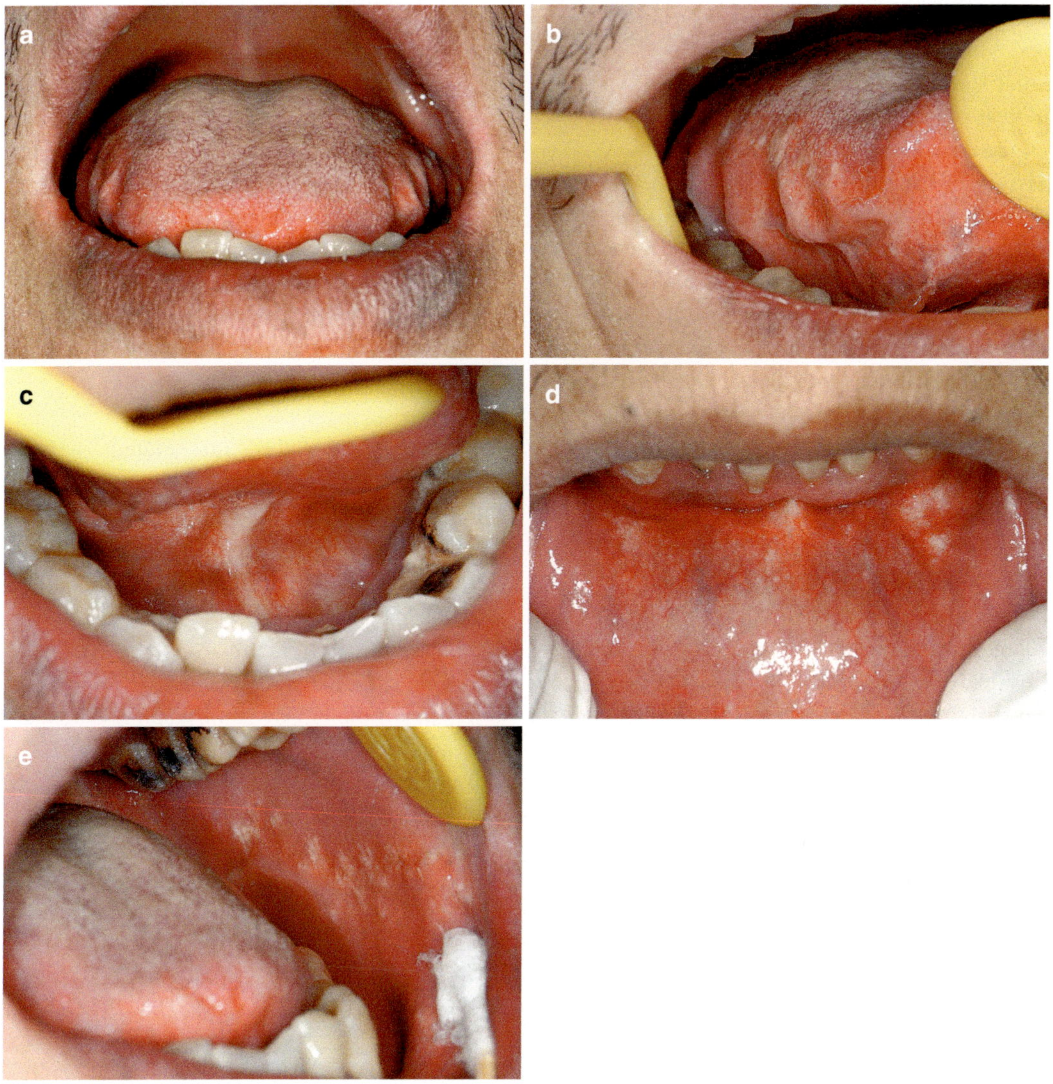

Fig. 10.7 (**a**) Increased tongue volume which cannot be extended outside the mouth. (**b**) Obvious teeth marks on the right lateral tongue. (**c**) Yellowish-white granular materials deposited in the frenulum of tongue. (**d**) Sporadic yellowish-white granular materials deposited in the lower labial mucosa. (**e**) Yellowish-white granular materials deposited in the left buccal mucosa

Age: 48 years
Sex: Male
Chief Complaints:
48-year-old man with limited movement of the tongue for 9 months
History of Present Illness:
A 48-year-old man presented to our clinic with unexpected limited movement of the tongue for 9 months. Eight months ago, hematoxylin and eosin staining had revealed submucous fibrosis of the tongue in a local hospital. The blood test of liver and kidney function showed normal results. Urine routine test revealed positive urinary protein. Serological test for HIV was normal. Toluidine red unheated serum test (TRUST) for syphilis was negative, but *Treponema pallidum* hemagglutination assay (TPHA) was positive. He denied the history of chewing betel nut.
Past Medical History: None
Allergy: None
Physical Examination:
Severe limited movement of the tongue was observed which cannot be extended outside the mouth. It appeared as increased tongue volume with firm texture and teeth marks. Yellowish-white granular materials were deposited in the bilateral tongue, lower labial mucosa, and buccal mucosa (Fig. 10.7).
Clinical Impression:
Oral amyloidosis
Laboratories and Imaging Studies:

1. Hematoxylin and eosin staining of the buccal mucosa and tongue biopsy revealed amyloidosis, and Congo red staining was positive.
2. Bone marrow aspirate revealed no typical changes.
3. Immunophenotype assay showed positive staining for CD138, PC, and Igκ, but negative for Igλ of plasmocytes, accounting for 20% of the karyocytes. So it was considered as plasma cell tumor infiltration.
4. Immunotyping of the cells revealed no significant changes in clonal B lymphocytes or plasma cells.
5. The results of cellular and humoral immunity assessment, chest X-ray, and abdominal ultrasound were normal.

Diagnosis:
Oral amyloidosis (associated with plasmacytoma?)
Diagnosis Basis:

1. The patients with increased tongue volume and firm texture.
2. Yellowish-white granular materials were deposited on the oral mucosa.
3. Results of the biopsy confirmed the diagnosis of amyloidosis.
4. Immunophenotype assay of bone marrow indicated plasma cell tumor infiltration.

Management:

1. Mix the triamcinolone acetonide and equal amount of water for injection or 2% lidocaine, intralesional multipoint low-dose injection.
2. She was transferred to the hematology department for further examination and therapy.

Case 95 Amyloidosis (Widespread Purple Bulla-Like Masses of the Oral Mucosa)

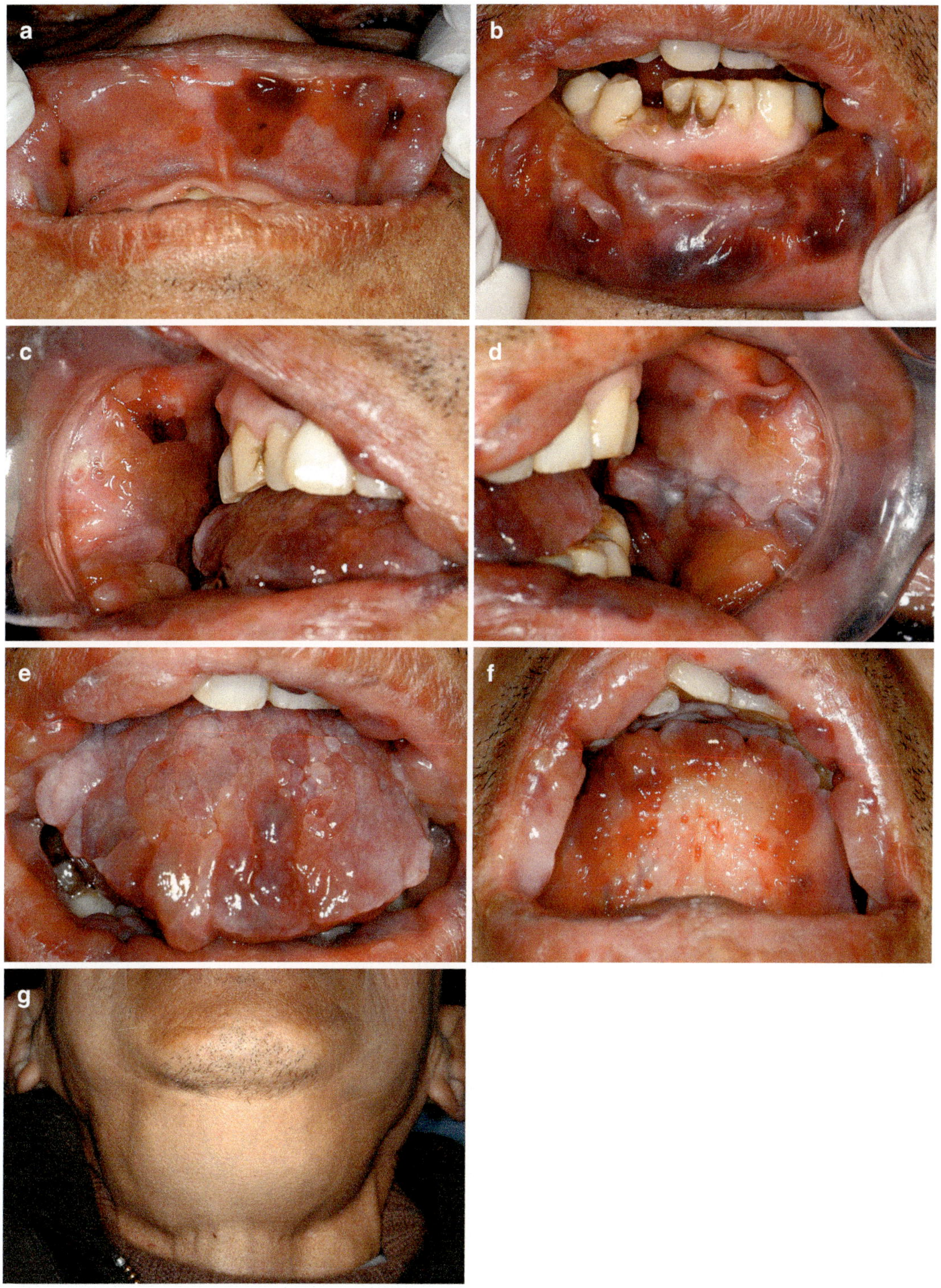

Fig. 10.8 (**a**) Purple bulla-like lesions on the upper lip. (**b**) Purple bulla-like masses on the lower lip. (**c**) Purple and red-purple bulla-like lesions on the right buccal mucosa. (**d**) Purple and red-purple bulla-like lesions on the left buccal mucosa. (**e**) Purple and red-purple bulla-like lesions on the dorsum of the tongue. (**f**) Purple and red-purple bulla-like lesions on the ventral tongue. (**g**) Swelling of the submandibular area (Reproduced from [34])

Age: 65 years
Sex: Male
Chief Complaints:
65-year-old man with inflexible tongue for 1 year
History of Present Illness:
A 65-year-old man presented with complaints of inflexible tongue and widespread masses on the oral mucosa for 1 year. The condition was getting worse in the past 6 months, with swelling of submandibular region for 5 months.
Past Medical History: Three months of gastrohelcosis and moderate anemia
Allergy: None
Physical Examination:
Multiple purple and red-purple bulla-like masses were observed on the buccal mucosa and lips. Some of them were soft. The tongue was enlarged, but a good range of movement. Lesions on the dorsum of the tongue were similar to those on the buccal mucosa, with atrophy of tongue papillae. However, papules on the ventral tongue were densely distributed, firm on palpation. A 7.5 × 4 × 3 cm^3 painless swelling was found in the submandibular region, poorly circumscribed. It was dense on palpation (Fig. 10.8).
Clinical Impression:
Oral amyloidosis?
Laboratories and Imaging Studies:

1. A routine blood test revealed anemia (hemoglobin, 73.00 g/L). The erythrocyte sedimentation rate (ESR) was significantly increased (48 mm/h).
2. Congo red staining of oral biopsy was positive.
3. The findings of contrast-enhanced CT revealed multiple osteolytic lesions in the skull (including parietal bone, occipital bone, and sphenoid bone) and mandible. The density of cervical vertebrae was uneven, indicating either multiple myeloma or metastatic tumor.
4. The results of cellular and humoral immunity assessment, chest X-ray, and abdominal ultrasound were normal.
5. The patient was suggested further inspections, including bone marrow aspiration, serum and/or urine protein electrophoresis, and immunofixation. But he refused these examinations and died of severe gastrorrhagia 2 months since the first visit.

Diagnosis:
Oral amyloidosis (associated with multiple myeloma?)
Diagnosis Basis:

1. The yellowish-white papule deposition was observed on the ventral surface of the tongue, firm on palpation.
2. Results of the biopsy confirmed the diagnosis of amyloidosis.
3. Swollen submandibular region.
4. The contrast-enhanced CT findings indicated multiple myeloma or metastatic tumor. No primary tumor was considered.
5. A routine blood test revealed moderate anemia.
6. The ESR increased significantly (48 mm/h).
7. The patients with gastric bleeding.

[Review] Amyloidosis
Amyloidosis is a group of diseases characterized by extracellular deposition of different kinds of fibrillar proteins, leading to tissue structure changes and dysfunction. All amyloid depositions have the similar fibrillar structure consisting of linear, aggregated fibrils with 7.5–10 nm in diameter [35, 36]. The most common site involved in oral cavity is the tongue, which manifests as a firm to rubbery macroglossia.

In the past, amyloidosis was classified with four typical forms: primary amyloidosis, secondary amyloidosis, familial amyloidosis, and localized amyloidosis. Primary amyloidosis referred to the deposition of fibrillar derived from monoclonal immunoglobulin light chains in major organs, such as the heart, kidney, and liver. Gastrointestinal tract and nervous system can also be involved. Secondary amyloidosis is often due to chronic inflammatory conditions, such as rheumatoid arthritis, chronic suppuration, familial Mediterranean fever, tuberculosis, and rickets. Familial amyloidosis is an autosomal dominant disease. Localized amyloidosis accounts for 9% of amyloidosis with a much more favorable prognosis [37].

New classification is based on the types of precursor protein which made the corresponding fibril deposition. Accordingly, the disease is designated as amyloid protein plus a suffix, in which A represents amyloid and the suffix specifies the protein. The most common types are immunoglobulin/light-chain related (AL) and familial transthyretin-associated (ATTR). Secondary amyloidosis is caused by amyloid derived from serum amyloid A, an acute-phase protein produced in response to chronic inflammation (AA).

AL amyloidosis is characterized by deposition of monoclonal immunoglobulin light chains. The presence of monoclonal paraprotein contains amyloid light chains in urine and serum, is also known as Bence-Jones protein (BJP). It often appears in urine of patients with myeloma, which may have the diagnostic significance [37]. Serum or urine BJP will be detected in up to 88% of individuals with primary systemic amyloidosis and 100% of patients with multiple myeloma [37]. The initial symptoms of AL amyloidosis are most frequently fatigue and weight loss, and the organs most commonly involved are the kidney and the heart. Renal amyloidosis may manifest as proteinuria and mild renal dysfunction, with profound edema and hypoalbuminemia. Cardiac lesions often present as congestive heart failure and thickened ventricle, and the ejection fraction is reduced.

AA amyloidosis occurs secondary to chronic inflammatory conditions such as tuberculosis or rheumatoid arthritis [38]. Renal deposition is the most common lesion that is often asymptomatic. Hepatomegaly and splenomegaly can be involved. In this condition, fibrils may be easy to deposit in the joints [39]. In addition, autonomy and sensory neuropathy, gastrointestinal hemorrhage, and spontaneous periorbital purpura are the uncommon features of AL and AA amyloidosis.

ATTR amyloidosis rarely affects the kidney and tongue, but peripheral sensory/motor and autonomic neuropathies are more common, as well as diarrhea and weight loss [37, 40].

Localized amyloidosis, which occurs without any evidence of systemic involvement, is much more rare than the others. In a review of 236 cases of amyloidosis, only 22 cases (9%) were localized. None of these individuals progressed to systemic amyloidosis in a follow-up of 10 years. They remained minimal dysfunction and symptom-free after being treated surgically [41].

The head and neck region is affected in 12–90% of amyloidosis patients, typically with the larynx and tongue affected [42]. The most common manifestations are hoarseness, nasal congestion, odynophagia, articulation problems, mandibular deformities, deglutition difficulties, airway obstruction, speech disorders, and hypogeusia. Amyloidosis involvement of the tongue is usually secondary to systemic diseases, consisting of tuberculosis, rheumatoid arthritis, and multiple myeloma. Macroglossia occurs in 26–83% of patients with multiple myeloma, often with enlarged tongue beyond the alveolar ridge, speech impairment, and dysphagia. Yellowish-white granular materials deposited along the lateral border can also be observed, as shown in Case 94 [37]. Oral amyloidosis could also present as widespread purple bulla-like masses of the oral mucosa, as shown in Case 95 [34].

The diagnosis of amyloidosis is made based on pathology. When stained with Congo red, the deposits of protein fibrils show apple-green birefringence on polarized light microscopy. Once the diagnosis has been made, an extensive workup for systemic disorders should be undertaken.

In AL amyloidosis, monoclonal paraprotein composed of amyloid light chains could be detected by immunofixation electrophoresis of serum or urine. Immunohistochemical staining of a bone marrow biopsy to search for κ- or λ-light chains should be performed to exclude plasma cell dyscrasia. Monoclonal immunoglobulin or immunoglobulin fragment may be produced by abnormal proliferation of a monoclonal group of plasma cells. The related disorders include multiple myeloma, solitary plasmacytoma, extramedullary plasmacytoma, paraproteinemia, and heavy-chain disease.

A variant transthyretin could be inspected by isoelectric focusing of the serum, which will separate variant from wild-type transthyretin. AA amyloidosis is suspected under chronic inflammatory condition in whom AL and ATTR amyloidosis have been excluded. Definite diagnosis is then made by immunohistochemical staining for the AA protein (Fig. 10.9).

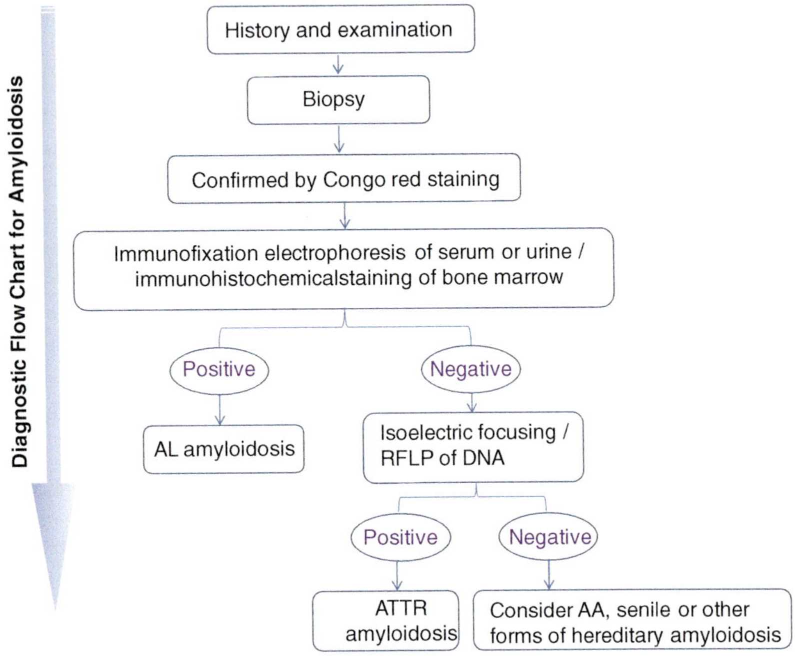

Fig. 10.9 Diagnostic flow chart for amyloidosis

Amyloidosis of the tongue is more related to multiple myeloma (MM) currently. MM accounts for approximately 10% of hematologic malignancies and tends to occur in middle-aged and elderly. The common clinical features are osteolytic bone lesions, anemia, hypercalcemia, renal failure, and infections.

The diagnostic criteria are 10% or more clonal plasma cells on bone marrow inspection or a biopsy that confirmed plasmacytoma and end-organ damage (hypercalcemia, renal insufficiency, anemia, or bone lesions) that is related to the underlying plasma cell disorder. In addition, the presence of 60% or more clonal plasma cells in the marrow could also be considered as myeloma regardless of the presence or absence of end-organ damage [43]. The serum or urine M protein is an abnormal immunoglobulin fragment or immunoglobulin light chain that is produced in excess by an abnormal monoclonal proliferation of plasma cells, typically in multiple myeloma. Therefore, an increase in single κ- or λ-light chain should be highly suspected of MM. In addition, autoimmune disease, infection, tumor, hepatitis, and cirrhosis are generally present increasing both κ- and λ-light chains. Among the patients with multiple myeloma, 15% may develop some form of amyloidosis [44]. A review study has found that anemia was present in 73% of patients with MM, the erythrocyte sedimentation rate increased in 84% (>20 mm/h), and lytic lesions in about 67% [45]. Enlarged submandibular glands present in about 40% of individuals with MM-associated amyloidosis [46, 47].

The median survival time for patients without MM was 15 months, compared to 5 months for those with MM [41]. Suspected patients with MM-associated amyloidosis should be performed with biopsy and Congo red staining as soon as possible. It is important to carry out comprehensive inspections for an early and accurate diagnosis, such as blood routine, erythrocyte sedimentation rate, urine routine, chest CT, abdominal ultrasonography, ultrasonic cardiogram, serum or urine M protein, and bone marrow biopsy.

There is no specific therapy for amyloidosis. The commonly used drugs include colchicine, melphalan, and prednisone. Once patients with secondary amyloidosis have some primary disorders, the underlying systemic diseases should be timely treated. In case of the localized form, intralesional triamcinolone acetonide multipoint low-dose injection could be used. Surgical and laser treatment could be employed [48].

AL amyloidosis is a subtype with poor prognosis if left untreated, with a median survival time of 1–2 years. The survival time of AA amyloidosis is affected by associated systemic diseases.

10.6 Florid Papillomatosis with Acanthosis Nigricans Maligna

Case 96 Florid Papillomatosis with Acanthosis Nigricans Maligna

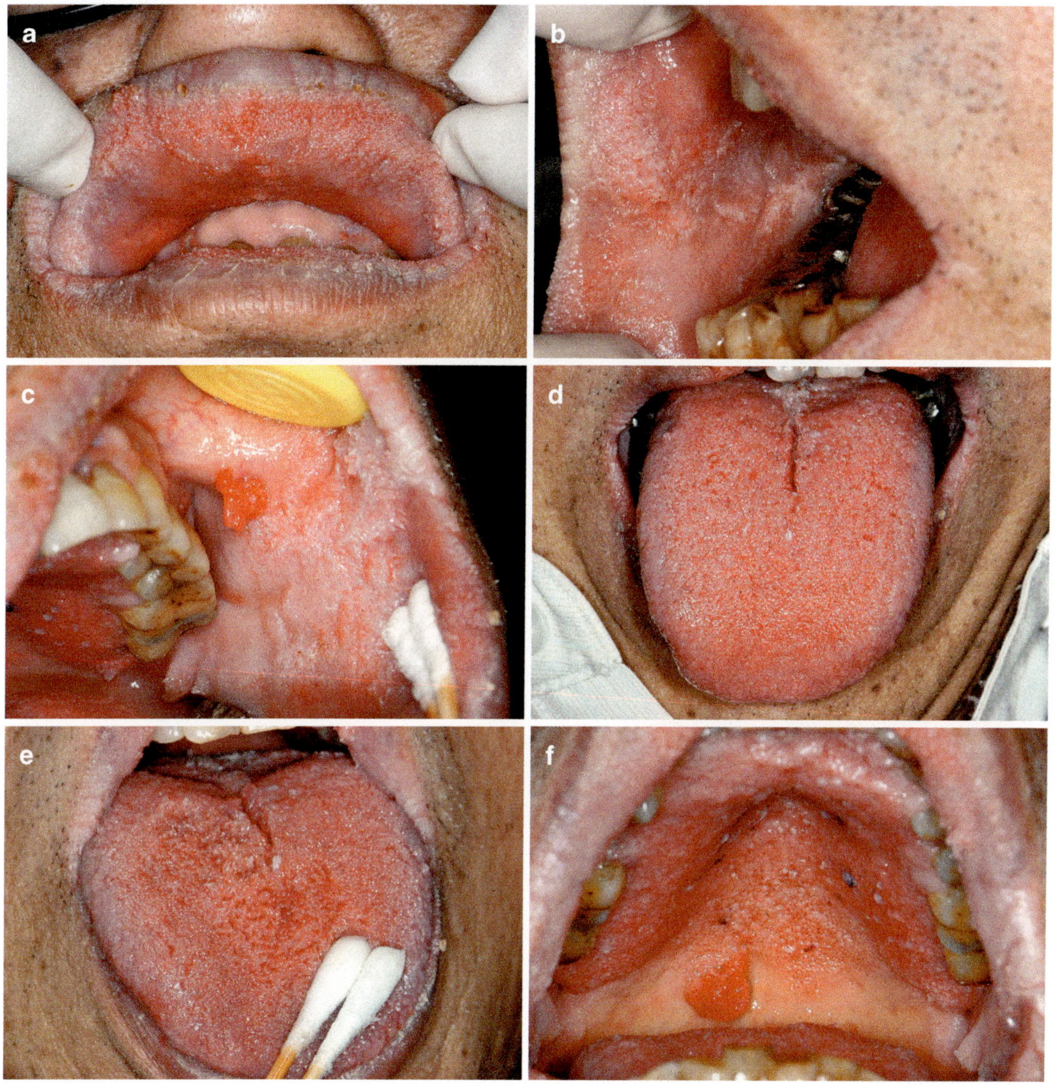

Fig. 10.10 (**a**) Widespread exuberant papillomatosis of the upper lip. (**b**) Widespread exuberant papillomatosis of the right buccal mucosa. (**c**) Widespread exuberant papillomatosis of the left buccal mucosa. (**d**) Widespread exuberant papillomatosis of dorsum of the tongue. (**e**) Widespread exuberant papillomatosis of dorsum of the tongue. (**f**) Widespread exuberant papillomatosis of the palate. (**g**) Multiple "wartlike" papillomatous on the insteps. (**h**) Hyperkeratotic soles with prominence of the papillomatous growths and hyperpigmentation. (**i**) Multiple "wartlike" papillomatous on the back of the hand. (**j**) Brownish hyperpigmentation of the axilla. (**k**) Brownish hyperpigmentation of the mammary areola

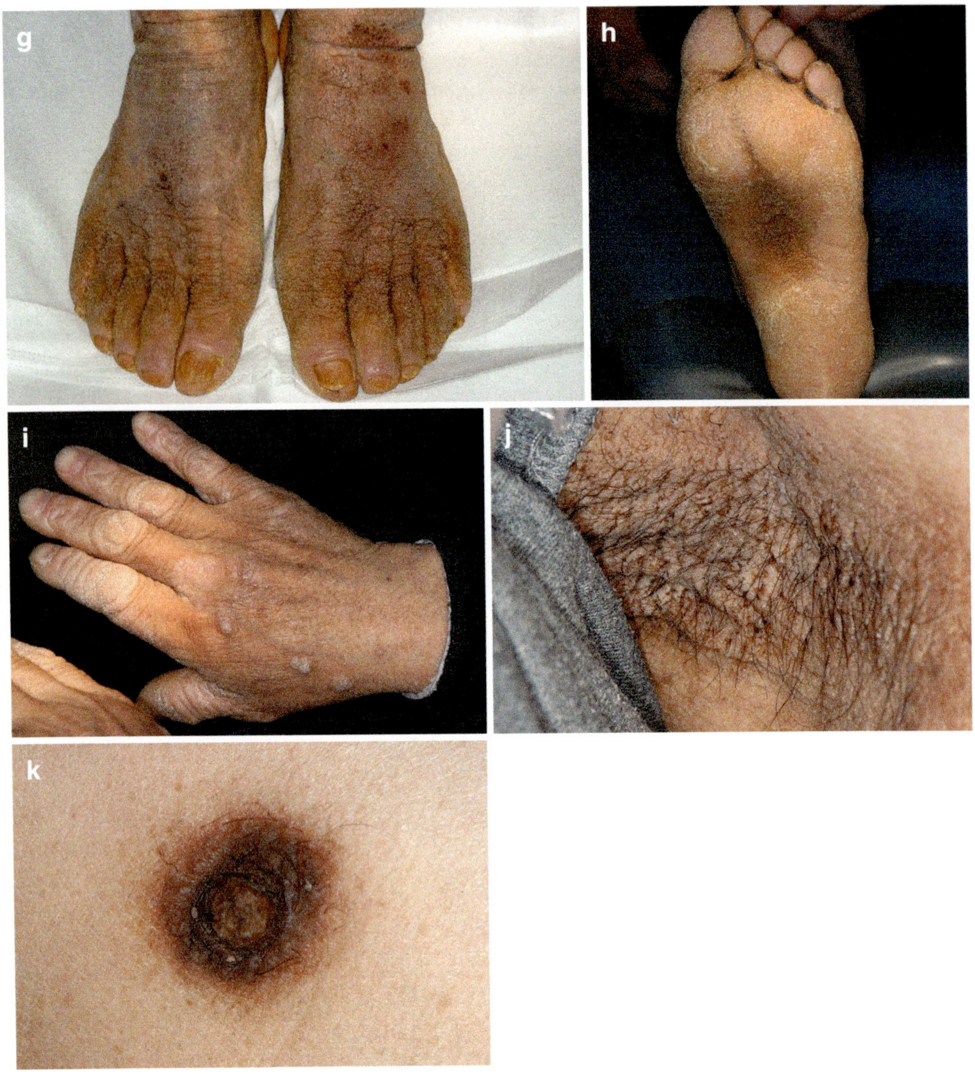

Fig. 10.10 (continued)

Age: 72 years
Sex: Male
Chief Complaints:
72-year-old man with oral verrucous lesions for 6 months
History of Present Illness:

A 72-year-old man presented to our clinic complaining of oral verrucous lesions, which appeared half a year ago. The verrucous neoplasm gradually increased in number and became widespread, almost involved the whole oral mucosa. During this period he also noticed cutaneous warty papule on his upper and lower limbs. Routine blood test, blood glucose, and liver and kidney function were normal. Serological tests for syphilis and HIV were normal.

Past Medical History: None
Allergy: None
Physical Examination:

Oral examination revealed exuberant papillomatosis of the tongue, buccal mucosa, lips, and palate. Lesions appeared as normal color, lithe papillomatous growths. Moreover, scarlet papillomatosis by an area of 1 × 1 cm is located at the anterior right buccal mucosa and posterior palate. Significant cutaneous physical findings included brownish hyperpigmentation and velvety thickening of the skin. There were multiple "wartlike" papillomatous involvements of the neck, axillae, and mammary areolae. In addition, extensive verrucous papules and plaques appeared on the upper limbs and insteps. The palms and soles were hyperkeratotic with prominence of the papillomatous growths and hyperpigmentation (Fig. 10.10).

Clinical Impression:

Widespread oral verrucous lesions (acanthosis nigricans?)

Laboratories and Imaging Studies:

1. Wartlike buccal and lingual lesions were biopsied. HE staining revealed papillomatosis, moderate hyperacanthosis, acanthosis, and irregular basal hyperpigmentation.
2. The dermatologists were called in for the consultation diagnosed as acanthosis nigricans.
3. Chest CT revealed tumor infiltration of the upper lobe of the right lung, enlarged hilar, and mediastinal lymph nodes.
4. Serum tumor marker results: carcinoembryonic antigen (CEA) 31.27 ng/ml (N, <5 ng/ml) and cytokeratin fragment (Cyfra211) 17.47 ng/ml (N, <5 ng/ml).
5. Bronchoscopy examination did confirm the diagnosis of a poorly differentiated pulmonary adenocarcinoma.

Diagnosis:

Florid papillomatosis with acanthosis nigricans maligna (associated with pulmonary adenocarcinoma)

Diagnosis Basis:

1. Widespread oral verrucous lesions with papillomatosis.
2. Extensive verrucous papules and plaques appeared on the upper limbs and insteps. The palms and soles were hyperkeratotic with prominence of the papillomatous growths and hyperpigmentation.
3. Diagnosis of a poorly differentiated pulmonary adenocarcinoma.

Management:

1. Topical use of compound chlorhexidine solution, oral rinse, 3 times daily.
2. He was transferred to the oncology department for further therapy.

[Review] Florid Papillomatosis with Acanthosis Nigricans Maligna

Acanthosis nigricans (AN) is a rare mucocutaneous condition characterized by the manifestations of thick velvety skin with hyperpigmentation and verrucous papillomatous lesions of undetermined cause. It may develop in response to tumor, drug, and genetic, metabolic, or endocrinological factors, and eight types were classified: benign AN, obesity-associated AN (pseudo AN), syndromic AN (syndrome associated with diabetes mellitus and autoimmune diseases), acral AN, unilateral AN, drug-induced AN (corticosteroids, nicotinic acid, diethylstilbestrol, insulin, etc.), mixed-type AN, and malignant AN. The majority (80%) of patients is either idiopathic or associated with benign conditions, which is reversible [49, 50]. Benign AN occurs to newborns or children frequently, it has a familial hereditary tendency, and it may fade with age. Obesity-related AN will improve with weight loss, and drug-induced AN is likely to resolve when the drug is ceased [51, 52]. Gastric adenocarcinoma is the most common underlying malignancy of malignant AN. Other malignant neoplasms affect gastrointestinal tract, ovaries, uterus, breast, and prostate [53].

Cutaneous AN typically manifests as hyperpigmented plaques that gradually thicken, leading to a velvety appearance. Neck, groin, and axillae are the predilection sites. And oral cavity can also be affected by florid papillary growths [51].

Florid cutaneous papillomatosis (FCP) is characterized by the rapid growth of multiple verrucous lesions that are difficult to distinguish them from viral warts. They may affect the trunk, face, and periorbital, ocular, and oral mucosa [49, 54]. Gastric adenocarcinoma is the most common underlying malignancy, often concomitant with FCP [55]. However, FCP has recently been thought to be a variant of malignant AN [54] or a term used to define verrucous papillomatous lesions of malignant AN [49].

FCP with malignant AN is an obligate paraneoplastic syndrome (PNS) [52]. Paraneoplastic syndrome (PNS) is the consequence of tumor inside, instead of local or metastasis occurrence, such as tumors of the lung, breast, ovaries, or lymphatic system. This syndrome is mediated by cytokines secreted by tumor or by an immune response against the tumor. Although the etiology and pathogenesis of PNS still remain unclear, the autoimmune abnormality is believed to the leading cause. Antigens expressed by tumor cells trigger various antibodies to start an antitumor immune response. Normal tissues expressing similar protein can then be attacked by these autoantibodies [56]. It is important to make early diagnosis if widespread verrucous lesions or multiple papillomatous lesions occur, in order to detect underlying malignancy as soon as possible. If malignant AN is suspected, computed tomography, serological tumor markers, and biopsy performed immediately should be the most effective.

Topical fade creams or cosmetic surgery can lighten skin cosmetically in less severe cases. Malignant AN may regress following tumor-specific therapy and usually worsens with cancer progression.

10.7 Focal Dermal Hypoplasia

Case 97 Focal Dermal Hypoplasia

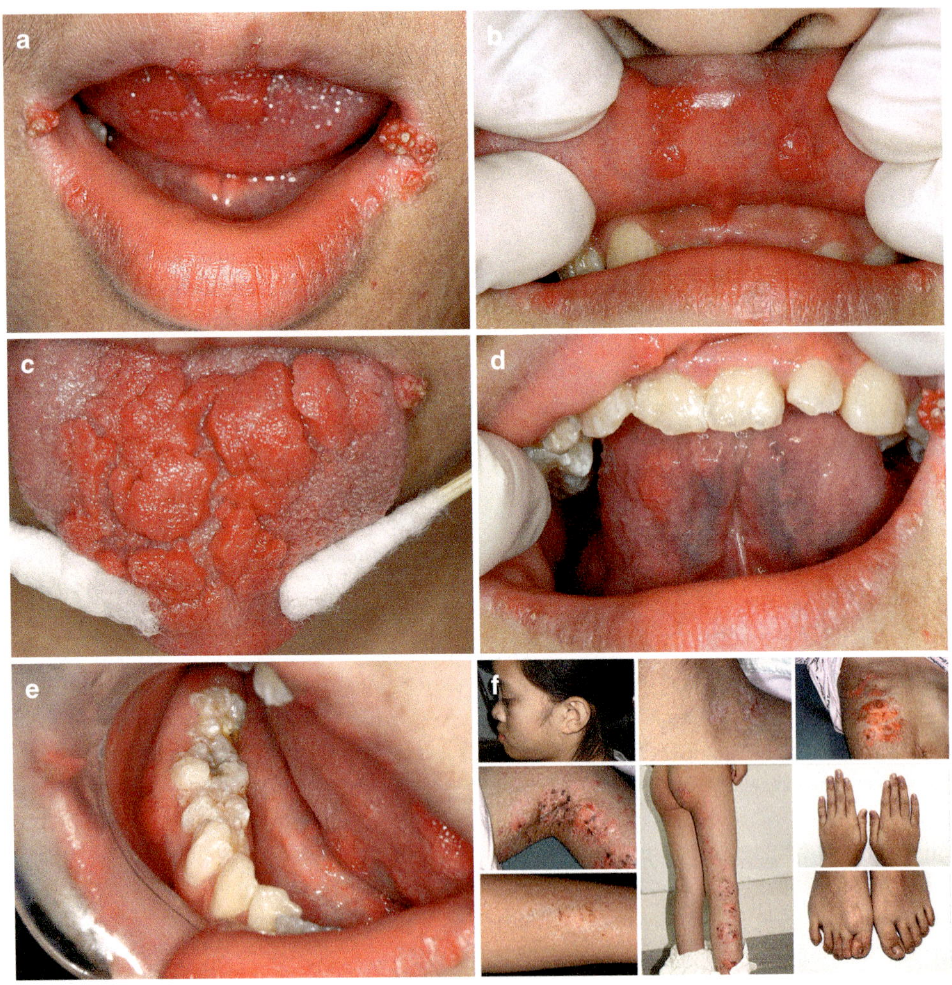

Fig. 10.11 (**a**) Raspberrylike papilloma over the corner of the mouth. (**b**) Raspberrylike papilloma on the upper lip. (**c**) Widespread raspberrylike papilloma on the tongue. (**d**) Raspberrylike papilloma on the ventral tongue and enamel hypoplasia of incisors. (**e**) Enamel hypoplasia of molars and papilloma on the gingiva. (**f**) Skin lesions: mid-face hypoplasia, skin hypopigmentation, red proliferation on the right abdomen (area was 5 × 8 cm^2), linear dermal atrophy along Blaschko's lines of the right legs, hypoplastic nails with longitudinal splitting, and partial absence of the fingernails and toenails (Reproduced from [57])

Age: 12 years
Sex: Female
Chief Complaints:
12-year-old girl with papillary lesions on the lips and tongue for 8 years
History of Present Illness:
A 12-year-old girl presented to our clinic with papillary lesions on the corner of the mouth for 8 years. Laser resection was performed repeatedly in other hospitals, while relapse easily suffered. Four years ago, painless papillomata appeared on the tongue without treatment, following red proliferation on the right abdomen. She also complained of translucent epidermis on the shoulders, arms, left side of the body, right abdomen, and both legs from birth, which was untreated.
Past Medical History: None
Allergy: None
Physical Examination:
Raspberrylike papillomas on the corner of the mouth, perioral skin, lips, and tongue were detected. There are also enamel hypoplasia, septal bone absorption of the premolar, and molars on the right mandible (Fig. 10.11a–e).
Reticulated and atrophic scars were located on the trunk and extremities. There was a red prominence with area of 5 × 8 cm^2 on the right abdomen. Fat herniation and hypopigmentation of her shoulders, arms, right abdomen, and legs were observed. These lesions followed Blaschko's lines. Hypoplastic nails with longitudinal splitting and partial loss of nails were also noted. The girl had midface hypoplasia (Fig. 10.11f).
Clinical Impression:
Multiple oral papillomas (congenital disorder?)
Laboratories and Imaging Studies:

1. The results of routine blood test, blood biochemistry, abdominal ultrasound, pre-transfusion test, stool routine, and both humoral and cellular immunities were normal.
2. No evidence of HPV-6, HPV-11, HPV-16, and HPV-18 infections was detected in the skin lesions by fluorescent Q-PCR analysis.
3. Biopsy from the dorsum of the tongue and left corner of the mouth showed evidence of papilloma.
4. Biopsy of papillary lesions on the right abdomen showed more likely to be focal dermal hypoplasia.
5. Mild septal bone absorption of the right mandibular was detected by oral X-ray.
6. Mild pulmonary valve stenosis was found by cardiac color Doppler imaging. Bone age was normal.

Diagnosis:
Focal dermal hypoplasia
Diagnosis Basis:

1. Multiple oral verrucous lesions with enamel hypoplasia
2. The typical cutaneous manifestations

Management:
Orthopedic surgery was suggested to remove the oral hyperplasia that greatly impacts on appearance, as well as obvious hyperplasia on the right abdomen. Regular follow-up visit and close observation were suggested.

[Review] Focal Dermal Hypoplasia
Focal dermal hypoplasia (FDH), also known as Goltz-Gorlin syndrome, could affect multiple systems such as the mucosa, skin, bones, and teeth, which arise from the mesoderm and ectoderm. It is more common in women (90%) [58, 59]. Mutation of *PORCN* (porcupine homolog) gene is closely associated with FDH, with an X-linked dominant manner [60]. To date, there are about 80 mutations of *PORCN* identified in FDH [61].

The clinical manifestations of FDH include [57]:

1. Skin abnormalities occur in over 95% patients of FDH, including atrophy, pigmentation, fat herniation, hypoplastic nails, and papilloma. These manifestations are often along Blaschko's lines. The dermal hypoplastic lesions are transparent at birth and slowly heal with crust formation with age. Papilloma is often located on the skin, oral cavity, perioral regions, esophagus, crissum, genitalia, and ocular areas, leading to corresponding malformation and dysfunction [62].

2. Skeletal involvement has different forms. Over 50% of the patients present with limb deformity, including syndactyly, oligodactyly, and camptodactyly. Osteopathia striata is also the typical presentation of skeletal system. X-ray inspection of metaphysis can help diagnose.
3. Craniofacial abnormalities, such as pointed chin and notched alae nasi, are characteristic of FDH.
4. Oral lesions affect the mucosa and teeth. Oral papilloma is one of the most common clinical features. Hypodontia, microdontia, and abnormal condition involving eruption, position, and number were also common [63–65].
5. Ocular abnormalities are present in approximately 15% of the patients, which tend to be asymmetrical. The severity ranges from mild appearance impairment to blindness. It is mainly presented by microphthalmia, following iris and chorioretinal coloboma, anophthalmia, and cornea abnormalities [66, 67].

The following systemic disorders are uncommon, with some of which causing fatal risk:

1. Gastrointestinal system. Hernia can occur at the locations of skin hypoplasia [68].
2. Kidneys and urinary system. Tissue defects such as hypoplastic kidneys, renal ectopia, horseshoe kidney, bifid ureter, and even absent kidney could occur [69–71].
3. Nervous system. Mental retardation is usually observed, as well as hydrocephalus and epilepsy [72].
4. Cardiovascular system. Cardiac ventricular septal defect, hypoplasia of pulmonary arteries/veins, ectopia cordis, and pulmonary valve stenosis may occur [73].
5. Reproductive system. They are predominantly found in females (90%). Uterus bicornis most commonly occurs, followed by septate hymen, athelia, and mammary hypoplasia [71, 74].

There is no gold standard for diagnosis of FDH. Typical clinical manifestations such as cutaneous, skeletal, ocular, and oral abnormalities offer clues for the clinical diagnosis. A comprehensive evaluation can help us to make an accurate diagnosis timely.

Other diseases with similar manifestations should be considered in the differential diagnosis:

1. Nevoid basal cell carcinoma syndrome. This is a multisystem disease caused by *PTC* (patched) mutations, including multiple-site basal cell carcinomas, jaw keratocysts, palmar/plantar dyskeratosis, bifid rib, and falx cerebri calcification [75].
2. Oculocerebrocutaneous syndrome. This is a rare congenital anomaly affecting the skin, eye, and central nervous system, with similar manifestations of FDH. And cerebral malformation is the key point to diagnose [76].
3. Rieger's syndrome. This is a rare autosomal-dominant disease characterized by ocular, dental, and periumbilical lesions. Dental dysplasia presents as midfacial hypoplasia, loss of incisors, and second premolars [77].
4. MIDAS syndrome. The typical signs are microphthalmia, dermal aplasia, and sclerocornea (MIDAS for short). Linear erythematous dysplasia occurs on the lower jaw skin, neck, and head, combined with microphthalmia, corneal opacities, and orbital cysts. Other features include corpus callosum hypoplasia, sclerocornea, chorioretinal malformation, hydrocephalus, seizures, mental retardation, and nail dystrophy. The disease-causing gene is located on Xp22.3, which is different from FDH [78].

Considering the multisystem involvement of FDH, the therapeutic goal is to improve function and cosmetic appearance of impaired system. Therapeutic principles for skin lesions are to facilitate healing and prevent infection. The pulse dye laser has been reported to reduce pruritus and erythema [79]. And photodynamic therapy can be used to treat refractory hyperplasia [80]. Severe systemic disorders should be treated by specialists. Orthopedic surgery is suggested to remove oral papilloma that seriously affected the appearance. Those with minor expression can expect to have a normal life span, and the degree of affected organ systems impacts an individual's mortality.

References

1. Hou M, Dai K, Peng J. Blood platelet disorders. 2nd ed. Beijing: Science and Technology Literature Press; 2013.
2. Guzeldemir E. The role of oral hygiene in a patient with idiopathic thrombocytopenic purpura. Int J Dent Hyg. 2009;7(4):289–93.
3. Javed F, Utreja A, Bello CFO, et al. Oral health status in children with acute lymphoblastic leukemia. Crit Rev Oncol Hematol. 2012;83(3):303–9.
4. Vardiman JW, Thiele J, Arber DA, et al. The 2008 revision of the World Health Organization (WHO) classification of myeloid neoplasms and acute leukemia: rationale and important changes. Blood. 2009;114(5):937–51.
5. Breed CD. Diagnosis, treatment, and nursing care of patients with chronic leukemia. Semin Oncol Nurs. 2003;19(2):109–17.
6. Wu J, Fantasia JE, Kaplan R. Oral manifestations of acute myelomonocytic leukemia: a case report and review of the classification of leukemias. J Periodontol. 2002;73(6):664–8.
7. Fatahzadeh M, Krakow AM. Manifestation of acute monocytic leukemia in the oral cavity: a case report. Spec Care Dentist. 2008;28(5):190–4.
8. Cooper CL, Loewen R, Shore T. Gingival hyperplasia complicating acute myelomonocytic leukemia. J Can Dent Assoc. 2000;66(2):78–9.
9. Demirer S, Ozdemir H, Sencan M, Marakoglu I. Gingival hyperplasia as an early diagnostic oral manifestation in acute monocytic leukemia: a case report. Eur J Dent. 2007;1(2):111–4.
10. Begon E, Blum L, Benramdane R, et al. Oral manifestation of T-cell leukemia/lymphoma. Arch Dermatol. 2010;146(7):804–5.
11. Audouin J, Comperat E, Le TA, et al. Myeloid sarcoma: clinical and morphologic criteria useful for diagnosis. Int J Surg Pathol. 2003;11(4):271–82.
12. Campidelli C, Agostinelli C, Stitson R, Pileri SA. Myeloid sarcoma: extramedullary manifestation of myeloid disorders. Am J Clin Pathol. 2009;132(3):426–37.
13. Papamanthos MK, Kolokotronis AE, Skulakis HE, Fericean AM, Zorba MT, Matiakis AT. Acute myeloid leukaemia diagnosed by intra-oral myeloid sarcoma. A case report. Head Neck Pathol. 2010;4(2):132–5.
14. Goteri G, Ascani G, Messi M, et al. Myeloid sarcoma of the maxillary bone. J Oral Pathol Med. 2006;35(4):254–6.
15. Soares AF, Aquino AR, Carvalho CH, Nonaka CF, Almeida D, Pinto LP. Frequency of oral mucositis and microbiological analysis in children with acute lymphoblastic leukemia treated with 0.12% chlorhexidine gluconate. Braz Dent J. 2011;22(4):312–6.
16. Meng W, Zhou Y, Zhang H, et al. Nasal-type NK/T--cell lymphoma with palatal ulcer as the earliest clinical manifestation: a case report with literature review. Pathol Oncol Res. 2010;16(1):133–7.
17. Jaffe ES. The 2008 WHO classification of lymphomas: implications for clinical practice and translational research. Hematology Am Soc Hematol Educ Program. 2009;2009:523–31.
18. Hong J, Park S, Baek HL, et al. Tumor cell nuclear diameter and CD30 expression as potential prognostic parameter in patients with extranodal NK/T--cell lymphoma, nasal type. Int J Clin Exp Pathol. 2012;5(9):939–47.
19. Yu WW, Hsieh PP, Chuang SS. Cutaneous EBV-positive gammadelta T-cell lymphoma vs. extranodal NK/T-cell lymphoma: a case report and literature review. J Cutan Pathol. 2012;40(3):310–6.
20. Pongpruttipan T, Sukpanichnant S, Assanasen T, et al. Extranodal NK/T-cell lymphoma, nasal type, includes cases of natural killer cell and alphabeta, gammadelta, and alphabeta/gammadelta T-cell origin: a comprehensive clinicopathologic and phenotypic study. Am J Surg Pathol. 2012;36(4):481–99.
21. Kawakami K, Ito R, Tono Y, et al. Orbital inflammatory lesion as an initial manifestation of systemic nasal type NK/T-cell lymphoma. J Clin Exp Hematopathol. 2012;52(2):137–9.
22. Li S, Feng X, Li T, et al. Extranodal NK/T-cell lymphoma, nasal type: a report of 73 cases at MD Anderson Cancer Center. Am J Surg Pathol. 2013;37(1):14–23.
23. Pacino GA, Serrat A, Redondo LM, Verrier A. Langerhans cell histiocytosis: clinical diagnostic features and current concepts. Med Oral. 1999;4(5):607–18.
24. Dagenais M, Pharoah MJ, Sikorski PA. The radiographic characteristics of histiocytosis X. A study of 29 cases that involve the jaws. Oral Surg Oral Med Oral Pathol. 1992;74(2):230–6.
25. Duncan WK, Post AC, McCoy BP. Eosinophilic granuloma. Oral Surg Oral Med Oral Pathol. 1988;65(6):736–41.
26. Hartman KS. Histiocytosis X: a review of 114 cases with oral involvement. Oral Surg Oral Med Oral Pathol. 1980;49(1):38–54.
27. Egeler RM, D'Angio GJ. Langerhans cell histiocytosis. J Pediatr. 1995;127(1):1–11.
28. Hernandez-Juyol M, Boj-Quesada JR, Gallego MS. Oral manifestations of Langerhans cell histiocytosis. Case study of a two-year-old boy. Med Oral. 2003;8(1):19–25.
29. Minguez I, Minguez JM, Bonet J, Penarrocha M, Sanchis JM. Oral manifestations of chronic disseminated histiocytosis. A report of 10 cases. Med Oral. 2004;9(2):152–4. 149–52.
30. Becelli R, Carboni A, Gianni C, Alterio A, Renzi G. A rare condition of Hand-Schuller-Christian disease. J Craniofac Surg. 2002;13(6):759–61.
31. Milian MA, Bagan JV, Jimenez Y, Perez A, Scully C, Antoniades D. Langerhans' cell histiocytosis restricted to the oral mucosa. Oral Surg Oral Med Oral Pathol Oral Radiol Endod. 2001;91(1):76–9.
32. Madrigal-Martinez-Pereda C, Guerrero-Rodriguez V, Guisado-Moya B, Meniz-Garcia C. Langerhans cell histiocytosis: literature review and descriptive analy-

sis of oral manifestations. Med Oral Patol Oral Cir Bucal. 2009;14(5):E222–8.
33. Zhang K, Zeng H, Chen WQ. Clinical features and diagnosis of langerhans cell hyperplasia. Ai Zheng. 2006;25(1):88–91.
34. Li Y, Liu N, Xu Y, et al. Widespread purple bulla-like masses of the oral mucosa. Oral Surg Oral Med Oral Pathol Oral Radiol. 2012;114(5):552–7.
35. Khan MF, Falk RH. Amyloidosis. Postgrad Med J. 2001;77(913):686–93.
36. Steciuk A, Dompmartin A, Troussard X, et al. Cutaneous amyloidosis and possible association with systemic amyloidosis. Int J Dermatol. 2002;41(3):127–32; discussion 133–4.
37. Fahrner KS, Black CC, Gosselin BJ. Localized amyloidosis of the tongue: a review. Am J Otolaryngol. 2004;25(3):186–9.
38. Angiero F, Seramondi R, Magistro S, et al. Amyloid deposition in the tongue: clinical and histopathological profile. Anticancer Res. 2010;30(7):3009–14.
39. Danesh F, Ho LT. Dialysis-related amyloidosis: history and clinical manifestations. Semin Dial. 2001;14(2):80–5.
40. Falk RH, Comenzo RL, Skinner M. The systemic amyloidoses. N Engl J Med. 1997;337(13):898–909.
41. Kyle RA, Bayrd ED. Amyloidosis: review of 236 cases. Medicine (Baltimore). 1975;54(4):271–99.
42. Kerner MM, Wang MB, Angier G, Calcaterra TC, Ward PH. Amyloidosis of the head and neck. A clinicopathologic study of the UCLA experience, 1955–1991. Arch Otolaryngol Head Neck Surg. 1995;121(7):778–82.
43. Rajkumar SV. Multiple myeloma: 2013 update on diagnosis, risk-stratification, and management. Am J Hematol. 2013;88(3):225–35.
44. Oliveira EV, Pozetti AC, Pozetti EM, Antonio JR, Michalany NS. Primary systemic amyloidosis associated with multiple myeloma. An Bras Dermatol. 2012;87(1):119–22.
45. Kyle RA, Gertz MA, Witzig TE, et al. Review of 1027 patients with newly diagnosed multiple myeloma. Mayo Clin Proc. 2003;78(1):21–33.
46. Prokaeva T, Spencer B, Kaut M, et al. Soft tissue, joint, and bone manifestations of AL amyloidosis: clinical presentation, molecular features, and survival. Arthritis Rheum. 2007;56(11):3858–68.
47. Chang SS, Lu CL, Tsay SH, Chang FY, Lee SD. Amyloidosis-induced gastrointestinal bleeding in a patient with multiple myeloma. J Clin Gastroenterol. 2001;32(2):161–3.
48. Thibault I, Vallieres I. Macroglossia due to systemic amyloidosis: is there a role for radiotherapy. Case Rep Oncol. 2011;4(2):392–9.
49. Bottoni U, Dianzani C, Pranteda G, et al. Florid cutaneous and mucosal papillomatosis with acanthosis nigricans revealing a primary lung cancer. J Eur Acad Dermatol Venereol. 2000;14(3):205–8.
50. Yeh JS, Munn SE, Plunkett TA, Harper PG, Hopster DJ, du Vivier AW. Coexistence of acanthosis nigricans and the sign of Leser-Trelat in a patient with gastric adenocarcinoma: a case report and literature review. J Am Acad Dermatol. 2000;42(2 Pt 2):357–62.
51. Tyler MT, Ficarra G, Silverman S Jr, Odom RB, Regezi JA. Malignant acanthosis nigricans with florid papillary oral lesions. Oral Surg Oral Med Oral Pathol Oral Radiol Endod. 1996;81(4):445–9.
52. Brinca A, Cardoso JC, Brites MM, Tellechea O, Figueiredo A. Florid cutaneous papillomatosis and acanthosis nigricans maligna revealing gastric adenocarcinoma. An Bras Dermatol. 2011;86(3):573–7.
53. Weger W, Ginter-Hanselmayer G, Hammer HF, Hodl S. Florid cutaneous papillomatosis with acanthosis nigricans in a patient with carcinomas of the lung and prostate. J Am Acad Dermatol. 2007;57(5):907–8.
54. Csete B, Moezzi M, Lengyel Z, Hodosi B, Zombai E, Battyani Z. Florid cutaneous papillomatosis leading to social exclusion. Br J Dermatol. 2005;153(3):667–9.
55. Janniger EJ, Schwartz RA. Florid cutaneous papillomatosis. J Surg Oncol. 2010;102(6):709–12.
56. Koyama S, Ikeda K, Sato M, et al. Transforming growth factor-alpha (TGF alpha)-producing gastric carcinoma with acanthosis nigricans: an endocrine effect of TGF alpha in the pathogenesis of cutaneous paraneoplastic syndrome and epithelial hyperplasia of the esophagus. J Gastroenterol. 1997;32(1):71–7.
57. Wang L, Jin X, Zhao X, et al. Focal dermal hypoplasia: updates. Oral Dis. 2014;20(1):17–24.
58. Goltz RW, Peterson WC, Gorlin RJ, Ravits HG. Focal dermal hypoplasia. Arch Dermatol. 1962;86:708–17.
59. Lasocki AL, Stark Z, Orchard D. A case of mosaic Goltz syndrome (focal dermal hypoplasia) in a male patient. Australas J Dermatol. 2011;52(1):48–51.
60. Grzeschik KH, Bornholdt D, Oeffner F, et al. Deficiency of PORCN, a regulator of Wnt signaling, is associated with focal dermal hypoplasia. Nat Genet. 2007;39(7):833–5.
61. Lombardi MP, Bulk S, Celli J, et al. Mutation update for the PORCN gene. Hum Mutat. 2011;32(7):723–8.
62. Quain RD, Militello G, Junkins-Hopkins J, Yan AC, Crawford GH. Erythematous atrophic macules and papules following the lines of Blaschko. Focal dermal hypoplasia (FDH), or Goltz syndrome. Arch Dermatol. 2007;143(1):109–14.
63. Baxter AM, Shaw MJ, Warren K. Dental and oral lesions in two patients with focal dermal hypoplasia (Goltz syndrome). Br Dent J. 2000;189(10):550–3.
64. Balmer R, Cameron AC, Ades L, Aldred MJ. Enamel defects and lyonization in focal dermal hypoplasia. Oral Surg Oral Med Oral Pathol Oral Radiol Endod. 2004;98(6):686–91.
65. Seoane J, Gibson RL, Almagro M, Pintos E. Oral manifestations associated with focal dermal hypoplasia. Dermatology. 2009;219(4):368–70.
66. Marcus DM, Shore JW, Albert DM. Anophthalmia in the focal dermal hypoplasia syndrome. Arch Ophthalmol. 1990;108(1):96–100.
67. Prenner JL, Ciaccia S, Capone A Jr, Trese MT. Retinal detachment in focal dermal hypoplasia. Eur J Ophthalmol. 2004;14(2):166–8.

68. Bhatia AM, Clericuzio CL, Musemeche CA. Congenital ventral hernia in association with focal dermal hypoplasia. Pediatr Dermatol. 1995;12(4):336–9.
69. Han XY, Wu SS, Conway DH, et al. Truncus arteriosus and other lethal internal anomalies in Goltz syndrome. Am J Med Genet. 2000;90(1):45–8.
70. Suskan E, Kurkcuoglu N, Uluoglu O. Focal dermal hypoplasia (Goltz syndrome) with horseshoe kidney abnormality. Pediatr Dermatol. 1990;7(4):283–6.
71. Lopez-Porras RF, Arroyo C, Soto-Vega E. Focal dermal hypoplasia with uterus bicornis and renal ectopia: case report and review of the literature. Case Rep Dermatol. 2011;3(2):158–63.
72. Kanemura H, Hatakeyama K, Sugita K, Aihara M. Epilepsy in a patient with focal dermal hypoplasia. Pediatr Neurol. 2011;44(2):135–8.
73. Smigiel R, Jakubiak A, Lombardi MP, et al. Co-occurrence of severe Goltz-Gorlin syndrome and pentalogy of Cantrell—case report and review of the literature. Am J Med Genet A. 2011;155A(5):1102–5.
74. Reddy J, Laufer MR. Congenital anomalies of the female reproductive tract in a patient with Goltz syndrome. J Pediatr Adolesc Gynecol. 2009;22(4):e71–2.
75. Kimonis VE, Goldstein AM, Pastakia B, et al. Clinical manifestations in 105 persons with nevoid basal cell carcinoma syndrome. Am J Med Genet. 1997;69(3):299–308.
76. Bleeker-Wagemakers LM, Hamel BC, Hennekam RC, Beemer FA, Oorthuys HW. Oculocerebrocutaneous syndrome. J Med Genet. 1990;27(1):69–70.
77. Prabhu NT, John R, Munshi AK. Rieger's syndrome: a case report. Quintessence Int. 1997;28(11):749–52.
78. Happle R, Daniels O, Koopman RJ. MIDAS syndrome (microphthalmia, dermal aplasia, and sclerocornea): an X-linked phenotype distinct from Goltz syndrome. Am J Med Genet. 1993;47(5):710–3.
79. Alster TS, Wilson F. Focal dermal hypoplasia (Goltz's syndrome). Treatment of cutaneous lesions with the 585-nm flashlamp-pumped pulsed dye laser. Arch Dermatol. 1995;131(2):143–4.
80. Liu J, Hsu PT, Vanderwielen BA, Teng JM. Treatment of recalcitrant excessive granulation tissue with photodynamic therapy in an eight-year-old patient with focal dermal hypoplasia syndrome. Pediatr Dermatol. 2012;29(3):324–6.

11 Oral Mucosal Pigmentation

Yu Zhou, Xin Jin, and Qianming Chen

Keywords
Melanoplakia · Vitiligo

Y. Zhou
State Key Laboratory of Oral Diseases, National Clinical Research Center for Oral Diseases, Department of Oral Medicine, West China Hospital of Stomatology, Sichuan University, Chengdu, Sichuan, China

X. Jin
College of Stomatology, Chongqing Medical University, Chongqing Key Laboratory of Oral Diseases and Biomedical Sciences, Chongqing, China

Q. Chen (✉)
Changjiang Scholars Program, Ministry of Education, Beijing, China

State Key Laboratory of Oral Diseases, National Clinical Research Center for Oral Diseases, Department of Oral Medicine, West China Hospital of Stomatology, Sichuan University, Chengdu, Sichuan, China
e-mail: qmchen@scu.edu.cn

Q. Chen, X. Zeng (eds.), *Case Based Oral Mucosal Diseases*,
https://doi.org/10.1007/978-981-13-0286-2_11

11.1 Melanotic Macule

Case 98 Melanotic Macule

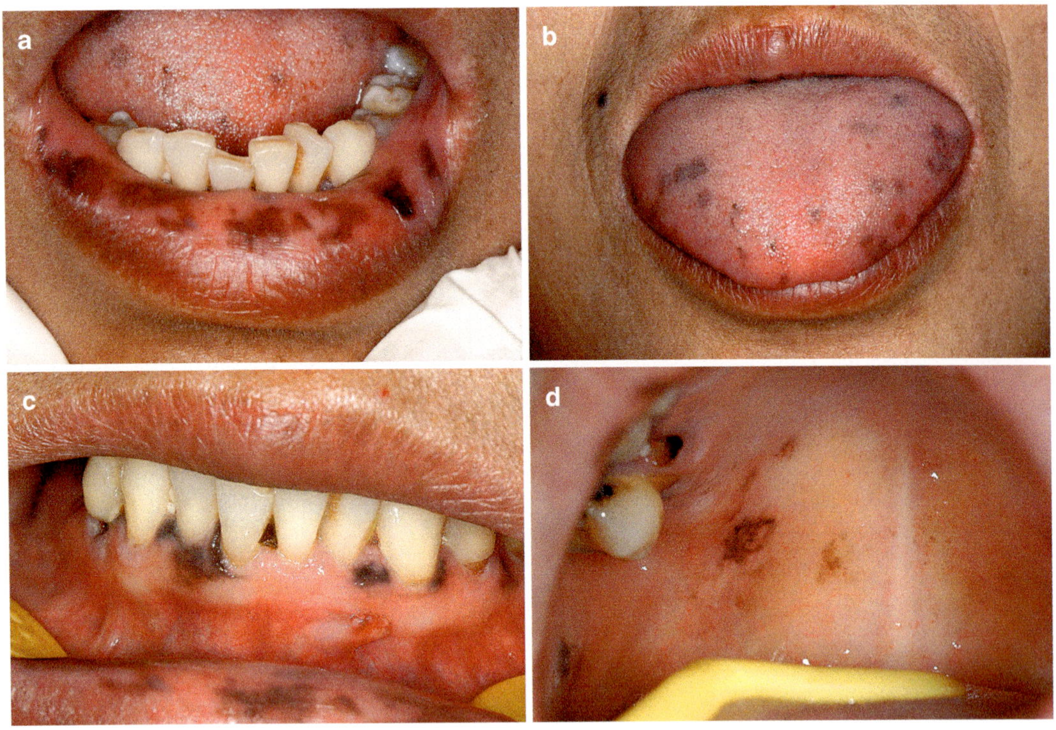

Fig. 11.1 (**a**) Scattered brownish black patches on the lower lip, which were flat, soft, and not erosive. (**b**) Scattered brownish black patches on the dorsum of tongue, which were flat, soft, and not erosive. (**c**) Scattered brownish black patches on the lower lip and gingiva, which were flat, soft, and not erosive. (**d**) Scattered brownish black patches on the hard palate, which were flat, soft, and not erosive

Age: 63 years
Sex: Female
Chief Complaints:
63-year-old woman with dark patch for 10 years
History of Present Illness:
Melanin patch occurs in the oral cavity 10 years ago and gradually increased. The patient had not felt discomfortable. She denies contacting heavy metal, having hematochezia, fatigue, or loss of weight.
Past Medical History: None
Allergy: None
Physical Examination:
Scattered brownish black patches were detected on the lips, dorsum of tongue, gingiva, hard palate, and buccal mucosa, which were flat, soft, and not erosive (Fig. 11.1).

Clinical Impression:
Melanotic macule?
Further Examination:

1. Normal serum content of heavy metal (lead, mercury)
2. No bowel polyps found during colonoscopy
3. No abnormalities in serum cortisol testing

Diagnosis:
Melanotic macule
Diagnosis Basis:

1. Multiple scattered flat black patches.
2. Rule out systemic disease and pigmentation induced by exogenous substances through asking the history and physical examinations.

Management:

Advise observing. If the patient is in a stable condition, he should have regular reexamination every 6 months. If the melanin patch enlarges, bulges or festers, he should have reexamination timely.

[Review] Melanotic Macule

Pigmentation of oral mucosa is divided into endogenous and exogenous pigmentation. The former includes melanoplakia, pigmentation polyposis syndrome, primary hypoadrenalism, polyostotic fibrous dysplasia, oral melanoacanthoma, pigmented nevus, malignant melanoma, etc. The latter includes pigmentation induced by heavy metal, drugs, chronic inflammation, smoking, etc.

Melanoplakia refers to melanin patch which is not related with pigmentation of oral mucosa induced by the systemic disease and exogenous substance. It is benign pigmentation. Oral melanoplakia is presented brown to black, scattered, homogeneous oval patch on the oral mucosa, whose border is clear. The patch is not higher than the mucosal surface and usually less than 1 cm in diameter. Labial mucosa is the most common location; gingiva, palate, and buccal mucosa can also be involved. It often occurs in middle age with predilection for female [1]. The etiology is not clear; some scholars have reported it has family history and may have a genetic predisposition [2]. It is benign lesion, doesn't require further treatment [3], but needs follow-up observation.

In order to diagnose oral melanoplakia, we need to exclude endogenous and exogenous mucosal pigmentation of melanin which is induced by the following disease or factors.

Pigmentation polyposis syndrome, also called Peutz-Jeghers syndrome, is a kind of autosomal dominant disease and associates with genetic mutation of STK11/LKB1. Its characteristics are small, multiple melanin spots on the oral mucosa and peripheral skin of the mouth, multiple gastrointestinal polyps, and has familial tendency. Melanin spot is often less than 1 mm. The lower lip is the most common location; nasal, colonic, rectal mucosa, and limb skin can also be involved (Figs. 11.2 and 11.3). A fading or a disappearance of the spots is usually observed in older age. The risk of cancerization of the gastrointestinal tract, pancreas, and thyroid are increased. Patients often have symptoms like chronic abdominal pain, emesis, diarrhea, anemia, melena, etc. The diagnostic needs colonoscopy examination. Besides the treatment of intestinal polyps, it also needs to be checked regularly preventing cancerization of other organs [4, 5].

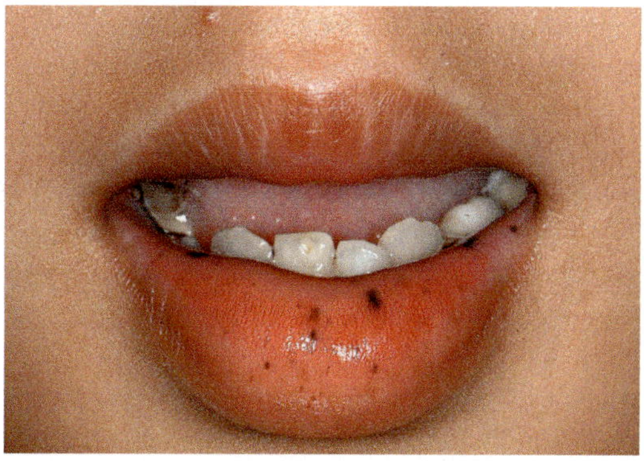

Fig. 11.2 Pigmentation polyposis syndrome: dozens of small black spots on the lower lip

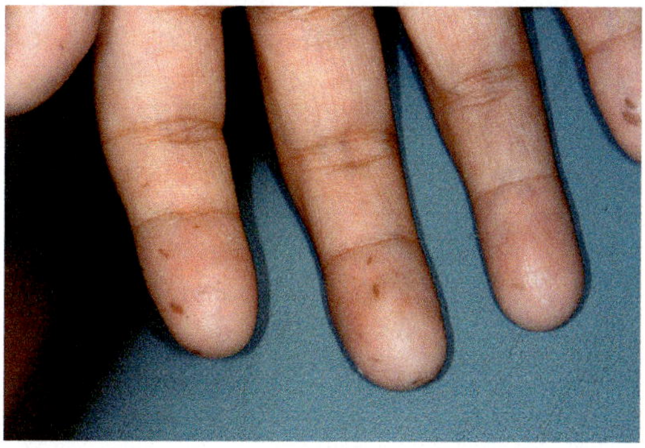

Fig. 11.3 Pigmentation polyposis syndrome: dozens of small black spots on the finger pulp

Laugier-Hunziker syndrome is a rare pigmentation disease on the lips, oral mucosa, skin, and nails (toenails), the course of the disease progresses slowly, and the lesion on the skin is often progressively severe. It is not easy to distinguish from Peutz-Jeghers clinically. In fact, they have obvious differences in onset time, skin lesion progression, abdominal manifestations, and genetic mutations. Vast majority of Laugier-Hunziker syndrome is sporadic cases and occurs in middle-aged adults. Pigmented spots gradually aggravate with age increasing and are not associated with colon polyps, the abdominal symptoms above, and the genetic mutations of STK11/LKB1 [6, 7].

Addison disease, also called primary hypoadrenalism, is caused by the damages of the bilateral adrenal glands induced by tuberculosis, autoimmune reaction, malignant tumor metastasis, lymphoma, leukemia, systemic fungal infections, etc. The gland damage causes insufficient secretion of adrenocortical hormone, which stimulates adenohypophysis to produce more adrenocorticotropic hormone (ACTH), leading to the melanocyte-stimulating hormone increase, finally manifesting as diffuse dark spots on the skin and oral mucosa. Pigmentation is one of the early symptoms and is also the most characteristic manifestation of the disease. Pigmentation is most obvious in the exposed parts and location where it is easily influenced by friction and can also be observed in mucous membrane. In addition, symptoms like fatigue, weakness, weight loss, the drop in blood pressure, appetite loss, mental disorders, etc., can also occur. This disease is more common among adults and is rarely found among the elderly and young children [8, 9]. The diagnosis of the disease needs to detect the basic level of cortisol in the blood and urine and the ACTH level in the blood and do ACTH excitation test.

Polyostotic fibrous dysplasia, also known as McCune-Albright syndrome, is a rare congenital disease found in children and adolescents. It shows a little higher rate among women compared to men. The course progresses slowly, and it has a tendency of self-limiting. The characteristics are the pigmentation on the oral mucosa or skin, multiple fibrous osteitis, and precocious puberty. Oral mucosa pigmentation is presented as brown spot, and the lip is the most common location [10]. The definite diagnosis needs clinical three major characteristics with bone X-ray film.

Other endocrine diseases associated with oral mucosa pigmentation include hyperfunction of thyroid, Nelson syndrome. The latter is progressive skin pigmentation of melanin and pituitary adenomas after the surgery of removal of bilateral adrenal for treating Cushing's syndrome. These oral mucosa pigmentation related with systematic disease generally do not need treatment, and the disappearance of oral dark spots may follow the treatment of the systematic disease [1, 11].

Hemochromatosis is a disease induced by iron metabolism disorder (disorder of iron metabolism) which is caused by the excessive accumulations of iron in the body. High-iron diet, much blood transfusion, or systemic disease can cause excessive accumulations of iron. This disease can also be found in the hemolytic disease like globin generation barrier anemia. Middle-aged men are easily affected and women are rarely affected. Clinical manifestations are the skin of the face, upper limbs, opisthenar, and armpit, perineal skin representing bronze-colored or gray black. There can be bluish-gray or bluish-black pigmented spots on the oral mucosa, usually observed in the junction between hard and soft palate. There are also clinical manifestations of abnormal liver function and diabetes. The disease can be diagnosed by abnormal liver function, blood glucose, pigmentation of the skin or mucosa, increased serum iron content, etc. [11, 12].

Oral melanoacanthoma is rare and presented as brown and brownish-black patch or plaque with clear boundary, which is similar to skin melanoacanthoma. The etiology is not clear. The buccal mucosa, lip, upper palate, tooth, and gingival mucosa are the most common locations. The average age is 28, and it has predilection for females. It may be associated with stimulated factors and is a benign disease without malignant potential [1].

Melanocytic nevus is divided into junctional nevus, intradermal nevus, and compound nevus and is rarely observed on the oral mucosa. It clinically is presented as small, slightly protuberant, brown, bluish-gray, or black papules with clear border. It is difficult to distinguish pigmented nevus from melanoma in early stage especially the lesion on the palate clinically.

Malignant melanoma is one of the high malignant degree tumors of oral and maxillofacial region. The skin and mucosa can be involved, and it can be observed more on the mucosa than the skin. Malignant melanomas of oral and maxillofacial region often originate from pigmented nevus, mainly malignant transformation from junctional nevus; also melanoplakia can be involved [13]. Ultraviolet ray, heredity, endocrine, chronic stimulation, and injury have a certain relationship with the incidence of malignant melanoma. It is more commonly found in people at the age of around 40. There is no significant difference in rates between genders. It represents the lesion of pigmented nevus or melanoplakia in the early stage. When it undergoes malignant transformation, it becomes bigger quickly, its pigment becomes deep, it has radiated extension, it ruptures (errhysis), satellite nodules occur surrounding it, and lymph nodes increase sharply. The palate, gingiva, and buccal mucosa are commonly involved in malignant melanoma (Fig. 11.4). It often presents as slightly elevated, bluish-brownlesions, with surface rupture and rapid growth. When alveolar process and the jaw bone are affected, it can cause teeth to loosen. Malignant melanoma often has early and extensive lymph node metastasis. First of all it metastasizes to submandibular lymph nodes and upper deep cervical lymph node groups. The rate of blood metastasis is high, it can amount to 40%, and it mainly metastasizes to the lung, liver, bone, brain, and other organs. The diagnosis is mainly based on its clinical manifestations. Because biopsy can promote tumor proliferation and metastasis, it is generally not suitable for biopsy. But because of the difficulties of diagnosis, frozen biopsy can be taken during the surgery. After making a definite diagnosis, it should complete the radical resection at the same time [14–16].

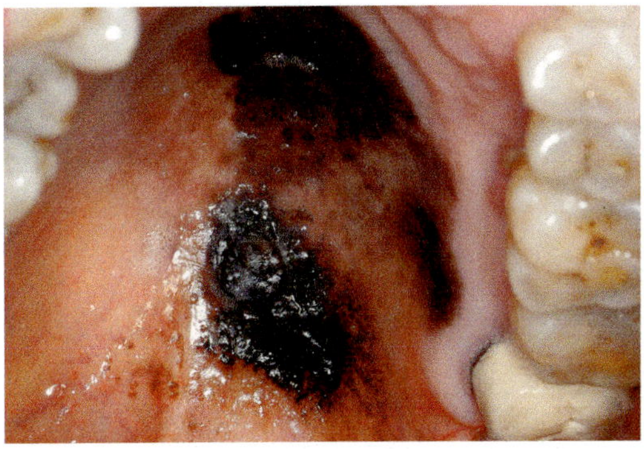

Fig. 11.4 Malignant melanoma on the palate

Some heavy metal poisoning, such as chronic lead poisoning, bismuth poisoning, and mercury poisoning, will form lead lines, bismuth lines, or mercury lines on gingival margin presenting black-blue and bluish-gray pigmentation band or gray-black and bluish-gray pigmented spots on the lips, tongue, and buccal membrane with inflammation of oral mucosa when the disease is severe. The diagnosis needs to measure heavy metal content in the blood and urine [11].

Excessive smoking can make oral mucosa representing brown to black; irregular melanin spots which can be found in 25–31% of smokers and the lips, buccal mucosa, and labial attached gingiva of the lower anterior teeth are mainly involved. Some reports have said it can fade after 3 years of quitting smoking [1, 3].

A variety of drugs such as diazepam, contraceptive drugs, antimalarial drugs, imidazole tetracycline, and cell inhibitors can cause oral membrane pigmentation. After stopping taking drugs, pigmented spots will sustain for some time. In addition, some gargle such as chlorine or the traditional Chinese medicine also can make the temporary pigmentation of oral mucosa.

Long-term inflammation of oral mucosa such as oral lichen planus and pemphigus can cause pigmentation on mucosa. The etiology is not clear, and the darker-skinned people are more commonly affected. Dark brown-colored area is adjacent to reticular, ulcerative, bullous lesion on the oral mucosa. In general, pigmentation turns for the better after inflammation is relieved [1].

Some other abnormal color diseases of the oral mucosa related to vascular lesions are common found in [3].

Kaposi's sarcoma mainly occurs in patients with HIV infection. Early lesions on infected patients may present as a flat or slightly raised brown, purple lesion. Advanced lesions appear as deep red or purple patches, nodules, and it may have ulceration, bleeding, and necrosis (Fig. 8.12).

Hemangioma is a benign lesion caused by vascular endothelial cell proliferation. Vascular malformation refers to the structural abnormalities of blood vessels without endothelial cell proliferation. Two kinds of lesions are involved in dysplasia and are often found in infants and young children. Hemangioma can be relieved with age increasing, and vascular malformation has no obvious change. The tongue is the most commonly affected on the oral mucosa. Two kinds of vascular lesions have similar clinical manifestations, and the lesions are flat or slightly raised. The color depends on the type of the blood vessels and depth of the lesion in the organization, ranging from dark red to purple. In general, the color fades when doing diascopic examination (Fig. 11.5).

Varix is abnormal swollen veins, and it is commonly found in the patients at the age of more than 60. The ventral of the tongue mucosa is the most common location in the oral. It is presented much bluish-violet, irregular, soft protuberance, and the color fades when doing diascopic examination (Fig. 11.6). If the vessel contains thrombus, it presented solid purple nodules, the color will not fade when pressing it, and thrombus are commonly found in lower lip and buccal mucosa.

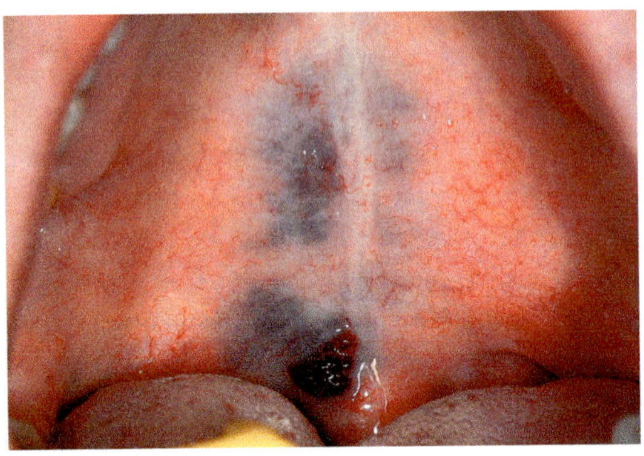

Fig. 11.5 Hemangioma on the palate

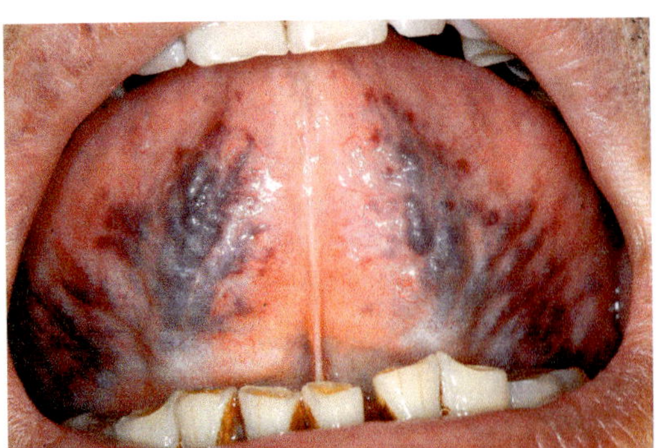

Fig. 11.6 Varicose veins on the ventral surface of tongue

Hemorrhagic diseases such as hematoma, petechia, and ecchymosis are generated by blood spilling into the soft tissue. The lesion is raised or flat, and the color will not fade when pressing it. It may occur after trauma or thrombocytopenic purpura; the color depends on the time after the blood spilled out of the vessel; because of the hemoglobin degradation, it will appear red, purple, blue, dark blue, etc. The color will gradually be normal in 2 weeks. If traumatic stimulated factors are unchecked, the platelet disease and blood coagulation disorders should be considered (Fig. 10.1).

The diagnosis of oral melanoplakia can be made after excluding the diseases above. At present, it is regarded as benign lesions, and conventional biopsy is not advocated. There is no effective therapy yet, so the observation and regular subsequent visit are suggested. If color or size of melanoplakia changes, especially if protrusion, ulceration, or bleeding of the surface appears, the patients should return immediately to rule out melanoma.

11.2 Oral Mucosal Depigmentation

Case 99 Oral Mucosal Depigmentation
Age: 41 years

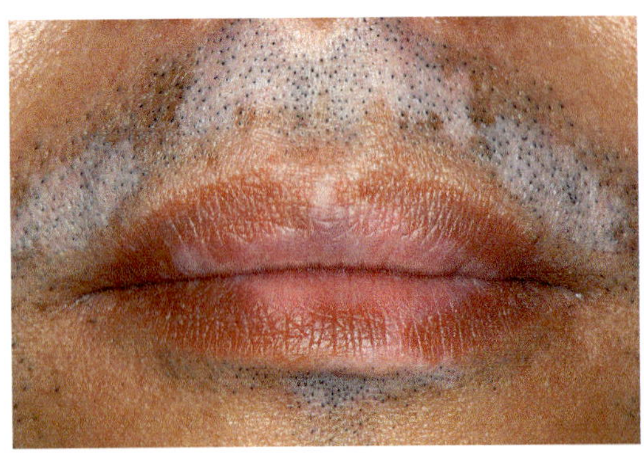

Fig. 11.7 The color of upper and lower lip is not uniform, with more color shallow white area. Upper and lower lip and lip red skin appeared with depigmentation area, which is around with brown pigmentation

Sex: Male
Chief Complaints:
41-year-old man with depigmentation of both the lips with dryness for 2 years
History of Present Illness:
Two years ago, the patient felt dryness of both the lips, and then he had depigmentation of both the lips.
Past Medical History: Vitiligo
Allergy: None.
Physical Examination:
Upper and lower lip appeared dry, with uneven color and pigment depigmentation area. The lips and the skin around the lips also appeared with depigmentation area, surrounded by brown pigmentation (Fig. 11.7).
Diagnosis: Vitiligo
Diagnosis Basis:
The color of the lips and skin becomes obviously shallow.
Management:

1. Medication
   Rp.: Vitamin E 100 mg × 60 tablets
   Sig.: topical use t.i.d.
   Compound ulcer paste 15 g × 2
   Sig.: topical use t.i.d.
2. Don't apply hormone agents on the lips and surrounding skin without doctor's advice.

[Review] Oral Mucosal Depigmentation
Oral mucosal depigmentation is often located in the labial mucosa and lips' skin.

Depigmentation of skin generally refers to vitiligo. Vitiligo is an acquired pigmentation disorder of the skin and mucous membranes. The actual pathogenesis of vitiligo still remains unknown and has been attributed to the inhibition of tyrosinase system or the destruction of melanocytes induced by immune dysfunction, nerve mental abnormality, and endocrine abnormality of the genetic qualities of an individual affected by a variety of internal and external factors, eventually resulting in depigmentation [17]. Literature has been reported that local use of glucocorticoid drugs can cause skin depigmentation [18]. The lip mucosa depigmentation found by the author clinically was caused by long-term excessive application of hormone drugs.

Vitiligo is significantly more prevalent in young adult patients, and its prevalence appears to be equal between men and women. It typically occurs in exposed and frictional areas (facial and forehead, cervical region, trunk, arms and legs). It is clinically characterized by the development of well-circumscribed, depigmented macules and patches with a pigmentation ring [17]. Vitiligo often involves the mucous membrane; 29% of the cases is only involving mucosa as a literature reported (70/241) [19]. Vitiligo frequently occurs at sites that are normally hyperpigmented, including the lips, perioral skin, labia, glans, and the inside mucosa of wrapping [20]. The course is chronic, sustainable life, while can sometimes be relieved itself. Association of vitiligo with other autoimmune diseases has been reported, such as pemphigus [21].

Histopathology showed a decrease of the density of melanocytes in the skin lesions or non-melanoma cells. Melanocytes on the pigmented edge of vitiliginous skin are larger [17].

The diagnosis of vitiligo is usually made according to the acquired white macules or patches with pigmentation margins and no self-conscious symptom.

It is refractory to medical therapy, with chronic course and little chance of recovery. After the patients are referred to the department of dermatology, therapeutic approaches such as surgery, phototherapy, agents for oral administration or topical use can be employed. However, there is no effective therapy for oral mucosal depigmentation [22].

References

1. Gondak RO, da SR, Jorge J, et al. Oral pigmented lesions: clinicopathologic features and review of the literature. Med Oral Patol Oral Cir Bucal. 2012;17(6):e919–24.
2. Ho KK, Dervan P, O'Loughlin S, et al. Labial melanotic macule: a clinical, histopathologic, and ultrastructural study. J Am Acad Dermatol. 1993;28(1):33–9.
3. Kauzman A, Pavone M, Blanas N, et al. Pigmented lesions of the oral cavity: review, differential diagnosis, and case presentations. J Can Dent Assoc. 2004;70(10):682–3.

4. Higham P, Alawi F, Stoopler ET. Medical management update: Peutz Jeghers syndrome. Oral Surg Oral Med Oral Pathol Oral Radiol Endod. 2010;109(1):5–11.
5. Daley TD, Armstrong JE. Oral manifestations of gastrointestinal diseases. Can J Gastroenterol. 2007;21(4):241–4.
6. Ma DL, Vano-Galvan S. Hyperpigmentation in Laugier-Hunziker syndrome. CMAJ. 2011;183(12):1402.
7. Wang WM, Wang X, Duan N, et al. Laugier-Hunziker syndrome: a report of three cases and literature review. Int J Oral Sci. 2013;4(4):226–30.
8. Chi AC, Neville BW, Krayer JW, et al. Oral manifestations of systemic disease. Am Fam Physician. 2010;82(11):1381–8.
9. Shah SS, Oh CH, Coffin SE, et al. Addisonian pigmentation of the oral mucosa. Cutis. 2005;76(2):97–9.
10. Collins MT, Singer FR, Eugster E. McCune-Albright syndrome and the extraskeletal manifestations of fibrous dysplasia. Orphanet J Rare Dis. 2012;7(Suppl 1):S4.
11. Meleti M, Vescovi P, Mooi WJ, et al. Pigmented lesions of the oral mucosa and perioral tissues: a flowchart for the diagnosis and some recommendations for the management. Oral Surg Oral Med Oral Pathol Oral Radiol Endod. 2008;105(5):606–16.
12. Pietrangelo A. Hereditary hemochromatosis: pathogenesis, diagnosis, and treatment. Gastroenterology. 2010;139(2):393–408, 408.e1–2.
13. Chan RC, Chan JY, Wei WI. Mucosal melanoma of the head and neck: 32-year experience in a tertiary referral hospital. Laryngoscope. 2012;122(12):2749–53.
14. Mihajlovic M, Vlajkovic S, Jovanovic P, et al. Primary mucosal melanomas: a comprehensive review. Int J Clin Exp Pathol. 2012;5(8):739–53.
15. Knight DA, Ngiow SF, Li M, et al. Host immunity contributes to the anti-melanoma activity of BRAF inhibitors. J Clin Invest. 2013;123(3):1371–81.
16. Bhullar RP, Bhullar A, Vanaki SS, et al. Primary melanoma of oral mucosa: a case report and review of literature. Dent Res J (Isfahan). 2012;9(3):353–6.
17. Alikhan A, Felsten LM, Daly M, et al. Vitiligo: a comprehensive overview. Part I. Introduction, epidemiology, quality of life, diagnosis, differential diagnosis, associations, histopathology, etiology, and work-up. J Am Acad Dermatol. 2011;65(3):473–91.
18. El Madani HA, Tancrede-Bohin E, Bensussan A, et al. In vivo multiphoton imaging of human skin: assessment of topical corticosteroid-induced epidermis atrophy and depigmentation. J Biomed Opt. 2012;17(2):026009.
19. Kanwar AJ, Parsad D, De D. Mucosal involvement in vitiligo: a comprehensive review of 241 cases. J Eur Acad Dermatol Venereol. 2011;25(11):1361–3.
20. Mchepange UO, Gao XH, Liu YY, et al. Vitiligo in North-Eastern China: an association between mucosal and acrofacial lesions. Acta Derm Venereol. 2010;90(2):136–40.
21. De D, Kanwar AJ, Saikia UN, et al. Colocalization of mucosal vitiligo and oral pemphigus vulgaris. Indian J Dermatol Venereol Leprol. 2012;78(1):111–3.
22. Korobko IV. Review of current clinical studies of vitiligo treatments. Dermatol Ther. 2012;25(Suppl 1):S17–27.

Other Oral Mucosal Diseases

12

Xin Jin and Xin Zeng

Keywords
Benign Lymphadenosis of the Oral Mucosa · Epithelial Pearls · Verruciform Xanthomatosis · Palate Perforation · Xerostomia

X. Jin
College of Stomatology, Chongqing Medical University, Chongqing Key Laboratory of Oral Diseases and Biomedical Sciences, Chongqing, China

X. Zeng (✉)
State Key Laboratory of Oral Diseases, National Clinical Research Center for Oral Diseases, Department of Oral Medicine, West China Hospital of Stomatology, Sichuan University, Chengdu, Sichuan, China

12.1 Benign Lymphadenosis of the Oral Mucosa

Case 100 Benign Lymphadenosis of the Oral Mucosa

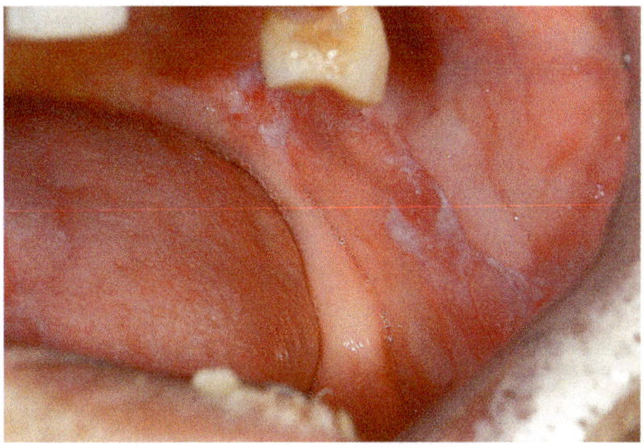

Fig. 12.1 Plaque-like mixed with papular lesions and striations from the left labial mucosa near commissure extending to the retromolar region

Age: 67 years
Sex: Female
Chief Complaints:
A 67-year-old woman with bilateral buccal irritative pain for 6 months
History of Present Illness:
A 67-year-old woman presented to our clinic claiming that she has felt pain at the bilateral buccal mucosa when taking in spicy or hot food for 6 months.

Q. Chen, X. Zeng (eds.), *Case Based Oral Mucosal Diseases*,
https://doi.org/10.1007/978-981-13-0286-2_12

Past Medical History: None
Allergy: None
Physical Examination:
Plaque-like mixed with papular lesions and striations were on the left buccal mucosa from labial mucosa near commissure extending to the retromolar region. Furthermore, soft, plaque-like, and slightly erosive lesions were detected on the left mandibular molar vestibule (Fig. 12.1).
Clinical Impression:
Oral lichen planus?
Laboratories Studies:
Tissue biopsy of papular-like lesion on left buccal is performed. Histological examination revealed lymphoid tissue proliferation in the lamina propria, the formation of lymphoid follicles, and the acanthosis of partial epithelium, supporting the diagnosis of benign lymphadenosis of the oral mucosa.
Diagnosis:
Benign lymphadenosis of the oral mucosa

Diagnosis Basis:

1. The clinical manifestations are similar to oral lichen planus.
2. The diagnosis was confirmed by tissue biopsy.

Management:

1. Medication.
   Rp.: Dexamethasone paste 15 g × 1
   Sig.: Topical use t.i.d.
2. Regular follow-up visit and close observation were suggested.

[Review] Benign Lymphadenosis of the Oral Mucosa

Benign lymphadenosis of the oral mucosa (BLOM) is a relatively rare disease of oral mucosa which usually is found on the mucosa of the lips, buccal mucosa, and also could be observed on the palate, tongue, and buccogingival sulcus, in the form of single or multiple lesions, with/without cutaneous lesions. BLOM may be regarded as a precancerous lesion which requires regular follow-up visit and close observation [1]. There are only few case reports and research articles about this disease, mostly from China.

The etiology of BLOM is not known. Some researchers considered BLOM as a proliferation disease of the regional humoral immune reaction mediated by B-lymphocytes. In the epithelium layer, the pathological changes of BLOM are characterized by parakeratosis, acanthosis, thickening of basement membrane, and liquefaction degeneration of basal cells, possibly accompanied with epithelium dysplasia. While, in lamina propria, inflammation cells widely infiltrate, lymphoid follicles are formed, along with capillary proliferation and swelling of endothelial cells [2].

BLOM usually occurs in lips, the so-called pruritic cheilitis, follicular cheilitis, or cheilitis of benign lymphadenosis. The major clinical features are labial lesions with regional intense itching, possibly with erosion, crust, and leak of yellow mucus, which is clinically indistinguishable from chronic cheilitis. Clinical manifestations of BLOM in other oral parts are lack of typical features, which is usually diagnosed as oral lichen planus, especially the buccal lesions. It could be confirmed by tissue biopsy (Fig. 12.2).

Studies showed that treatment method of local resection or ^{32}P topical application is effective, with a good prognosis [2]. Clinically, the symptomatic approach is sufficient. Management is similar to that of erosive OLP if the lesion is widespread. Close observation and regular follow-up visit are required.

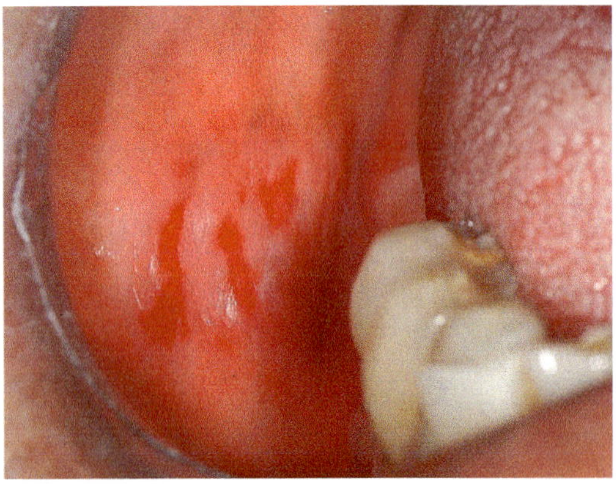

Fig. 12.2 Benign lymphadenosis of the right buccal mucosa: irregular hyperemia with whitish lesions on the right buccal mucosa

12.2 Epithelial Pearls

Case 101 Epithelial Pearls

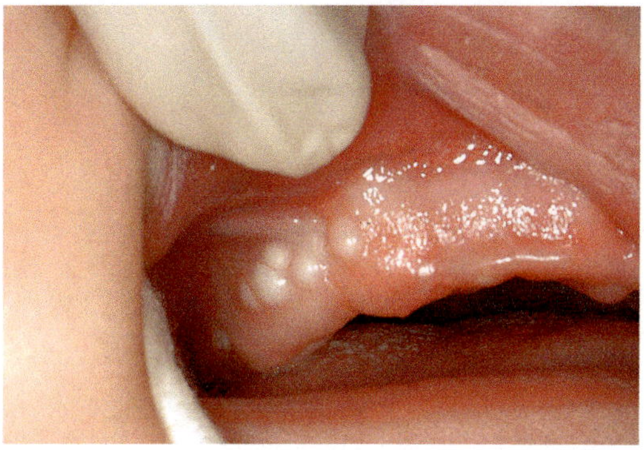

Fig. 12.3 Papules with diameter varied from 2 to 3 mm on the posterior maxillary buccal gingiva, with smooth surface and solid texture

Age: 40 days
Sex: Male
Chief Complaints:
A 40-day-old male infant with gingival papules for 2 days
History of Present Illness:
His parents found several white papules on the right maxillary gingiva by accident 2 days ago, without difficulty in feeding and sleeping.
Past Medical History: None
Allergy: None
Physical Examination:
Six white nodular papules with diameter varied from 2 to 3 mm on the posterior maxillary buccal gingiva. The borders are well-demarcated, with smooth surface and solid texture (Fig. 12.3).
Clinical Impression:
Epithelial pearls
Diagnosis Basis:

1. The patient is a 40-day-old newborn infant.
2. The clinical feature is white gingival papules.

Management:

1. Explain and observation was suggested. Do not puncture the papules nor do other treatment.

[Review] Epithelial Pearls
Epithelial pearls are pinhead-shaped or globular white/yellowish-white papules on the gingiva in 4–6-week-old newborn infants. It is also called "the horse teeth" due to the appearance similar to the newly erupted teeth. It could also be observed along the palatal midline.

The epithelial pearls are elevated firm papules, and the diameter varies from 1 to 3 mm. According to a clinical observational study comprised of 517 newborn infants, the incidence of epithelial pearls is 43.7%. There was no significant relationship between the incidence rate of the epithelial pearls and factors such as baby's sex, mother's age, the course of the pregnancy, trouble at birth, the period of pregnancy, baby weight at birth, etc. [3].

The earliest morphological sign of tooth formation is the appearance of the primary dental lamina, which are stripes of thickened epithelium marking the future tooth rows, underlying along the horseshoe-shaped dental arches [4]. During the cap stage, enamel organ is widely connected with dental laminae. In the late bell stage, the dental lamina (including the lateral lamina) disintegrates, by the invasion of mesenchymal cells, and is gradually resorbed, leaving the developing teeth completely separated from the epithelium of the oral cavity. However, in some cases, these epithelial cells are not resorbed and persist as epithelial islands within the jawbone as well as in the gingiva. Microscopically, these islands look like glands, so referred to as cell rest of Serres. These epithelial remnants have the capacity to proliferate, keratinize, and form pinhead-shaped or globular white papules within the jawbone as well as in the gingiva, so-called epithelial pearls. When approaching or breaking through the oral mucosa, these epithelial pearls could be automatically resolved by the friction caused by baby sucking or feeding [5].

Epithelial pearls are asymptomatic, not harmful to baby sucking or primary tooth development, and usually resolve spontaneously several months after birth, and no treatment is indicated. Additionally, parents should be well-informed that puncturing the papules is avoided; otherwise, these damages would lead to infections, even neonatal septicemia due to the weak immunity, vulnerable oral mucosa, and the richness of blood supply of newborn babies.

In the differential diagnosis of epithelial pearls, natal/neonatal teeth should be considered. The primary tooth eruption is present at the age of 6 months. Natal teeth are present at birth, and neonatal teeth (less common) erupt during the first month of life. The morbidity of natal and neonatal teeth ranges from 1:3500 to 1:2000. It most commonly occurs in the mandible incisor area, followed by the maxillary incisor region; cuspid or molar regions may also be seen. The exact etiology for the premature eruption is unknown. Autosomal dominant inheritance or endocrine disturbances could be the cause.

Usually, natal teeth or neonatal teeth are conical, loose, and small, with enamel hypoplasia. Palpation shows soft, sometimes firm like normal teeth (Fig. 12.4). They are almost exclusively limited to the oral mucosa due to the underdeveloped roots. The infants are at risk of swallowing or inhaling because of the tooth mobility. Ulceration (Fig. 12.5) and breastfeeding difficulties are other common complications, which would affect nutrient intake.

If the tooth is extremely loose, extraction is indicated. If there was no obvious loosening of tooth, then grinding off the sharp tooth edge, feeding with spoon, or treatment of ankyloglossia is suggested, to reduce friction. Management of natal and neonatal teeth requires thorough clinical and radiology tests, to distinguish it from prematurely erupted primary teeth or supernumerary teeth. The supernumerary teeth should always be extracted, but it depends on local or general complications and parental opinion. If the extraction is performed, dentures are required for patients since 3 years old, in order to prevent secondary tooth eruption difficulties [6].

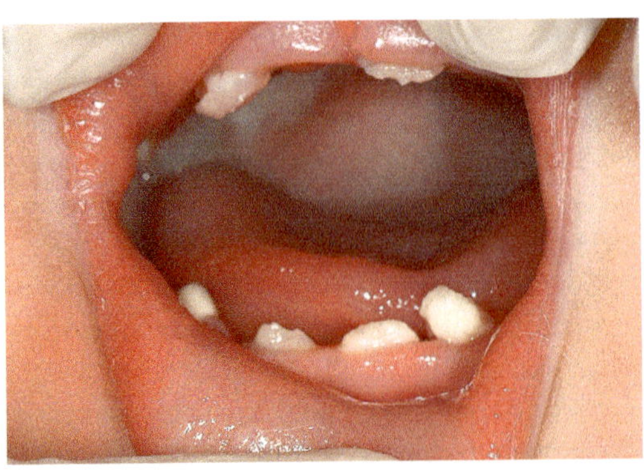

Fig. 12.4 Natal teeth of 3 months of age: erupted teeth exhibiting variable shape, loose, with enamel hypoplasia

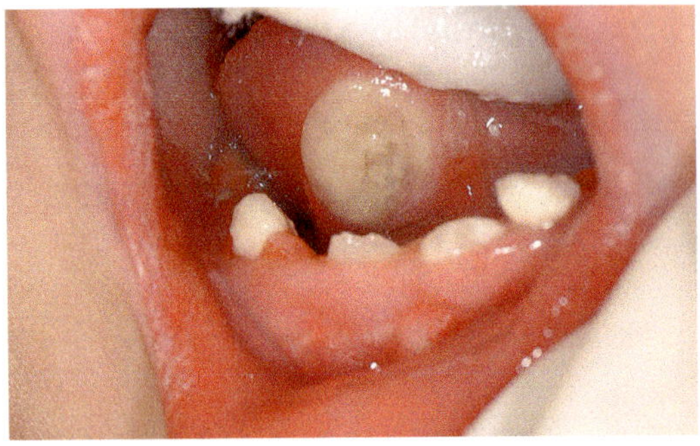

Fig. 12.5 Natal teeth of 3 months of age: ulceration on the corresponding ventral tongue

12.3 Verruciform Xanthomatosis

Case 102 Verruciform Xanthomatosis

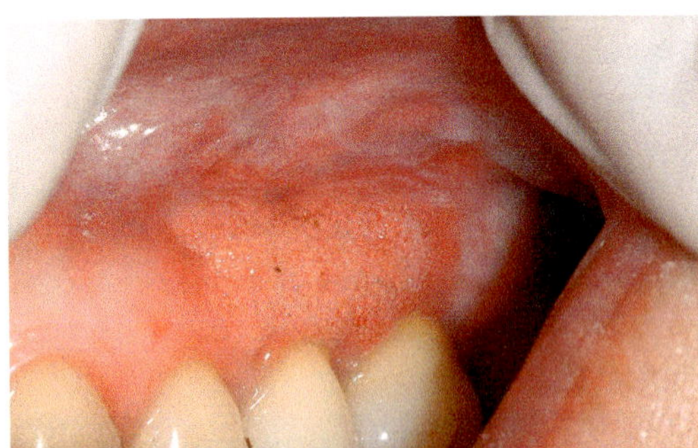

Fig. 12.6 A well-defined papillary plaque on the left maxillary gingiva, with rough and slightly hyperplastic surface

Age: 49 years
Sex: Female
Chief Complaints:
A 49-year-old woman with left maxillary gingival pain when taking food for 6 months

History of Present Illness:
A 49-year-old woman presented to our clinic claiming that she felt rough and painful gingiva when taking food for 6 months.
Past Medical History: None
Allergy: None
Physical Examination:
A well-demarcated papillary reddish plaque with size of 1.5 cm × 1 cm was detected on the left maxillary gingiva. The lesion is slightly hyperplastic, with rough surface. White striae could be observed on the left lateral ventral tongue and buccal mucosa (Fig. 12.6).
Clinical Impression:
Gingival hyperplasia?

Laboratories Studies:

1. Blood routine and blood sugar level: normal.
2. Tissue biopsy of the lesion on the left maxillary gingiva is performed. Histopathology exam proved the diagnosis of gingival verruciform xanthomatosis.

Diagnosis Basis:

1. The clinical manifestation showed papillary reddish lesion on the gingiva.
2. Tissue biopsy confirmed the diagnosis.

Management:

1. Resection of the lesion is suggested.
2. During a follow-up of 1 year, there is no relapse.

[Review] Verruciform Xanthomatosis (VX)
Verruciform xanthomatosis (VX) is a rare benign mucocutaneous papillary disease, with the oral mucosa as predilection site. About 75% of oral cases are located on the hard palate, the gingiva, or the alveolar ridge (Fig. 12.7). It may also affect the skin and genital mucosa, such as the vulva, scrotum, and penis. VX primarily affects middle-aged without gender predilection [7, 8].

VX manifests as an asymptomatic solitary, slow-growing, and slightly raised lesion with a rough granular, plaque-like, papular, verrucous, papillary, or cauliflower-like surface and sharply delineated margins. It appears as pink, red, yellow, white, or gray in color, with up to 2 cm in diameter [9]. VX combined with lichen planus has been reported (Fig. 12.7).

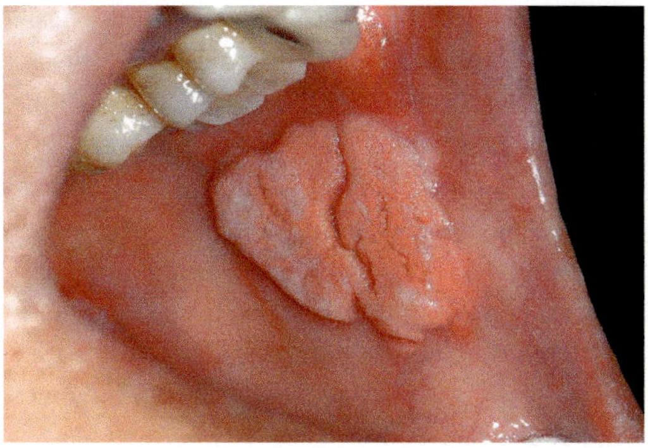

Fig. 12.7 VX with oral lichen planus on the left buccal mucosa

The differential diagnosis includes papilloma, verruca vulgaris, verrucous carcinoma, squamous cell carcinoma, and verrucous leukoplakia. The pathological changes presented as foamy macrophages and papillary proliferation with brightly eosinophilic parakeratin, keratin squames, and neutrophilic exocytosis, which can differentiate VX from others [9, 10].

The etiology of VX remains unclear. The characteristic foamy cells are found to be macrophages after scavenging excessive accumulation of lipids. One popular view is that epithelial damage results in the breakdown of phospholipid-rich cell membranes. Macrophages swallow the released lipids, which become lipid-laden or foamy in appearance [7]. An immunologic pathogenesis has also been suggested due to the predominant T-cell infiltration and decreased Langerhans cell numbers compared to normal tissue. Additionally, VX has been reported to combine with chronic inflammation such as pemphigus vulgaris, lichen planus, discoid lupus erythematosus, psoriasis, and graft-versus-host disease; thus, some researchers hold the opinion that immunological factors are predominant in VX [7, 9]. Poor clearance of lipid-rich interstitial fluid and obstruction of lipophage migration occur in the setting of lymphedema, which is suggested as an essential role in the pathogenesis of VX [11]. Others suggested that VX is also associated with HPV and EB virus infections [12]. A recent study revealed that local stimuli or trauma accompanied with galectin-7 overexpression is considered to induce cholesterol synthesis, epidermal apoptosis, and subsequent lipid incontinence via HMG-CoA synthase 1(HMGCS1). The excessive lipid scavenged by macrophages and the formation of lipophage are the characteristic feature of VX [13].

VX is a benign disease with good prognosis and low relapse rate. The treatment for oral VX is often surgical resection.

12.4 Palate Perforation

Case 103 Palate Perforation (Invasive Fungal Infection Related?)

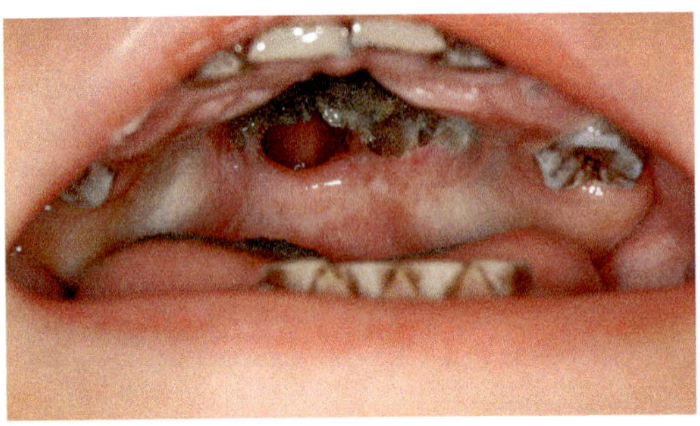

Fig. 12.8 Palatal ulcer and necrosis on the posterior part of the hard palate, part of the bone tissue exposed and blackened, with a 9 mm in diameter perforation at the mid-right

Age: 16 months
Sex: Male
Chief Complaints:
A 16-month-old boy with palate ulcer for 1 month
History of Present Illness:
A 16-month-old boy presented to our clinic with a complaint of gradually extending palatal ulcer for 1 month. He was diagnosed with acute lymphocytic leukemia (ALL) 2 months ago and was being treated with chemotherapy and corticosteroid therapy in stable condition. Forty-five days ago, the blood culture demonstrated *Candida parapsilosis*, suggesting the complication of fungal septicemia during his hospitalization. Serologic tests for syphilis and HIV were negative. Chest X-ray and abdominal ultrasound examination results were normal. Microbiological culture of the secretion from the palatal lesion revealed negative result.
Past Medical History: ALL
Allergy: None
Physical Examination:
A 30 mm × 20 mm palatal ulcer in the posterior part of the hard palate was observed, with well-defined borders. In the lesion area, part of the bone tissue is exposed and blackened, with a 9 mm in diameter perforation filled with food debris located at the mid-right. The surrounding tissues were soft (Fig. 12.8).
Clinical Impression:
Palate perforation (invasive fungal infection related?)

Diagnosis Basis:

1. Local soft and hard tissue defect on the palate.
2. Diagnosis of ALL with the complication of fungal septicemia. But diagnosis of invasive fungal infection-related palate perforation requires tissue biopsy.

Management:

1. Medication.
   Rp.: Sodium bicarbonate solution (2%) 250 mL × 1
   Sig.: Rinse t.i.d.
   Nystatin liniment 15 g × 1
   Sig.: Topical use t.i.d.
2. Regular follow-up visit and close observation were suggested. Biopsy would be performed after the chemotherapy session, followed by the palatoplasty considered.

Case 104 Palate Ulcer and Perforation Related to Mucormycosis

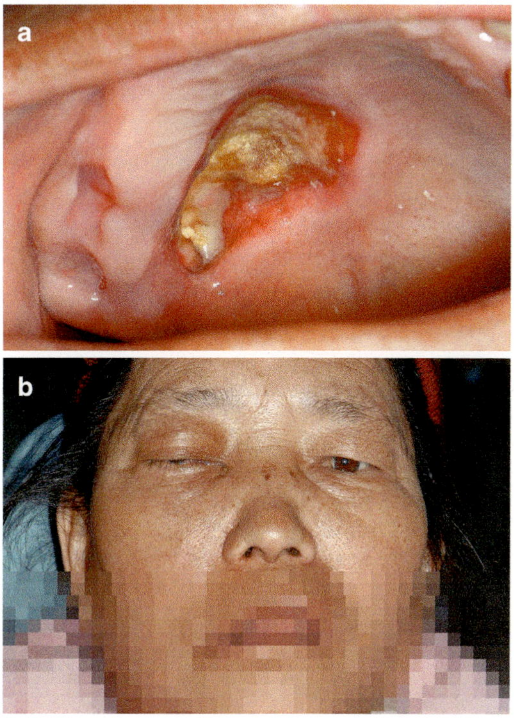

Fig. 12.9 (**a**) Deep ulcer on the posterior hard palate, with congestive margin and yellowish pseudomembrane, the central part of the ulcer with bone loss formed a perforation. (**b**) Swelling on the right side of the cheek and right orbital region, with difficulty in opening the eyes

Age: 57 years
Sex: Female
Chief Complaints:
A 57-year-old woman with an ulcer on the right side of the palate for 20 days
History of Present Illness:
A 57-year-old woman was referred to our clinic from the Department of Infectious Diseases, with the main complaint of a 2 cm ulcer on the right palate, expanding in size gradually for the past 20 days. History revealed that her maxillary posterior teeth (seven teeth altogether) were extracted in a dental clinic 38 days ago. One week after the tooth extraction, she had flu-like symptoms, with eyelid pain and blurred vision of her right eye, followed by slight fever and right orbital swelling. Then she had been diagnosed with type 2 diabetes mellitus and right orbital cellulitis based on the high blood glucose level (33.9 mmol/L) in the local hospital. After cefixime, levofloxacin and hypoglycemic agents were prescribed; orbital swelling and blurred vision were improved slightly. Fourteen days ago, she was hospitalized in the Department of Infectious Diseases. Her blood glucose level was under control. Blood routine examination showed the decreased RBC count (3.32 × 1012/L) and HGB level (101 g/L), with normal liver and kidney function. Serological tests for HBV, HCV, syphilis, and HIV are all clear. CT scan and MRI indicated the right nasal sinusitis, involving the right maxillofacial and temporal soft tissue, the right mastoid region, and frontal lobe brain tissues, mainly due to the diffusion of nasal sinusitis. Nasal secretion smear demonstrated G+ bacillus and coccus, and saliva smear revealed yeast-like fungi. The level of fungal G test (beta-glucan antigenemia assay) is 95.99 pg/mL. Thus, she was diagnosed with right orbital and facial cellulitis (suspected deep fungal infection) and was under antibiotic therapy.
Past Medical History: Hypertension and diabetes
Allergy: None
Physical Examination:
Oral examination showed a 1.8 cm × 4 cm deep ulcer in the posterior region of the right hard palate, with congestive margin and yellowish pseudomembrane. The central part of the ulcer with bone loss formed a perforation. Extraoral examination revealed swelling on the right side of the cheek and right orbital region, with difficulty in opening the eyes (Fig. 12.9).
Clinical Impression:

Palate ulcer and perforation (invasive fungal infection related?)

Laboratories and Imaging Studies:

1. Tissue biopsy of the palatal ulcer margin was performed. Histopathology exam showed chronic inflammation, with pseudoepitheliomatous hyperplasia in the epithelial layer. Plasmocytes, monocytes, and lymphocytes are

infiltrated surrounding the submucosal vessels and salivary glands. Localized lymphadenia, bone trabecula, and blood clot were also observed.
2. Tissue biopsy of the nasal lesion was performed. Histopathology exam revealed severe chronic inflammation in the nasal and sinus mucosa, localized erosion, and interstitial edema accompanied with inflammatory polyps. Extensive inflammatory exudation and necrosis, sporadic bone chips with multifocal abscess, and localized fungi (*Mucorales*?) were observed.
3. The nasal secretion culture demonstrated *Mucorales*.

Diagnosis:
Palate ulcer and perforation related to mucormycosis

Diagnosis Basis:

1. Local soft and hard tissue defect on the palate.
2. History of tooth extraction with uncontrolled hyperglycemia.
3. CT scan and MRI indicated the right nasal sinusitis and diffused in surrounding multiple sites.
4. Fungal G test (beta-glucan antigenemia assay)—early exam for fungal infection—with level of 95.99 pg/mL (negative, <60 pg/mL; susceptive, 60–100 pg/mL; positive, >100 pg/mL) suggested consideration of fungal infection.
5. Tissue biopsy of the nasal mucosal lesion revealed severe chronic inflammation in the nasal and sinus mucosa, and localized fungi were noticed (*Mucorales*?).
6. The nasal secretion culture demonstrated *Mucorales*.
7. Antifungal therapy (amphotericin B) is effective, resulting in relief of facial and orbital swelling.

Management:

1. Medication.
   Rp.: Sodium bicarbonate solution (2%) 250 mL × 1
   Sig.: rinse t.i.d.
2. Continue the antifungal therapy in the Department of Infectious Diseases. The debridement for the necrotic tissue and palatoplasty could be considered if the infection is under control.

[Review] Palate Perforation
Palate perforations are rear oral lesions without unified definition. Palate perforation denotes a collection of lesions manifesting as hard or soft palate tissue necrosis, even localized tissue defect. The etiology is complicated; the main causes are discussed as follows:

12.4.1 Infections

Syphilis is caused by *Treponema pallidum*. Tertiary syphilis is characterized by a painless localized granuloma (gumma) which presents on the hard palate. The gumma begins as a swelling that eventually ulcerates and then goes through repeated phases of healing and breakdown. Bone destruction of the hard palate may occur with palatal perforation and, in some cases, oral nasal fistula [14]. In infants with congenital syphilis, gumma and palate perforation could also be observed. The diagnosis of syphilis is performed by a combination of social or STD history, family history, and serological testing indicating positive antibody formation to the *Treponema*.

Other bacterial infections which could induce palate perforation such as lepriasis (*Mycobacterium leprae* infection), pulmonary tuberculosis (*Mycobacterium tuberculosis* infection), rhinoscleroma (*Rhinoscleroma bacillus* infection), and actinomycosis (*Actinomyces* infection) are reported [15–22].

A mold is a group of fungi that grow in the form of hyphae. Molds which induce palate perforation include *Mucorales*, fungal genus *Aspergillus*, *Paracoccidioidomycosis brasiliensis*, etc. Oral/facial invasive fungal infections (IFI) are rare in the healthy population, while the incidence of opportunistic IFI is growing in patients with specific conditions such as immunosuppression, bone marrow transplantation, acquired immunodeficiency syndrome, and diabetes. The definition of deep fungal infection or invasive fungal infection is still controversial. Some researchers considered that all fungal infection could be invasive. However, the term deep fungal infection should be used only to characterize systemic, generalized, deep-seated, visceral and severe, life-threatening fungal infections, in contrast to superficial, local, benign, self-limiting fungal diseases [23]. Several case reports demonstrated that palate perforation was caused by mucormycosis or aspergillosis in children who had acute lymphoblastic leukemia (ALL) under chemotherapy [24–26], such as the case 103 in this unit. In case 104, the palate perforation of the patient with diabetes was also proved to be related to opportunistic deep fungal infection based on several tests and effective antifungal treatment.

12.4.2 Systemic Disorders

Wegener's granulomatosis (WG) is a systemic disease characterized by necrotizing granulomas and extensive small vessel vasculitis. WG is widely thought to be an autoimmune disease. Patients present with symptoms based on the affected organs, including the respiratory tract, kidney, and skin. Necrotizing granulomatous ulcers in the soft palate or pharynx are common oral lesions, which are less common located in the gingiva and other parts. Deep pain-free oral ulcers expand rapidly with specific bad breath. Ulceration and osteonecrosis on the palate would result in the exposure of the underlying bone and finally palatal perforation. Cutaneous manifestations include palpable purpura, erythema, necrotic nodules, papules, and ulcers [27].

Crohn's disease (CD) is a chronic recurrent granulomatous inflammatory disease which occurs in the digestive tract. CD can affect any part of the gastrointestinal (GI) tract, but the terminal ileum (TI), with rich lymphoid tissue, is the susceptible area. The lesions are often segmental with "skip" areas of normal regions; therefore, CD is also known as regional enteritis or segmental ileitis. Oral lesions could be observed in the buccal, labial, gingival, and laryngeal mucosa, manifestations of which are "knife-cut" linear ulcers with a rolled edge, hyperplastic folds, and nodular or granular hyperplasia. Other oral features include diffuse lip swelling, erythematous and granular gingivitis, and minor or major recurrent aphthous stomatitis. In a case report of a patient suffering from CD for 4 years, with the intraintestinal condition worsened, she has developed saddle nose deformity, alar collapse, and palatal perforation as extraintestinal manifestations of the disease [28].

Extranodal natural killer/T-cell lymphoma (ENKL), nasal type, is a rare disease related to EB virus infection. A case report of ENKL presents a palatal perforation in a 21-year-old man, who was diagnosed through immunophenotyping after excluding bacterial osteomyelitis, invasive fungal infection, and Wegener's granulomatosis [29]. Other disorders such as maxillary sinus carcinoma and mucoepidermoid carcinoma may induce palate perforation as well [30, 31].

12.4.3 Development Defect

Cleft palate is the birth defects which could cause palate perforation. Its embryologic basis is a failure of the mesenchymal masses of the lateral palatine processes to meet and fuse with each other, with the nasal septum, and/or with the posterior margin of the median palatine process or primary palate. Congenital palate perforation is common birth defects in children [32].

12.4.4 Drug Abuse

Cocaine abuse increased worldwide, with reported cases of palate perforations increased. The drug can result in direct irritation and ischemia of the nasal and palatal mucosa. A case report presented a 48-year-old female with 15 mm × 17 mm palate perforation without signs of infection. Medication and lifestyle history revealed her alcohol intake for decades, cocaine usage for 1 year, and marijuana consumption for 10 years [33]. In a systematic review, no particular gender predilection was observed, though females represented a little over half of the total cases (58.33%). Regarding the location, more lesions were located in the hard palate, less in soft palate [34]. Additionally, abuse of heroin and anesthetics also may induce palate perforation.

12.4.5 Trauma

Edge tools such as chopsticks, iron pole, or iatrogenic materials puncture the palate, thus causing tissue defect. Such cases reported are accidentally caused as a complication of orotracheal intubation [35, 36].

Since the causes of the palate perforation are numerous, clinicians should determine the underlying causes (e.g., development defect, trauma, infection, systemic disorders, and drug abuse) for the lesions in order to take specific treatment. In the case of infection-induced palate perforation, anti-infection therapy should be the first step, followed by the debridement for all the necrotic tissue and palatoplasty once the infection is under control, in order to recover the structure and function of the palate [37]. For the patients with non-infection causes, clinicians should promptly control the original underlying conditions such as tumors and immune-related disorders. For patients with obvious risk factors such as drug or medication abuse and trauma, removal of these factors and the following reconstructive surgery are recommended.

12.5 Xerostomia

Case 105 Xerostomia and Sjögren's Syndrome

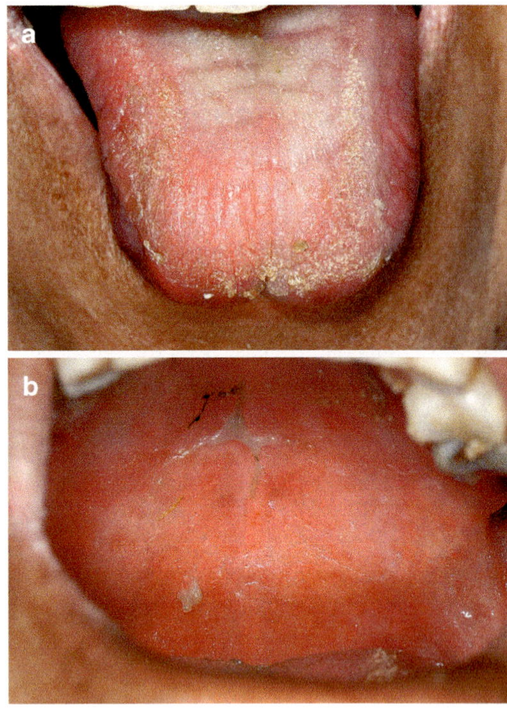

Fig. 12.10 (**a**) Dry appearance and atrophic dorsum of the tongue, accompanied by irregular fissures. (**b**) Dry and rough appearance of the palate

Age: 50 years
Sex: Female
Chief Complaints:
A 50-year-old woman with dry mouth for 5 years
History of Present Illness:
A 50-year-old woman presented to our clinic with a subjective feeling of dry mouth without obvious precipitating factors. It was getting worse gradually with difficulties in swallowing

and eating. She also claimed dry eyes and joint pain. Drug treatment was actually ineffective.

Past Medical History: Stomach illness

Allergy: None

Physical Examination:

Oral examination showed that the mucosa is dry, and no saliva drainage was observed when pressing the major salivary gland. Dry appearance and atrophic area were noted on the dorsum of the tongue, accompanied by irregularly fissured lines (Fig. 12.10).

Clinical Impression:

Xerostomia, Sjögren's syndrome?

Laboratories and Imaging Studies:

1. Blood routine, liver and kidney function, and blood sugar level are normal. Rheumatoid factor (RF) was found to be greatly increased (1100 IU/mL), and antinuclear antibodies (ANAs) (++++), anti-SSA (++), and anti-SSB (++) were strongly positive.
2. Dynamic salivary scintigraphy of the salivary gland function showed severe impaired function of the salivary gland.
3. The diagnosis of xerophthalmia was made by Department of Ophthalmology.

Diagnosis:

Xerostomia, Sjögren's syndrome

Diagnosis Basis:

1. Patients with symptoms suggestive of SS: long-lasting dry mouth, dry eye, and joint pain.
2. Clinical diagnosis of xerostomia and xerophthalmia.
3. Serological examination showed strongly positive of anti-SSA (++) and anti-SSB (++).
4. Dynamic salivary scintigraphy showed severe damage of salivary gland function.

Management:

1. Medication.
   Rp.: Lusun capsules 0.3 g × 81 tablets
   Sig.: 0.6g p.o. t.i.d.
   Anethol trithione 25 mg × 48 tablets
   Sig.: 25 mg p.o. t.i.d.
   Sodium bicarbonate solution (4%) 250 mL × 1
   Sig.: Rinse t.i.d.
   Nystatin liniment 15 g × 1
   Sig.: Topical use t.i.d.
2. The patient was referred to a rheumatologist for further treatment.

[Review] Xerostomia

Xerostomia is a symptom with multiple causes, not an independent disease. The diagnosis could be made once a subjective complaint of patients is dry mouth [38, 39]. Ten percent of the general population experiences long-lasting oral dryness. Complaints of dry mouth are more prevalent in older people, which more than 25% are affected [40]. In the majority of the cases, it results from salivary gland hypofunction. However, clinicians encounter numbers of patients with symptoms of xerostomia in the clinic of oral medicine.

The causes of xerostomia are complicated. Medication is the most common cause of dry mouth; approximately 64% of xerostomia is related to medication use. Hundreds of medicines could induce xerostomia [41]. Medications with anticholinergic activity (e.g., atropine and scopolamine) are antagonists of some acetylcholine receptors and thus inhibit salivary secretion and induce dry mouth. Antihypertensive agents (reserpine, methyldopa) could suppress sympathetic nervous system, resulting in the interference of saliva secretion. Antidepressants, especially tricyclic antidepressants (TCAs), could induce xerostomia due to the similar function as that of atropine. Other medications include parasympatholytic agents, antithyroid medicine, sedative, diuretic agents, and alpha- and beta-receptor-blocking drugs. Some Chinese herbal medicines, even some plants such as gingko, *Urtica dioica*, dandelion, chilis, and garlic, could induce oral dryness [42, 43].

Many salivary gland diseases and hypoplasia could lead to dysfunction which triggers xerostomia. In the case of acute purulent parotitis, swelling epithelium and narrowed or even blocked duct decrease the salivary secretion. When the acute condition turns into chronic disease, glandular tissue is damaged and replaced by fibrotic connective tissue and adipose tissue, markedly decreasing the salivary flow. Besides, salivary gland tumors, sialolith, cystic fibrosis, undersized salivary glands, and glandular hypoplasia all can be the causes of xerostomia [44, 45].

Radiation therapy (RT) of the head and neck regions is another common cause of xerostomia. Ionizing radiation can injure the major and minor salivary glands; this can lead to atrophy, even death of the secretory components. When the radiation dose is in excess of 52 Gy, RT will lead to rapid and remarkable damage [46, 47]. Previous studies considered that these damages are permanent and irreversible. However, recent researches revealed that secretory function could not recover with the dose higher than 30 Gy, while the function could gradually return when the dose is lower than 25 Gy, which needs to be further confirmed [48].

Numerous systemic disorders will lead to salivary gland dysfunction. Patients with diabetes mellitus are vulnerable to xerostomia due to the increased plasma osmotic pressure and polyuria which lead to excessive water loss.

Sjögren's syndrome (SS) is a chronic autoimmune disease characterized by progressive destruction of exocrine glands leading to mucosa and conjunctiva dryness, accompanied with various autoimmune disorders. Dry mouth and dry eye caused by dysfunction of salivary and lacrimal glands are the major clinical manifestations, and dryness of other mucosal areas such as the nasopharynx, skin, and vulva could also be affected due to the damage in other exocrine glands and organs. Signs of systemic autoimmune disease include purpuma, arthralgias, myositis, interstitial pulmonary fibrosis, and polyneuritis [49]. The etiology of SS is unclear. Serologic test showed positive autoantibodies, suggesting SS is an autoimmune disease. SS is classified as primary or secondary. Primary Sjögren's syndrome occurs only in the presence of exocrine gland destruction, whereas secondary SS occurs accompanied with autoimmune diseases such as rheumatoid arthritis. Xerostomia is the early symptom of SS, with various degrees depending on the destruction level of salivary glands. Oral examination indicates little or no saliva drainage from bilateral parotid gland ducts.

Salivary gland lesions are reported to occur in 4–8% of HIV-positive patients. The damages commonly manifest as repeating salivary gland enlargements and xerostomia. Salivary gland dysfunction is common in patients with chronic hepatitis C, with prevalence ranging from 10% to 33%, in which saliva flow rate is obviously decreased and xerostomia is induced. Furthermore, hyperthyroidism, sinusitis, graft-versus-host disease, ganglia lesion, and disorders in the central nervous system could result in xerostomia [50–52].

Psychological conditions such as anxiety or fear, especially depression, also may give rise to subjective symptoms of dry mouth. Bergdahl et al. examined the depressive symptoms in 94 subjects with a sensation of a dry mouth. The results showed that individuals with a subjective dry mouth condition were significantly more depressive, indicating that subjective dry mouth may be of psychological origin. The underlying mechanisms are as follows: (1) degradation of catecholamine in the adrenal medulla reduces blood flowing to the salivary glands, affecting the saliva flow rate; (2) psychological stress diminishes taste perception and reduces the activity of glandular motor nerves, incapacitating the saliva draining from glandular acini; and (3) blockade of acetylcholine M receptors induces xerostomia [53].

Oral dryness may also be caused by mouth breathing due to nasal disorders. Mouth breathing accelerates the evaporation of saliva, leading to xerostomia. Because of the dry mouth, patients always wake up during the night [54].

It is controversial that age is a risk factor of xerostomia. Although it was previously thought that salivary function declined with age, it is recently accepted that salivary gland secretion is similar between elderly and younger patients. It is likely that numerous systemic diseases and medications contribute significantly to dry mouth in older people [55].

Clinical manifestations are various. Hyposalivation, saliva pool disappeared and no saliva drainage observed when pressing the major salivary gland, does exist in some patients complaining of dry mouth. However, other patients whose clinical signs are not obvious may need psychological counseling.

Management of underlying disorders such as salivary gland diseases and systemic or psychological conditions is the first step in treatment of the dry mouth. The side effects of medications may be alleviated by alternative drugs or altering the doses or dosage forms. Prophylaxis for radiation-induced xerostomia includes:

1. Radioprotective agents, such as amifostine, could reduce the damage caused by RT and thus decrease the incidence of xerostomia in patients undergoing head and neck radiotherapy. Amifostine use has been approved by FDA, but the decreased sensitivity of tumor cells makes its application controversial.
2. Precise radiation is critically important for protecting salivary gland tissue, especially parotid glands from radiotherapy.
3. Submandibular gland transposition, preventing exposure of the gland, has been reported being effective for preventing post-RT xerostomia.

A night guard device that covered the dental arch and the hard palate is reported by Yamamoto K et al. to be used for the management of sleep-related xerostomia [56].

Symptomatic treatments should be adopted. The commonly used drugs include:

1. Pilocarpine and cevimeline belong to cholinomimetic drugs; they are effective for salivary stimulation. But the side effects, such as excessive sweating, flushing, and urinary and gastrointestinal disturbances, should be the concern. The use of pilocarpine and cevimeline is contraindicated in patients with uncontrolled asthma, angle-closure glaucoma, cardiovascular diseases, Parkinson's disease, or chronic obstructive pulmonary disease. Common dose of pilocarpine is 5–10 mg orally 3–4 times daily, while cevimeline is 30 mg orally three times daily.
2. Anethole trithione is a cholagogue that has been shown in clinical trials to increase salivary secretion. Usual dose is 25 mg orally three times daily.
3. Mucolytic agents such as bromhexine HCl (30 mg orally three times daily) and ambroxol hydrochloride (8–16 mg orally three times daily) could reduce viscosity of saliva in patients with xerostomia.
4. Chinese herbal medicines such as Zhibai Dihuang pills, nourishing yin and clearing heat, and lusun capsules, inducing saliva and slaking thirst, are both effective in treating dry mouth.

Approaches such as oral rinses with sodium bicarbonate solution and topical use of nystatin liniment are suggested to prevent and treat fungal infection.

Daily symptomatic approaches such as sipping water throughout the day are necessary for patients with xerostomia. There are a number of oral rinses, mouthwashes, gels, spray, and artificial saliva available for dry mouth patients to relieve discomfort and substitute partially the function of saliva. The use of room humidifiers, particularly at night, may lessen discomfort markedly. Chewing sugar-free gums or lozenge can be effective in stimulating salivary flow, thus improving symptoms.

In patients with a subjective sensation of dry mouth without local or systemic disorders, the combination of psychological counseling and management similar to that of burning mouth syndrome is recommended.

References

1. Li S, Yu S. Study of the benign lymphadenosis of oral mucosa. J Mod Oral Med. 2007;4:340–2.
2. Cheng B, Chen X. Clinicopathological features and immunohistochemical analysis of the benign lymphadenosis of oral mucosa. J Compr Stomatol. 1998;14(2):99–101.
3. Tonouchi K, Ohta K, Tomizawa M, et al. A clinical observation of epithelial pearls in newborn babies. 1 Appearances and continuous changes. Shoni Shikagaku Zasshi. 1990;28(3):786–97.
4. Thesleff I, Tummers M. Tooth organogenesis and regeneration. BTI-StemBook. 2008.

5. Arnold WH, Rezwani T, Baric I. Location and distribution of epithelial pearls and tooth buds in human fetuses with cleft lip and palate. Cleft Palate Craniofac J. 1998;35(4):359–65.
6. Mhaske S, Yuwanati MB, Mhaske A, et al. Natal and neonatal teeth: an overview of the literature. ISRN Pediatr. 2013;2013:956269.
7. Shahrabi FS, Treister NS, Khan Z, et al. Oral verruciform xanthoma associated with chronic graft-versus-host disease: a report of five cases and a review of the literature. Head Neck Pathol. 2011;5(2):193–8.
8. Bhalerao S, Bhat P, Chhabra R, et al. Verruciform xanthoma of the buccal mucosa: a case report with review of the literature. Contemp Clin Dent. 2012;3(Suppl 2):S257–9.
9. Oliveira PT, Jaeger RG, Cabral LA, et al. Verruciform xanthoma of the oral mucosa. Report of four cases and a review of the literature. Oral Oncol. 2001;37(3):326–31.
10. Cheng YS, Wright J, Lucente J, et al. Oral and maxillofacial pathology case of the month. Verruciform xanthoma. Tex Dent J. 2010;127(1):126–7. 130–131.
11. Lu S, Rohwedder A, Murphy M, et al. Verruciform xanthoma: localized lymphedema (elephantiasis) is an essential pathogenic factor. J Cutan Pathol. 2012;39(3):391–4.
12. Maldonado-Cid P, Noguera-Morel L, Beato-Merino MJ, et al. Verruciform xanthoma associated with reactivation of Epstein-Barr virus. Actas Dermosifiliogr. 2013;104(5):445–6.
13. Fujimoto N, Asano C, Ono K, et al. Verruciform xanthoma results from epidermal apoptosis with galectin-7 overexpression. J Eur Acad Dermatol Venereol. 2013;27(7):922–3.
14. Bains MK, Hosseini-Ardehali M. Palatal perforations: past and present. Two case reports and a literature review. Br Dent J. 2005;199(5):267–9.
15. Boldsen JL. Leprosy in medieval Denmark – osteological and epidemiological analyses. Anthropol Anz. 2009;67(4):407–25.
16. Thomas M, Emmanuel M. A case of advanced lepromatous leprosy with rhino-oro-laryngological involvement in the post-elimination era. Indian J Lepr. 2009;81(2):81–2.
17. Dhawan AK, Verma P, Sharma S. Oral lesions in leprosy revisited: a case report. Am J Dermatopathol. 2012;34(6):666–7.
18. Baruah B, Goyal A, Shunyu NB, et al. Tuberculosis of nose and palate with vanishing uvula. Indian J Med Microbiol. 2011;29(1):63–5.
19. Gaafar HA, Gaafar AH, Nour YA. Rhinoscleroma: an updated experience through the last 10 years. Acta Otolaryngol. 2011;131(4):440–6.
20. Nimare K, Shukla RK. A rare case of rhinoscleroma. Indian J Otolaryngol Head Neck Surg. 1999;52(1):74–5.
21. De D, Dogra S, Kanwar AJ, et al. Actinomycosis presenting as a destructive ulcerated plaque on the palate and gingiva. J Am Acad Dermatol. 2011;65(6):1235–6.
22. Garg R, Schalch P, Pepper JP, et al. Osteomyelitis of the hard palate secondary to actinomycosis: a case report. Ear Nose Throat J. 2011;90(3):E11–2.
23. Hof H. IFI = invasive fungal infections. What is that? A misnomer, because a non-invasive fungal infection does not exist. Int J Infect Dis. 2010;14(6):e458–9.
24. Barrak HA. Hard palate perforation due to mucormycosis: report of four cases. J Laryngol Otol. 2007;121(11):1099–102.
25. Karabulut AB, Kabakas F, Berkoz O, et al. Hard palate perforation due to invasive aspergillosis in a patient with acute lymphoblastic leukemia. Int J Pediatr Otorhinolaryngol. 2005;69(10):1395–8.
26. Castro LG, Muller AP, Mimura MA, et al. Hard palate perforation: an unusual finding in paracoccidioidomycosis. Int J Dermatol. 2001;40(4):281–3.
27. Kasifoglu T, Cansu D, Korkmaz C. Clinical images: perforation of the nasal septum and palate due to Wegener's granulomatosis. Arthritis Rheum. 2008;58(8):2564.
28. Oghan F, Pekkan G, Ozveren O. Saddle nose deformity, palatal perforation and truncus arteriosus in a patient with Crohn's disease. J Craniomaxillofac Surg. 2012;40(1):17–9.
29. Bhatt VR, Koirala B, Terjanian T. Extranodal natural killer/T cell lymphoma, nasal type presenting as a palatal perforation and naso-oral fistula. BMJ Case Rep. 2011;2011:bcr1120103511.
30. Nishimura G, Sano D, Tanigaki Y, et al. Maxillary sinus carcinoma: the only symptom was neck lymph node swelling. Auris Nasus Larynx. 2006;33(1):57–61.
31. Kolude B, Lawoyin JO, Akang EE. Mucoepidermoid carcinoma of the oral cavity. J Natl Med Assoc. 2001;93(5):178–84.
32. Dixon MJ, Marazita ML, Beaty TH, et al. Cleft lip and palate: understanding genetic and environmental influences. Nat Rev Genet. 2011;12(3):167–78.
33. Padilla-Rosas M, Jimenez-Santos CI, Garcia-Gonzalez CL. Palatine perforation induced by cocaine. Med Oral Patol Oral Cir Bucal. 2006;11(3):E239–42.
34. Silvestre FJ, Perez-Herbera A, Puente-Sandoval A, et al. Hard palate perforation in cocaine abusers: a systematic review. Clin Oral Investig. 2010;14(6):621–8.
35. Bartlett E, Mahabir RC, Verheyden CN. Traumatic palatal perforation after orotracheal intubation: a case report and a review of the literature. Cleft Palate Craniofac J. 2013;50(5):614–7.
36. Vincent RD Jr, Wimberly MP, Brockwell RC, et al. Soft palate perforation during orotracheal intubation facilitated by the GlideScope videolaryngoscope. J Clin Anesth. 2007;19(8):619–21.
37. Samanta DR, Senapati SN, Sharma PK, et al. Hard palate perforation in acute lymphoblastic leukemia due to mucormycosis-a case report. Indian J Hematol Blood Transfus. 2009;25(1):36–3.
38. Hay KD, Morton RP. Optimal nocturnal humidification for xerostomia. Head Neck. 2006;28(9):792–6.
39. Fox PC. Salivary enhancement therapies. Caries Res. 2004;38(3):241–6.

40. Orellana MF, Lagravere MO, Boychuk DG, et al. Prevalence of xerostomia in population-based samples: a systematic review. J Public Health Dent. 2006;66(2):152–8.
41. Ciancio SG. Medications' impact on oral health. J Am Dent Assoc. 2004;135(10):1440–8; quiz 1468–1469.
42. Abebe W. An overview of herbal supplement utilization with particular emphasis on possible interactions with dental drugs and oral manifestations. J Dent Hyg. 2003;77(1):37–46.
43. Sreebny LM, Schwartz SS. A reference guide to drugs and dry mouth – 2nd edition. Gerodontology. 1997;14(1):33–47.
44. Ono K, Tanaka T, Inoue H, et al. Small salivary gland size in patients with xerostomia of unknown etiology. Arch Oral Biol. 2009;54(4):369–73.
45. Fox PC, et al. Dent Assist. 2008;77(5):18, 20, 44–48; quiz 50–51.
46. Sciubba JJ, Goldenberg D. Oral complications of radiotherapy. Lancet Oncol. 2006;7(2):175–83.
47. Dirix P, Nuyts S, Van den Bogaert W. Radiation-induced xerostomia in patients with head and neck cancer: a literature review. Cancer. 2006;107(11):2525–34.
48. Li Y, Taylor JM, Ten HRK, et al. The impact of dose on parotid salivary recovery in head and neck cancer patients treated with radiation therapy. Int J Radiat Oncol Biol Phys. 2007;67(3):660–9.
49. Kassan SS, Moutsopoulos HM. Clinical manifestations and early diagnosis of Sjogren syndrome. Arch Intern Med. 2004;164(12):1275–84.
50. von Bültzingslöwen I, Sollecito TP, Fox PC, et al. Salivary dysfunction associated with systemic diseases: systematic review and clinical management recommendations. Oral Surg Oral Med Oral Pathol Oral Radiol Endod. 2007;103(Suppl: S57):e1–15.
51. De Vita S, Damato R, De Marchi G, et al. True primary Sjogren's syndrome in a subset of patients with hepatitis C infection: a model linking chronic infection to chronic sialadenitis. Isr Med Assoc J. 2002;4(12):1101–5.
52. Ooi SE, Tsai CY, Chou CT. Interstitial lung disease and xerostomia as initial manifestations in a patient with human immunodeficiency virus infection. J Microbiol Immunol Infect. 2005;38(2):145–8.
53. Bergdahl M, Bergdahl J, Johansson I. Depressive symptoms in individuals with idiopathic subjective dry mouth. J Oral Pathol Med. 1997;26(10):448–50.
54. Napenas JJ, Brennan MT, Fox PC. Diagnosis and treatment of xerostomia (dry mouth). Odontology. 2009;97(2):76–83.
55. Ship JA, Pillemer SR, Baum BJ. Xerostomia and the geriatric patient. J Am Geriatr Soc. 2002;50(3):535–43.
56. Yamamoto K, Nagashima H, Yamachika S, et al. The application of a night guard for sleep-related xerostomia. Oral Surg Oral Med Oral Pathol Oral Radiol Endod. 2008;106(3):e11–4.

Ethical Approval

Ethical approval was given by the West China Hospital of Stomatology Institutional Review Board with the following reference number: WCHSIRB-D-2014-148.

Q. Chen, X. Zeng (eds.), *Case Based Oral Mucosal Diseases*,
https://doi.org/10.1007/978-981-13-0286-2

Printed by Printforce, the Netherlands